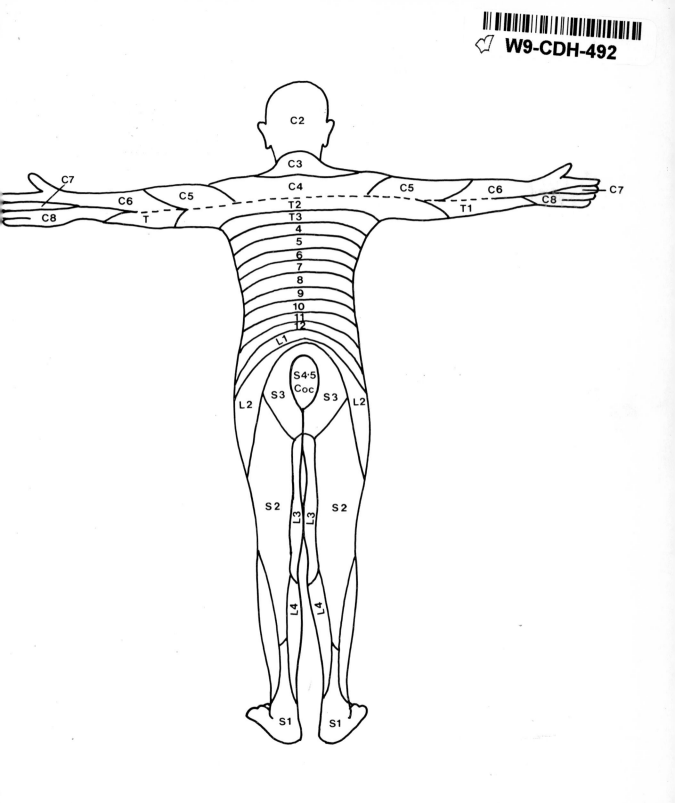

THIRD EDITION

PRACTICAL ORTHOPEDICS

THIRD EDITION

Practical Orthopedics

LONNIE R. MERCIER, M.D.

Clinical Instructor
Department of Orthopedic Surgery
Creighton University School of Medicine
Omaha, Nebraska

CONTRIBUTORS

FRED J. PETTID, M.D.

Associate Professor of Family Practice
Department of Family Practice
Creighton University School of Medicine
Omaha, Nebraska

DEAN F. TAMISIEA, M.D.

Clinical Instructor in Radiology
Creighton University School of Medicine
Omaha, Nebraska

JOHN J. HEIECK, M.D.

Assistant Clinical Professor
Department of Surgery
Creighton University School of Medicine
Omaha, Nebraska

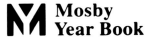

Mosby
Year Book

St. Louis   Baltimore   Boston   Chicago   London   Philadelphia   Sydney   Toronto

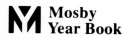
Mosby Year Book

Dedicated to Publishing Excellence

Sponsoring Editor: Kevin M. Kelly
Assistant Director, Manuscript Services: Frances M. Perveiler
Production Project Coordinator: Karen Halm
Proofroom Manager: Barbara Kelly

1   2   3   4   5   6   7   8   9   0   CL   MA   95   94   93   92   91

Library of Congress Cataloging-in-Publication Data
Mercier, Lonnie R., 1942-
    Practical orthopedics / Lonnie R. Mercier.—3rd ed.
        p.   cm.
    Includes bibliographical references.
    Includes index.
    ISBN 0-8151-5865-3
    1. Orthopedics.   I. Title.
    [DNLM: 1. Orthopedics.   WE 168 M555p]
RD731.M43   1991
617.3—dc20
DNLM/DLC   91-6271
for Library of Congress   CIP

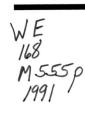
MOSBY—YEAR BOOK PRIMARY CARE SERIES

SERIES EDITORS

CHARLES E. DRISCOLL, M.D.

Professor and Head
Department of Family Practice
University of Iowa College of Medicine
Iowa City, Iowa

PAUL M. FISHER, M.D.

Associate Professor
Department of Family Medicine
Medical College of Georgia
Augusta, Georgia

JOSEPH E. SCHERGER, M.D., M.P.H.

Clinical Professor
Department of Family Practice
School of Medicine
University of California, Davis
Davis, California

FORTHCOMING TITLES

Goldstein and Goldstein/PRACTICAL DERMATOLOGY

Fleming and Barry/PRACTICAL MANAGEMENT OF SUBSTANCE
ABUSE

Pfenninger/OFFICE PROCEDURES FOR PRIMARY CARE

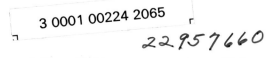

FOREWORD

In 1981, I started a family medicine practice in Weeping Water, Nebraska. My inpatient practice was in Papillion, Nebraska, a suburb of Omaha. It quickly became clear to me that one of the most important consultant relationships that I would need to develop would be with an orthopedist. There is a great deal of musculoskeletal disease in primary care.

I checked out the informal grapevine at the hospital to find out who was the best person for orthopedic referrals. There was uniformity of opinion. That person was Lonnie Mercier, M.D. I was told that Dr. Mercier was in solo practice, but that he was more available than most of the orthopedic groups. The OR nurses told me that he was a wonderful surgeon. The ER staff said that he was good in a crisis situation. More than one person commented that, "He is so nice. You wouldn't guess that he is a surgeon."

I soon found that all of this was true. Before long, Dr. Mercier was seeing the Weeping Water High School football stars whose injuries were beyond my skills. He was pinning the hips of my elderly patients with femoral fractures. And he was teaching me a great deal more about orthopedics than I had learned in my residency. Often this education occurred by telephone with me describing the findings of a patient or an x-ray.

One day in the hospital, I mentioned to Lonnie that I had not found the usual orthopedic textbooks to be very helpful. They tend to concentrate on severe fractures and surgical treatments. He told me that he knew of a book which might be helpful and promised to leave it at the nurse's station for me to pick up the next day. In his typically humble fashion, he failed to mention the book's author. The next day, as promised, I found a package at the nurse's station. It contained a copy of the first edition of *Practical Orthopedics.*

I was impressed that a person in full-time solo practice would write a textbook. Lonnie said that this seemed like the obvious thing to do after teaching many family medicine residents who had completed orthopedic rotations in his office. He felt that there was a need for a practical book about common orthopedic problems seen by primary care physicians.

Within a week of having the book in my office library, I received a call from the Weeping Water High School football coach. On two occasions in practice, his star running back had "cut to the outside of the field" and fallen to the ground. Each time the young athlete told the coach, "My ankle just gave out." When I examined the student, he had tenderness behind the lateral malleolus. I had no idea what was wrong. I opened *Practical Orthopedics* to the chapter on the ankle and learned for the first time about subluxing peroneal tendons. This was the first of many new diagnoses and treatments that I learned about from the book. I found it easy to use, nicely illustrated, and never lacking the answer that I was looking for.

In 1983, I left Weeping Water and joined the faculty at the Medical College of Georgia. The first edition of *Practical Orthopedics* quickly became the book I referred to most in my teaching of residents. My copy, in fact, suffered the ultimate compliment of a good book: it was stolen by a resident who intended to borrow it.

Lonnie Mercier, M.D., was right in his assessment that there is a need for such a book. This has become one of the most widely read primary care medical books published by Mosby–Year Book. The third edition is fully updated with a greatly expanded section on radiology ("Is this bump on this bone normal or not?"), and new advice on differential diagnosis. Like its two earlier editions, this book is an indispensable part of any family physician's, general internist's, or general pediatrician's library. Owning this book is like having your favorite orthopedic consultant on the telephone for a quick "curb-side consultation."

PAUL M. FISCHER, M.D.
Associate Professor
Department of Family Medicine
Medical College of Georgia
Augusta, Georgia

PREFACE TO THE THIRD EDITION

Publication of this edition of Practical Orthopedics reflects the positive response to the first editions. We have retained the previous format, dividing the text into two general sections. The first deals with musculoskeletal disorders by anatomical region and the later chapters discuss the arthritides, infection, roentgenographic diagnosis, and other areas of interest.

In revising the text, new disorders and viewpoints have been added and older material updated. In particular, discussions on advanced imaging techniques and disorders in the workplace have been broadened. Also appearing for the first time are sections on the role of exercise in health and algorithms for the evaluation and treatment of common disorders.

Perhaps the most helpful changes are those that are symptom based: that is, the addition of summaries based on the differential diagnosis of common presenting complaints. A considerable number of new illustrations also have been added.

We would again like to thank the many people who helped in the preparation of the manuscript and illustrations, as well as those who contributed roentgenograms and advice. We hope this edition continues to meet its goals for primary care physicians, residents, and students.

LONNIE R. MERCIER, M.D.

PREFACE TO THE FIRST EDITION

The stimulus to write this book was our participation in the orthopedic training of students and residents whose primary fields of interest are those other than orthopedic surgery. We were frequently asked to recommend an appropriate text for them to study but we found that none was available that met their needs. Most orthopedic surgery books are either too detailed or not complete enough to have any practical value in general medicine. We discovered, also, that no book existed that could be used as a current, practical guide and clinical reference by practicing physicians in the daily care of their patients. This book was undertaken to meet these needs.

In presenting a useful overview of orthopedic disorders, we have tried to discuss, in some depth, those conditions that are encountered frequently in daily practice. By emphasizing certain common features of these disorders, it is hoped that the fundamental concepts can be applied in the diagnosis and treatment of other musculoskeletal conditions.

The text is divided into two general sections. The first deals with musculoskeletal disorders by anatomical region. The later chapters discuss the arthritides, infection, injuries, and other common problems of interest, including a particularly useful chapter on radiologic aspects of orthopedic disease. The reader interested in sports medicine is directed to the index, where he will find references to discussions throughout the text on treatment of patients with athletic injuries.

The practice of orthopedics is, in a sense, rehabilitative medicine. It has as its goals improvement in the level of function of the patient and the diminution of pain. We hope you will find this book helpful in meeting these goals.

LONNIE R. MERCIER, M.D.
FRED J. PETTID, M.D.

CONTENTS

CHAPTER 1

Physical Examination

The diagnosis of disorders of the musculoskeletal system begins with a complete history and physical examination. The history is of special significance because physical findings are often minimal. Its importance cannot be overemphasized. Other additional early testing is usually unnecessary.

HISTORY

Birth History

The history of the pediatric patient should include several important points. It should first be determined whether fetal movements were experienced by the mother during pregnancy. Absence or weakness of these movements by the fourth or fifth month of gestation may indicate neuromuscular disease in the newborn. Any maternal diabetes, toxemia, drug ingestion, fetal distress, or prematurity are noted.

The type of delivery should also be noted. This is important because certain disorders such as congenital hip dysplasia are more common following breech delivery.

The condition of the child at birth and immediately after delivery should be ascertained. The presence of any jaundice, cyanosis, or difficulty with the delivery that might predispose the infant to brain damage is also recorded.

The physical and mental development of the child is then determined, and any deviation from normal progress is noted (Table 1–1).

Family History

A review of the family history is important not only for certain obvious musculoskeletal problems such as polydactyly but also for those disorders that may not be so obvious such as scoliosis and tuberculosis. Other family members may even need to be examined.

Past History

The general health of the patient is recorded, as well as any recent weight loss or gain. The patient's exact occupation should be determined and any relevant military history noted, especially if a disability rating resulted from time spent in the service. All chronic renal, metabolic, pulmonary, and previous orthopedic disorders should be assessed in view of the initial complaint.

Present Illness

The nature of the onset of symptoms, whether gradual or sudden, should be established. If an

1

TABLE 1–1.

Normal Milestones*

Age (mo)	Milestone
1–2	Holds up chin
6–8	Sits alone
8–10	Stands with support
10–12	Walks with support
14	Walks without support
24	Ascends stairs one foot at a time

*Note: there is frequently a wide variation in physical development, but if a child cannot walk unsupported by 18 months of age, a neuromuscular disorder should be suspected.

injury is involved, the exact date and place of the injury are recorded. This is frequently an important fact in determining injury liability. If the problem seems job related, other information regarding the work history may be helpful: (1) whether the symptoms may have been caused by the work or simply developed while working, (2) if the patient missed any work due to the problem, and (3) if the patient has ever been on light duty as a result of the disorder. The chief complaint should also be evaluated in relation to any previous similar symptoms or other musculoskeletal complaints. In addition, it should be noted whether the patient has had any other recent, seemingly unrelated illness or symptoms such as fever or chills. The results of any prior treatment or tests should also be ascertained.

The exact location and nature of any pain should be determined. In addition, the following important facts are noted: (1) the relationship of the pain to normal daily activities; (2) whether the pain is worse in the morning or late in the day; (3) whether coughing, sneezing, or other similar activities aggravate the pain; (4) whether the pain improves with rest; and (5) whether the pain remains well localized or is radicular in nature. If the pain is radicular, it should be determined whether the radiation follows any dermatome or peripheral nerve pattern. The effect of any home remedies on the pain should also be assessed.

Weakness and numbness are less common symptoms and may be extremely subjective. (Weakness is more often due to pain than actual motor loss.) An attempt should be made to document them, however. The following information should be ascertained: (1) whether the weakness is generalized or involves specific muscles or muscle groups; (2) whether there is any loss of sphincter control; and (3) whether the numbness follows a dermatome, peripheral nerve, or stocking/glove pattern. The pain and numbness that follow specific dermatome nerve patterns are often very diagnostic, but the numbness that follows a stocking or glove type of distribution frequently indicates psychosomatic illness. It should also be determined whether the symptoms are worse at night or during the day. The pain from carpal tunnel syndrome, for example, is characteristically most severe at night.

When deformity is the initial complaint, the following information should be obtained: (1) whether the patient or someone else first noticed the deformity; (2) whether it is increasing or decreasing; and (3) whether it is associated with any recent injury, joint swelling, or stiffness. The amount of actual disability that the deformity causes the patient is also of considerable importance.

(It should also be recorded whether or not the patient will be released to work and, if so, on what date. If this is clearly discussed with the patient and recorded in the chart, future correspondence with the employer or insurance companies is simplified.)

EXAMINATION

Valuable information can frequently be gained by merely observing the gait, general posture, and stance of many patients. This is especially helpful in the child who may otherwise be difficult to ex-

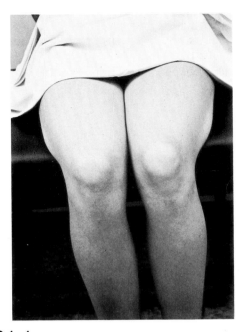

FIG 1–1.
Proper attire for knee examination. Both lower extremities are completely exposed.

amine. The height and weight of the patient are recorded, and all examinations are performed with the affected area completely exposed (Fig 1–1). The patient should always be viewed in profile as well as from the front and back.

The specific affected area is then inspected, and any swelling, discoloration, or areas of tenderness are noted. Palpation should be gentle but persistent. Every attempt should be made to describe affected areas according to their exact anatomic location. Movements or maneuvers that exacerbate the pain are recorded. Any muscle atrophy is noted and compared with measurements of the opposite extremity. Muscle power is tested in a similar manner. Alterations in skin temperature or perspiration are also noted.

Active and passive ranges of joint motion are carefully measured, and the patient is observed for any crepitus or resistance to movement. During the examination, adjacent joints may need to be stabilized in order to properly measure the affected joint (Fig 1–2).

Measurements of limb length and circumference are also made when indicated, and a complete neurologic examination is performed when neuromuscular disease is suspected.

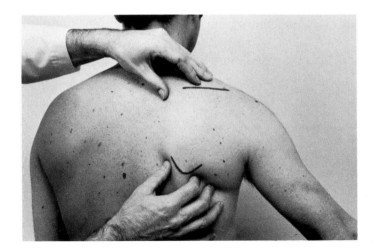

FIG 1–2.
True glenohumeral motion is measured by first stabilizing the scapula to prevent scapulothoracic motion. This is accomplished by prohibiting movement of the palpable spine and inferior angle.

ORTHOPEDIC TERMINOLOGY

General

Ankylosis: restriction of motion in a joint (synostosis)

Antalgic gait: gait pattern in which the weight is quickly removed from the affected extremity due to pain

Arthrodesis: surgical stiffening of a joint (fusion)

Arthroplasty: to restore motion and function to a joint

Coxa: hip bone or joint (os coxae)

Cubitus: elbow

Effusion: escape of fluid into a cavity

Functional: nonorganic, not due to a structural defect

Genu: knee or knee joint

Hallux: great toe

Orthopedic: "straight child"

Paresthesia: abnormal sensation, such as burning and tingling

Pes: foot

Pollex (pollicis): thumb

Radicular: spinal nerve involvement

Spondylitis: inflammation involving the spinal column

Spondylolisthesis: slipping of a vertebra, usually due to spondylolysis

Spondylolysis: dissolution or loosening of a vertebra

Spondylosis: disease, usually degenerative, of a vertebra

Sprain: injury to joint ligament or capsule

Strain: injury to muscle or tendon

Subluxation: incomplete dislocation

Talipes: talus (ankle) plus pes (foot)

Note: when referring to fingers, it is best to use a name (thumb, index, long, ring, and small) rather than a number

Motion

Flexion: bending of a joint

Extension: straightening of a joint

Abduction: movement away from the middle line (in the hand, the long finger is the middle line)

Adduction: movement toward the middle line

Pronation: to rotate the forearm in such a way that the palm looks backward when the arm is in the anatomic position

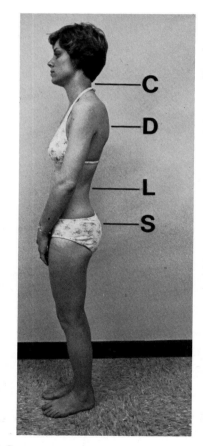

FIG 1–3.
A mild kyphosis is normally present in the dorsal *(D)* and sacral *(S)* spine. Lordosis is normally present in the cervical *(C)* and lumbar *(L)* spine.

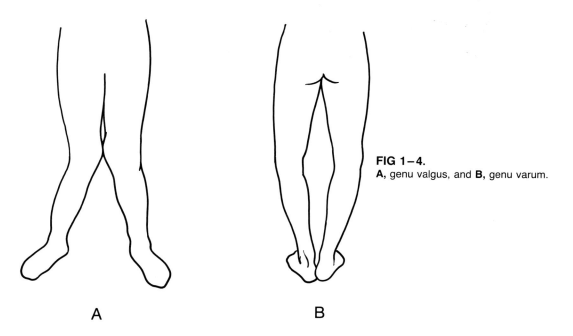

FIG 1–4.
A, genu valgus, and **B,** genu varum.

Supination: to rotate the forearm in such a way that the palm looks forward when the arm is in the anatomic position

Eversion: turning outward (in the foot, valgus, eversion, and pronation are frequently synonymous)

Inversion: turning inward (in the foot, varus, inversion, and supination are frequently synonymous)

Deformity

Kyphosis: curvature of the spine with posterior convexity (Fig 1–3)

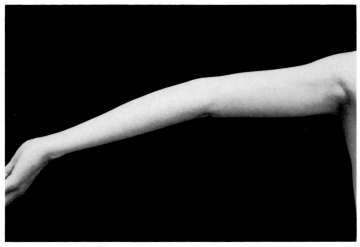

FIG 1–5.
Recurvatum of the elbow.

Lordosis: curvature of the spine with anterior convexity

Scoliosis: abnormal lateral curvature of the spine

Equinus: plantar flexion of the foot

Calcaneus: dorsiflexion of the foot

Planus: flat; abnormally low arch

Cavus: hollow; abnormally high arch

Varus: the distal part angulates toward the midline of the body (Fig 1−4)

Valgus: the distal part angulates away from the midline of the body

Recurvatum: backward bending or hyperextension (Fig 1−5)

CHAPTER 2

Fractures: General Management

Most fractures are easily recognized both clinically and roentgenographically (Fig 2–1). A satisfactory end result in the treatment of these injuries will depend not only on reduction of the fracture and maintenance of that reduction but also on restoration of the function of the injured extremity. These goals are reached by appreciating both the bony and soft tissue structures involved.

TERMINOLOGY

Fracture: a break in the continuity of a bone

Open ("compound"): fracture in which there is an open wound of the skin and soft parts that leads into the fracture

Closed ("simple"): fracture that does not have an open wound in the skin

Comminuted: fracture with multiple fragments (Fig 2–2)

Avulsion ("chip"): small fracture near a joint that usually has a ligament or tendon attached

Impacted: fracture whose ends are driven into each other

Displaced: fracture whose ends are separated

Greenstick: incomplete fracture that usually occurs in children

Pathologic: fracture that occurs because the bone is weakened by some abnormal condition

Intra-articular: fracture that involves the joint surface of a bone

Fatigue: fracture that results from repeated minor stresses

Torus: "buckle" fracture caused by compression of the cortex, most common in the distal portion of the radius of the child

Occult: clinical condition that suggests a fracture. Roentgenograms 2 to 3 weeks later may show the fracture line or new bone formation

Epiphyseal: fracture of the growth plate, usually in a long bone

Apposition: amount of end-to-end contact of the fracture (Fig 2–3)

Alignment: rotational or angular position

Nonunion: failure of bony healing

Malunion: healing in an unsatisfactory position

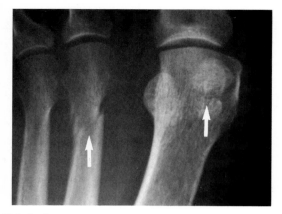

FIG 2–1.
Fracture of the second metatarsal neck and a bipartite tibial sesamoid *(arrows)*. The fracture is distinguished from the bipartite sesamoid or accessory bone by its sharp, pointed edges and irregular margin.

Dislocation (luxation): disruption in the continuity of a joint

Subluxation: partial disruption in the continuity of a joint (an incomplete dislocation)

Fracture-dislocation: dislocation that occurs in conjunction with a fracture of the joint (Fig 2–4). If incomplete, it is called a fracture-subluxation

Note: Fractures do not dislocate, they displace (shorten, angulate, etc). They are thus described according to the type, place in the bone, amount of displacement, and angulation (Fig 2–5). Rotation (torsion) is often difficult to visualize roentgenographically but relatively easy clinically. Rotation is usually described in reference to the distal fragment, as is angulation.

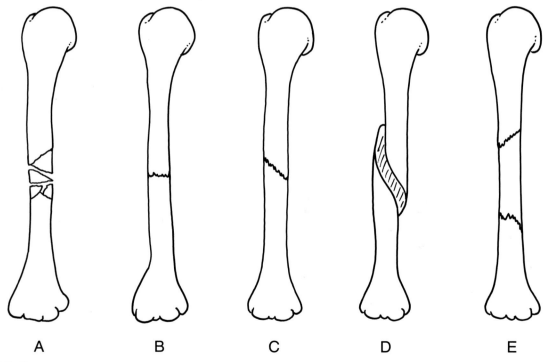

A B C D E

FIG 2–2.
Midshaft fractures of the humerus. **A,** comminuted. **B,** transverse, undisplaced. **C,** oblique, undisplaced. **D,** spiral. **E,** segmental.

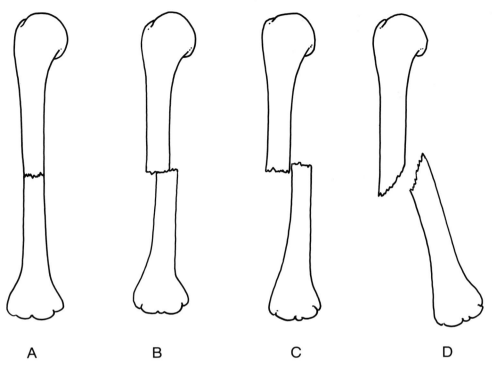

FIG 2–3.
Apposition and alignment of midshaft fractures of the humerus, anteroposterior (AP) view. **A,** perfect end-to-end apposition, perfect alignment, **B,** 50% end-to-end apposition, perfect alignment. **C,** side-to-side (bayonet) apposition, slight shortening, perfect alignment. **D,** no apposition, approximately 30-degree angulation.

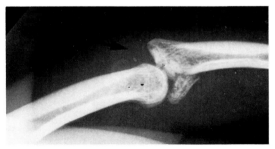

FIG 2–4.
A fracture-subluxation of the proximal interphalangeal joint with the middle phalanx subluxed dorsally.

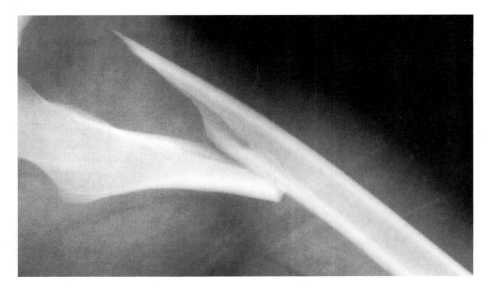

FIG 2–5.
A lateral view of a fracture of the upper portion of the femur. The fracture is closed. It is described as a closed, displaced spiral fracture of the proximal third of the femur with 20 to 30 degrees' angulation, apex anterior, and shortening of 1 to 2 cm.

GENERAL CONSIDERATIONS

Initial Care

All major long-bone fractures should be splinted before the patient is transported. Careless handling of the extremity that further damages the soft tissue should be avoided, but it is wise to correct any significant rotational or angular malalignment before applying a splinting device. This is done by gentle traction in the long axis of the limb. Do not, however, pull the protruding bone

ends of an open fracture back into the wound.

A variety of splinting devices are available that make transfer of the patient to the hospital more comfortable (Fig 2–6). Their use should be only temporary, however, until the diagnosis is confirmed roentgenographically. If definitive treatment of the fracture is to be delayed, a well-padded plaster splint or soft dressing such as the "Robert Jones" dressing should be applied. This

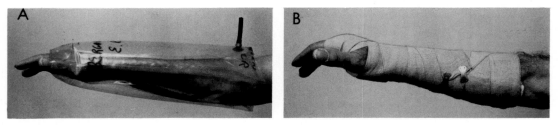

FIG 2–6.
A, temporary splint used for transfer. **B,** well-padded bulky dressing reinforced with plaster splints that should be applied as soon as possible. An elastic bandage alone should never be used. It does not immobilize, nor does it "reduce" swelling. It may, in fact, do more harm by further compressing the already compromised lymphatic and venous drainage systems.

TABLE 2–1.
Occasional Neurovascular Complications of Common Injuries

Bony Injury	Lesion	Prominent Early Findings
Anterior shoulder dislocation	Circumflex axillary nerve injury	Mid-deltoid numbness
Spiral fracture of humerus	Radial nerve injury	Wrist drop
Avulsion fracture of medial epicondyle	Ulnar nerve injury	Numbness of small finger, weak finger abduction, adduction
Severe elbow fracture	Brachial artery injury	Severe pain, pain on passive finger extension
Fractured distal radius, ulna	Median or ulnar nerve injury	Numbness, motor loss
Posterior dislocation of hip	Sciatic nerve injury (usually peroneal portion)	Foot drop, weak extensor hallucis longus, numbness on dorsum of foot or great toe
Fracture of upper fibula	Peroneal nerve injury	Same
Fracture of upper tibia	Compartment syndrome	Severe pain, pain on passive stretch of involved compartment muscles

dressing is made by applying several layers of cast padding or cotton roll to the extremity. Plaster splints are added, and the entire dressing is wrapped with elastic bandage.

The extremity is then elevated above the level of the heart, and ice is applied to control swelling. The neurologic and circulatory status of the extremity distal to the injury should always be checked and recorded (Table 2–1). A complete neurologic examination is usually unnecessary. If the patient can extend the thumb and flex and spread the fingers, the major nerves of the upper extremity are functioning; if the patient can flex and extend the toes, the major nerves to the lower extremity are intact. If a neurologic or vascular impairment is present, it is often relieved by reduction of the fracture or dislocation. If a neurologic impairment persists following the reduction, it is usually treated by simple observation and exercises to prevent contractures. The prognosis is generally good for complete recovery. Circulatory impairment that persists requires immediate vascular evaluation. The initial neurologic examination is particularly important because if a deficit is discovered only *after* treatment, it may not be able to be determined whether it was present before or occurred as a result of treatment.

DEFINITIVE FRACTURE CARE

Fracture healing is mainly a local event and is influenced very little by generalized disease or advanced age. When a fracture occurs, the periosteum and other soft tissues are damaged, and there is an outpouring of blood and exudate. The fibrin from this hematoma helps form a mesh that holds all of the elements of the fracture together. Cellular differentiation and tissue organization occur and lead to the formation of a soft, stabilizing callus that encompasses the fracture ends. Eventually, this callus matures into mineralized bone.

To encourage this sequence of healing, the bone ends must be kept in apposition, sufficient blood supply must be maintained, and the bone fragments must be adequately immobilized. Otherwise, fibrous tissue may form instead of callus and lead to nonunion. While healing bone does have some ability to "bridge" a gap, especially in the young whose callus-generating periosteum is so active, distraction of the bone ends is to be avoided. Conversely, compression of the fractured bone ends tends to stimulate fracture healing in many cases. Also, bones such as the clavicle and tibia, which are subcutaneous and have less surrounding soft tissue and blood supply, tend to heal more slowly, while fractures in the vascular metaphysis of any bone heal more rapidly. Open fractures or those with soft-tissue interposition will also heal more slowly because these factors compromise the local environment. Another element that influences healing is the type of fracture. Spiral shaft fractures, for example, tend to heal much more readily than do transverse shaft fractures because of the large amount of bone surface and hematoma available in the spiral fracture.

It is in consideration of these various local factors that decisions regarding the treatment of all fractures are made. These decisions are based on the goals of fracture treatment: (1) alignment of the bones in both the angular and rotational planes, (2) restoration of proper length, (3) restoration of apposition of the bone ends, and (4) adequate immobilization.

Many fractures require no treatment or, at most, simple restriction of activity with a sling or crutches (Table 2–2). The remaining fractures are usually treated by one of four general methods: (1) open or closed reduction with internal fixation, (2) continuous traction usually followed by cast immobilization, (3) closed reduction with external skeletal fixation, or (4) closed reduction followed by cast immobilization.

Open or Closed Reduction With Internal Fixation. Closed rather than open treatment of most fractures is usually preferred in order to avoid stripping the soft tissue and periosteum and devascularizing the bone ends. Closed treatment also decreases the chance of infection. There are several fractures, however, in which accurate anatomic positioning of the fragments and rigid internal fixation are beneficial: (1) displaced joint fractures, especially the weight-bearing joints; (2) fractures that cannot be reduced or held by closed methods; (3) fractures of the lower extremity in the elderly in order to allow early activity; (4) certain epiphyseal fractures that could result in a growth disturbance if not accurately reduced; and (5) joint fractures in which early motion would be helpful to prevent stiffness.

Continuous Traction. Traction is a means of aligning the bone ends and maintaining the reduction, especially if the fracture is comminuted or unstable. It is usually applied by a skeletal traction pin because prolonged skin traction may cause blisters. Skin traction is sufficient in the very young because their fractures stabilize sooner and require less time in traction. After enough healing has occurred to maintain length and alignment, a plaster cast is applied.

External Fixation. External skeletal fixation is a means of fracture treatment that utilizes multiple pins usually placed above and below the fracture site. The fracture is then reduced, and the pins are incorporated into an outrigger or plaster cast. This method is useful in compound fractures with soft tissue damage that require exposure of the fracture site. It is particularly helpful in Colles' fractures that are losing position.

TABLE 2–2.

Common Fractures Not Requiring Plaster Immobilization*

Fracture	Treatment
Impacted surgical neck of humerus	Shoulder immobilizer
Undisplaced radial head fracture	Sling
Undisplaced olecranon	Sling
Undisplaced patella	Knee immobilizer
Shaft of fibula	Crutches
Base of fifth metatarsal	Hard sandal
Stress fracture	Avoid offending activity
Toe phalanges (undisplaced)	Tape to adjacent toe
Undisplaced calcaneus	Crutches

*These fractures are stable and should not shift if the extremity is moved. A soft compression dressing for the first 2 to 3 days may be helpful in some cases.

The Elements of Closed Reduction

Most common fractures are able to be treated by manual reduction and immobilization, but in order for this procedure to be successful, certain mechanical aspects of the fracture should be understood. Whenever a bone has been broken and the fractured ends separate, the soft tissue (mainly periosteum) on the side opposite the direction of displacement will rupture and allow the fracture to angulate and rotate (Fig 2–7). The tissue on the side to which the displacement occurs remains intact, although it may be stripped off of the bone. This intact soft tissue forms a "hinge" that can be used in the treatment of many fractures to help guide the displaced distal fragment or fragments into place and to help maintain that position.

There are many methods used to place bones back into their original position. Most of these require that the distal fragment be placed into apposition to the proximal one. Some fractures require only a "push" back into place (Fig 2–8). Others need a more complicated maneuver that incorporates traction and manipulation of the fragments (Fig 2–9). The nature of the fracture and its displacement will determine which is necessary.

Before any reduction is attempted, each fracture should be thoroughly studied and a complete mental plan developed. This should include every detail in the manipulation, including

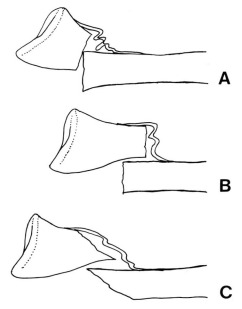

FIG 2–8.
A, an epiphyseal fracture that simply requires that the distal fragment be gently pushed back into place. **B,** a transverse fracture that may be reduced by simple traction. **C,** an oblique "toggle" type of fracture that will require a more complicated manipulation. Even though the fracture fragments are not shortened, they must be angulated in order to accomplish the reduction. Simple traction would only tighten the soft-tissue hinge and prevent reduction of this fracture.

where the operator will be positioned, how the extremity will be grasped and held, and where the assistant should be positioned. In general, most reductions are accomplished as follows: (1) a variable amount of traction is applied to the distal fragment with countertraction on the proximal fragment. (2) The deformity is increased if necessary, and rotational malalignment is then corrected. (3) The distal fragment is then reduced and the angular deformity corrected. The periosteal hinge will usually prevent overreduction.

Utilization of this manipulative method and the soft-tissue hinge applies only to transverse or short oblique fractures that are stable after their irregular bone ends are engaged. It does not work with long oblique or spiral fractures or

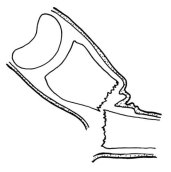

FIG 2–7.
A typical fracture with an intact "periosteal hinge" on the concave side.

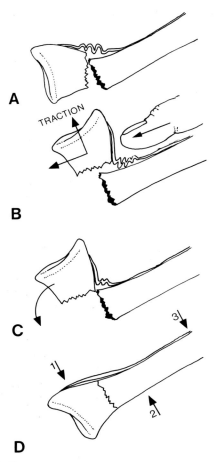

FIG 2–9.
A, typical Colles' fracture. **B,** the distal fragment is disimpacted, and the deformity is increased. Thumb pressure and traction are applied, and the distal fragment is pushed distally to reduce the dorsal cortex **(C).** The reduction is completed by volar pressure and held with three-point cast molding *(arrows)* to keep the soft-tissue hinge tight **(D).**

with markedly comminuted ones because their ends cannot be engaged to prevent shortening.

Questions often arise as to what constitutes an adequate reduction. In general, the following principles are valid:

1. Rotational deformity should always be completely corrected at any age.

2. In adults, angular deformity should also be completely corrected, especially in fractures of the fingers, forearm, and lower extremities.

3. In children, some angular deformity (15 to 20 degrees) that is close to a joint and in the same plane of motion as that joint will correct if sufficient growth remains.

4. Perfect apposition is not always necessary for normal healing.

5. Fractures involving the weight-bearing joints require exact reduction.

6. Slight shortening in the upper extremity is often acceptable, but proper length in the lower extremity is preferable.

Anesthesia

Adequate anesthesia can usually be obtained by direct infiltration of the fracture hematoma on the extensor side under sterile conditions with 5 to 10 mL of a local anesthetic. If a local anesthetic is to be used, the procedure should be undertaken soon after the injury. Otherwise, the hematoma may clot, and the anesthetic will not spread through the fracture as well. Regional anesthetics are also helpful because they eliminate the need to add more volume of fluid to an already swollen area. Digital or metacarpal blocks work well for finger fractures.

The intravenous or Bier block is useful in forearm and wrist fractures, although the movement of the extremity required to perform the block is sometimes uncomfortable. An intravenous line is always established in the other upper extremity in the event of a complication. Light sedation is then administered. Diazepam is favored because of its additional anticonvulsant activity. A small needle is then inserted into an appropriate distal vein on the injured extremity, and a double tourniquet is applied to the upper portion of the limb. The extremity is then exsanguinated up to the tourniquet with an elastic wrap or, if this is painful, simply elevated for 3 minutes to empty the venous system. The proximal tourniquet is then inflated above the systolic blood pressure, and any elastic wrap is removed. The venous system is then filled, depending on the size of the patient, with 30 to 50 mL of a 0.5% solution of lidocaine mixed with nonbacteriostatic normal saline. The needle is then removed from the involved extremity. After a few minutes, the fracture will be able to be manipulated. If the proximal tourniquet becomes painful, it can be released after the lower one has been inflated because the lower tourniquet is now in an area that has adequate anesthesia.

After the procedure has been completed, the tourniquet is slowly and intermittently released in order to avoid the undesirable central nervous system (CNS) and cardiovascular side effects that occasionally occur when the anesthetic enters the circulation. These are early CNS irritability followed by sedation. Seizures, tremors, and bradycardia have even rarely been reported. Both tourniquets should not be released until at least 20 minutes have passed after the lidocaine injection even if the procedure takes less time.

External Immobilization

Casts are applied for three reasons: (1) to immobilize the ends of a fracture, (2) to allow ambulation, and (3) to hold the position of reduction. A cast never completely immobilizes a fracture. If properly applied, however, it provides enough relative immobilization to allow the fracture to heal.

A variety of materials are available for casting. Plaster of Paris continues to be popular because it is easy to work, it has a long shelf life, and it is relatively low in cost. Synthetic casting materials are becoming increasingly popular because of their light weight and strength. A disadvantage for the generalist using these materials is that they have a relatively short shelf life of 2 to 3 months in some cases and they are also more expensive. Less material is usually needed than for plaster, however. Originally, these materials were touted as being able to be worn while swimming and bathing. While the cast material, padding, and stockinette are synthetic and do not "hold" water, the padding itself is difficult to dry completely even with a blow dryer. It tends to hold some moisture against the skin that can cause the skin to become macerated. Thus, it is not recommended that even these materials be allowed to get wet. If they are chosen, be certain to turn the packages occasionally so that the material does not become dry. Commonly used sizes, are 2-, 3-, and 4-in. stockinettes; 3- and 4-in. cast paddings; and 2-, 3-, 4-, and 5-in. plaster or lightcast rolls.

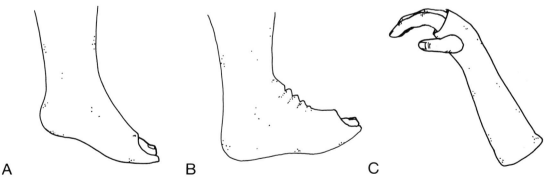

A   **B**   **C**

FIG 2–10.
Proper joint positions for casting. **A,** the ankle is in too much equinus. If the position is changed to the proper position of 90 degrees after the padding or plaster has been applied, a painful cast ridge may develop **(B). C,** proper position and length of the short arm cast. Note that the metacarpophalangeal joints should be able to be completely flexed to a right angle and the cast should not extend beyond the distal palmar crease or too far down on the small finger. The patient should also be able to fan the fingers. The elbow joint is usually casted at 90 degrees and the knee at 30 degrees if they are included in the cast.

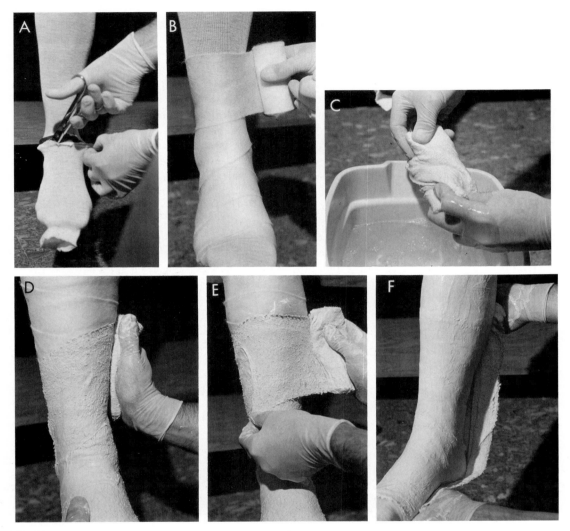

FIG 2–11.
The cast. **A,** a stockinette may first be applied. Any folds in front should be trimmed. **B,** beginning at one end, cast padding is added while overlapping each roll by half. **C,** the plaster is removed from the water after the bubbles cease. The ends are pinched shut, and the roll is gently squeezed to expel excess water. Less water or excess wringing causes faster drying. Using the larger sizes may help avoid premature drying of the roll. Wet plaster makes a smoother cast. **D,** beginning at one end, the plaster is pushed onto the extremity by using gentle pressure by the thenar eminence against the middle of the roll. The roll should remain in contact with the limb and is usually not lifted from it. Additional rolls are started where the last one ended. The roll is applied so that the opening side faces the operator and not the extremity. Rolling is continuous, and each layer is rubbed so that all layers fuse together. The short leg cast (SLC) should always extend under the metatarsal heads for support. **E,** tucks or pleats are taken as often as necessary to guide the roll and to accommodate any tapering of the limb. The stockinette is folded back and incorporated into the cast. **F,** reinforcing splints five to ten layers thick applied to the sides or back add a great deal of strength without adding much weight. They are particularly useful above the ankle where the cast is weakest and breakage is most common.

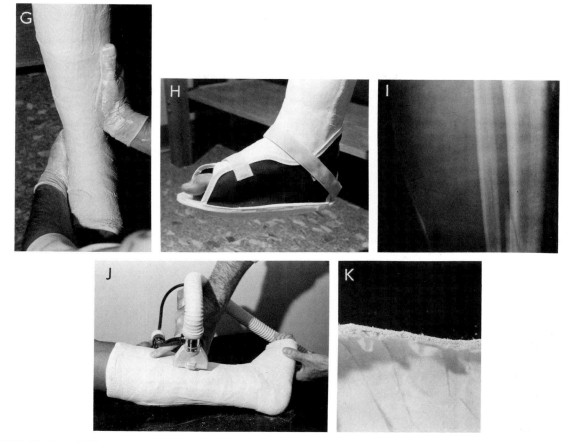

FIG 2-11 (cont'd.).
G, the cast is molded with the flat surface of the hands, if necessary, and trimmed, especially at the small toe. **H,** cast boots function better than walking heels. There are fewer repairs and a better gait. Wait 48 hours for the cast to cure before allowing weight bearing on plaster (1 hour for lightcast). **I,** roentgenogram of a portion of an SLC showing a cast of even thickness without excessive padding between the cast and the skin. **J,** casts are removed with the cast saw and spreader. The cast is removed by cutting down through both sides (a sharp saw blade works better than a dull one). Do not saw back and forth with the blade. It is better to pick the blade up and move it every time the plaster is cut through. Counterpressure with the thumb and/or index finger on the cast will prevent the blade from injuring the underlying skin. **K,** the sectioned cast showing even, fused plaster that is properly contoured and molded. It is as thick at the end as it is in the middle. The use of wider rolls will result in a more even cast than the use of many small rolls. Two 4-in. rolls of plaster will suffice for an adult short arm cast (or two 2-in. rolls of lightcast). Three 6-in. rolls are necessary for an adult SLC (or three 4-in. rolls of lightcast).

Bivalved splints (usually anterior and posterior) are occasionally preferred by some physicians to circular casts as primary care in order to avoid possible circulatory and swelling complications. These are sometimes called "sugar tong" if the unit is continuous. The splint system, shaped like an elongated "U," is held in position by gauze or an elastic bandage. It can be easily loosened or tightened if needed.

Whenever a cast is used, the extremity should always be held in the position of function while the cast is being applied, unless the extremity must be positioned otherwise, such as for maintenance of fracture position (Fig 2–10). Casts are always applied in the same orderly sequence. The assistant holds the extremity in the proper position, and a single layer of stockinette, although not always necessary, may be applied (Fig 2–11). Cast padding is then applied, beginning at one end and proceeding to the other to a double thickness by overlapping the roll 50% each turn. Do not overpad because the cast will be loose, but do place an extra piece of padding over bony prominences or other areas of concern (peroneal nerve at the fibular neck, ulnar styloid, both malleoli, and the olecranon process).

The plaster roll is then placed in lukewarm water and left until the bubbling ceases. Plaster sets more slowly in cold water, thus allowing more time to work. Warmer water causes plaster to set more quickly. Never use hot water. After removal from the water, the ends of the plaster are pinched together, and the roll is gently twisted. This removes some of the water but not the plaster. The plaster roll is then applied to the limb in the same manner as the cotton was, that is, starting at one end and going up and down the extremity while overlapping by 50% each turn. Moderate tension is used during the application, with greater tension being used on the proximal fleshy part of the extremity. Tucks or pleats are taken frequently to allow the plaster to be smooth and even on parts of the extremity that taper. This also avoids ridges or transverse creases. The roll is applied by pushing it with the thenar eminence and should be kept close to or on the extremity at all times.

The cast should be of uniform thickness, about 0.6 cm. No two turns should be made at the same spot, except at the ends of the cast. Thus, the plaster is applied evenly end to end and will not be any thicker at the fracture site than elsewhere. Each layer should be applied moist to allow each turn to bond to the next layer. If this does not occur, a cast results that is several individual layers thick rather than one single thickness. The plaster should be worked and smoothed during the application of each layer.

While the plaster is setting, it is contoured and molded with the flat of the palm or thenar eminence to apply the proper three-point fixation. Overzealous rubbing while in the late drying phase may cause the plaster to crumble while it is setting.

Lightcast is easier to apply in that tucks and reinforcing splints are not necessary. Always wear gloves because the bonding material adheres to the skin and is difficult to remove. Use *cool* water for lightcast.

As a general rule, a cast should immobilize one joint above and below the fracture, although short arm casts are often used for wrist fractures and short leg casts for ankle fractures. Two rolls of 4-in. plaster or 2-in. lightcast are sufficient for a short arm cast. Three rolls of 6-in. plaster or 4-in. lightcast are adequate for a short leg cast.

If the fracture is inherently stable, the cast merely acts as a splinting device. Fractures that require reduction use the cast to hold the reduction by maintaining three-point tension on the soft tissue hinge, two of the points being the operator's hands that mold the cast into a flat appearance. The third point is a wide area of the proximal portion of the cast. It is unnecessary to apply direct pressure there.

Aftercare

Following cast application, the extremity is elevated above the horizontal level of the heart, and ice is applied for 48 to 72 hours. The patient is closely observed for signs and symptoms of circulatory obstruction or acute compartmental syndrome. (Excessive pain may be the only early clue.) Hospitalization may even be necessary in some cases. The cast must be split and spread at the earliest sign of circulatory embarrassment. If discomfort secondary to swelling is the only problem, spreading the plaster alone is usually sufficient, but if there is concern for the circulatory status of the extremity, the entire cast, cotton, and every bit of stockinette should be split completely down to the skin and spread apart. If the problem persists, the entire cast should be removed, although this is usually unnecessary. Plaster "splits" more easily to relieve swelling than lightcast does. It needs to be cut on only one side and spread. The opposite side will usually crack and keep the split open. Fiberglass must be cut slightly on the opposite side. Otherwise, it "springs" back.

It is often difficult to differentiate among fracture pain, compartment syndrome, arterial injury, and nerve palsy, especially in an anxious patient. Peripheral nerve testing will usually rule out nerve palsy, and if peripheral pulses are present, arterial injury is unlikely. A compartment syndrome should be suspected if there is (1) pain on passive stretching of the muscles of the affected compartment, (2) sensory loss, and (3) tenseness of the involved compartment. Arterial injury or compartment syndrome secondary to swelling in a tight cast could lead to Volkmann's ischemic contracture if untreated (Fig 2–12). This is a rare complication and most commonly occurs following severe elbow injuries, high tibial fractures, and metatarsal fractures.

Movement of all joints that are not immobilized is encouraged as soon as possible. Fewer vasomotor disturbances, less swelling, and a

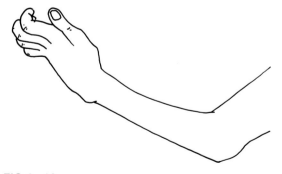

FIG 2–12.
Drawing of a typical Volkmann's ischemic contracture. Contractures and severe muscle loss are the usual end result. The deformity will often persist in spite of prolonged attempts at reconstructive surgery and therapy.

faster recovery will result. Painful pressure sores may develop rapidly under a cast. *Remember:* the pain will subside when tissue necrosis has occurred. These pressure areas, although rare in a properly padded cast, should be treated or at least evaluated before skin necrosis occurs. If a "window" must be cut in a cast or it must be split, the window or padding should always be replaced to prevent edema of the soft tissue from swelling through the hole or the split section. If a cast has been properly applied, it should not require changing during the course of treatment, even after swelling subsides. If the cast telescopes, however, and there is danger of losing the position of the fracture, it should be changed.

Roentgenograms are repeated at weekly intervals for 2 to 3 weeks mainly to assess the state of the reduction. Healing changes may not be visible for some time. The length of time required for complete healing varies with the age of the patient, the nature and site of the fracture, and the specific bone involved. As a rule, fractures in children and fractures near the ends of the bone (metaphysis) heal more rapidly than do those in the relatively avascular midshaft (diaphysis).

The determination as to when a cast may be removed is not made on the basis of the roentgenogram alone. Roentgenographic evidence of complete healing may lag several weeks behind true clinical union. In general, the cast may be removed when sufficient time has passed for the particular bone under treatment to heal. This varies with each bone. Clinical and roentgenographic assessments are made after the cast has been removed, and if the fracture has no motion and is not tender to palpation, pressure, or stress, then sufficient healing has probably occurred to allow the cast to be left off. If any doubt exists, a removable protective splint may be applied for another 2 to 3 weeks, and gradual resumption of limited activity is allowed. If motion, tenderness, or swelling is present, suggesting a slow union, another circular cast is applied, and the fracture is reassessed in 2 to 3 weeks.

Rehabilitation

It is important that the patient be kept informed of the entire treatment plan from start to finish. This should include what to expect after the cast has been removed: stiffness for several weeks, swelling, callous bumps, increased hair on the arms and legs in youngsters, or a temporary limp. These usually subside in a few weeks. It is equally important not to let the patient become active too quickly after the cast has been removed. Allow some time for the bone to regain its strength (4 to 6 weeks).

Rehabilitation is actually begun at the time of the injury by controlling excessive soft-tissue swelling. Scar formation is thus diminished, and earlier normal function is the end result once the fracture has healed. Early motion is encouraged, and after the initial pain and swelling have subsided, the patient is instructed to use any joints that are not immobilized by the cast and perform some meaningful tasks at home or work.

Following cast removal, active mobilization of joints that were immobilized by the cast is begun. A repetitive exercise that the patient may perform at home is preferable to most forms of physical therapy. Exercise in a swimming pool is an excellent method of restoring strength, mobility, and confidence following many injuries. Most extremities are able to regain most of their motion and strength within 4 to 6 weeks after the cast has been removed but it is not uncommon for some stiffness, weakness, and swelling to persist longer. Formal physical therapy is usually unnecessary.

A bone scan may remain positive up to 2 years following cast removal and signify ongoing fracture remodeling and strengthening. Wait at least 2 months after cast removal before allowing most sports activities.

Additional Principles

1. Always obtain comparison roentgenograms of the opposite extremity whenever a questionable fracture is present, especially in a child.
2. Always obtain roentgenograms in at least two planes at right angles to each other and include a joint above and below the area of injury. Obtain oblique views whenever necessary.
3. When one bone of a two-bone set (forearm, lower part of the leg) is fractured and becomes shortened or angulated, always look for injury to the other bone or a dislocation.
4. Be certain to correct both rotational and angular malalignment in the reduction.
5. Take stress roentgenograms whenever necessary.
6. Don't be satisfied with one diagnosis (always look for a second injury).
7. Reduce the fracture as soon as possible. There is little to be gained by "waiting for the swelling to go down." The swelling will probably only increase because of the deformity.
8. Avulsion fractures near a joint should always be carefully evaluated for instability and tendon function.
9. The measure of success is the usefulness of the extremity and not just the roentgenographic appearance.

FRACTURES IN CHILDREN

Fractures in children differ from those in adults in many respects. They are usually less complicated and, with a few exceptions, are always treated with closed methods. Nonunion is rare due to the active periosteum and abundant blood supply surrounding the bone of the growing child. The principles of treatment are similar to those in adults. However, the fact that in children the bone continues to grow after the fracture has healed will allow for some correction and realignment of minor deformities.

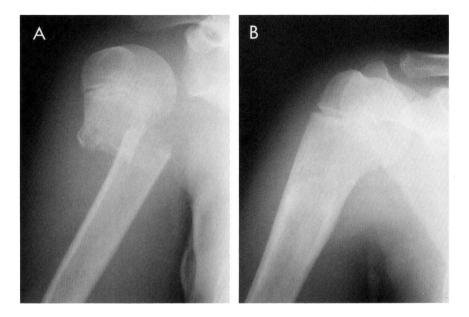

FIG 2–13.
A, fracture of the upper portion of the humerus in a patient aged 6 years. An attempt was made to reduce the fracture, but the position could not be improved and was accepted. **B,** the same patient approximately 10 months later. Although the two roentgenograms are not in the same rotation, the remodeling is obvious.

Principles of Treatment

1. Mild angular deformities will frequently correct themselves with growth. The amount of correction depends on the amount of angulation, the age of the child, and the distance of the fracture from the end of the bone. The closer the fracture is to the end of the bone and the younger the patient, the greater the amount of angulation that is acceptable (Fig 2–13). Correction is also more complete if the angulation is in the same plane of motion as the nearest joint. Angular deformities that are not in the same plane of motion as the nearest joint will persist, however.

2. Rotational malalignment does not correct itself.

3. Fractures of the midshaft of the bone will not realign.

4. Apposition and mild shortening are of little importance in the young child. Bayonet (side-to-side) apposition is perfectly acceptable in long bone fractures in boys under 12 years of age and girls under 10 years. Slight shortening with reduction may actually be desirable in the leg because acceleration of growth occurs following a displaced fracture. The tibia and femur may overgrow up to 1 cm following a displaced fracture. Thus, some slight overlapping of these bones is occasionally desirable.

5. Physical therapy after the fracture has healed is usually unnecessary and may even be unwise in the child. Forceful manipulation of the extremity will only cause more swelling and stiffness.

6. A tender growth plate following an injury usually means that a fracture is present. Therefore, the injury should be treated as a fracture. "Sprains" are rare in children.

7. Nonunion is almost impossible in children.

8. Malposition may not be correctable after 7 to 10 days. Attempts to manipulate the fracture after that may damage the growth plate.

Note: *Remodeling* is the process of smoothing off of the sharp bone ends. It occurs in adults as well as children. Only children who have growth left, however, have the ability to straighten or *realign* mild fracture deformities.

The Epiphyseal Plate

Two types of epiphyses exist in growing bones: the pressure epiphysis and the traction epiphysis (apophysis). Pressure epiphyses occur at the ends of long bones and contribute to the longitudinal growth of the bone. Traction apophyses, such as the iliac crest and trochanters of the hip, contribute primarily to the contour of the bone and little to actual longitudinal growth. They are present at the origin of major muscles and respond to traction rather than to pressure.

The epiphyseal plate itself consists of several zones or layers (Fig 2–14). The zone nearest the joint is the germinal cell layer. Moving away from the joint are the zone of proliferation, the zone of hypertrophic cartilage, and the zone of provisional calcification. Epiphyseal fractures may be catergorized according to the type of injury, the relationship of the fracture line to the germinal cell layer, and the prognosis. Salter's classification is commonly used.

Most epiphyseal fractures occur irregularly through the weakest zone, the zone of hypertrophic cartilage. They are usually transverse and do not travel vertically across the germinal cell layer. These fractures are classified by Salter as type I or type II fractures, and the prognosis for normal healing is good (Fig 2–15). Manipulative reduction is usually successful. Overzealous attempts to correct minor persistent deformities during the reduction should not be made because these mild deformities will usually correct themselves with growth. Further damage to the growth plate may be caused by overaggressive treatment.

Fractures that do traverse the growth plate vertically (type III, type IV) may disturb the growth so that angular deformity will result from continued growth. Cross-union may occur across the epiphyseal plate. These fractures are also frequently intra-articular, and accurate reduction is mandatory to prevent growth disturbance from occurring and to restore the joint surface. Sur-

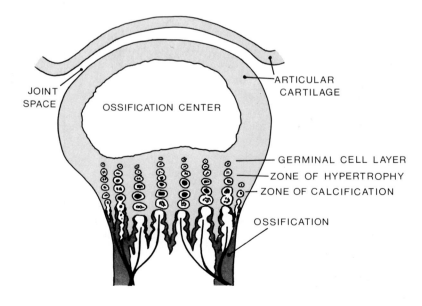

FIG 2–14.
The epiphyseal plate. Most epiphyseal fractures occur through the zone of hypertrophic cartilage.

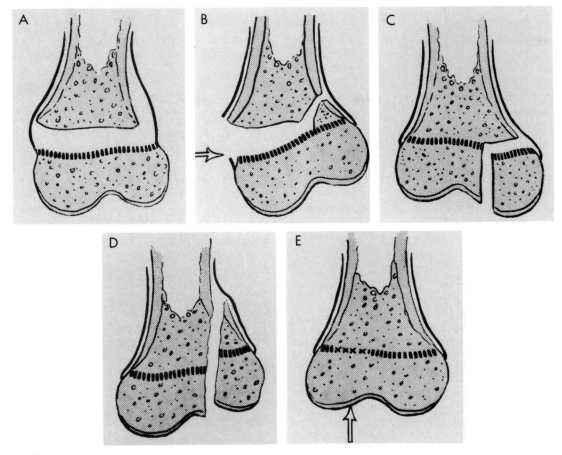

FIG 2–15.
Epiphyseal fractures. **A,** type I; **B,** type II; **C,** type III; **D,** type IV; **E,** type V crushing fracture. (From Salter RB, Harris WR: *J Bone Joint Surg [Am]* 1963; 45:609. Used by permission.)

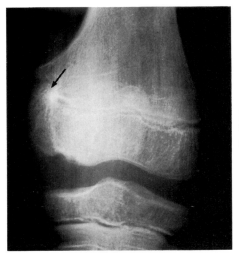

FIG 2–16.
Salter type V crush fracture that resulted in a complete bony bridge *(arrow)* being formed in the medial aspect of the lower femoral epiphysis.

gery is usually necessary in order to accomplish these goals. Type V fractures are crush injuries that have a poor prognosis (Fig 2–16). Frequently, no definite fracture line is visible.

FRACTURES REQUIRING SPECIAL CARE

Most of the fractures described throughout this text can be safely managed by the generalist using nonoperative means. There are, however, several common fractures that are fraught with complications even when treated by one familiar with them. Many fractures will also require surgical intervention or specialized closed treatment. These fractures should always be referred to a surgeon who is trained in their treatment. Some of the more common injuries include the following: (1) all open fractures. These need meticulous cleaning and debridement to prevent osteomyelitis or gas gangrene. (2) Intra-articular fractures. These require accurate reduction to prevent the onset of traumatic arthritis. (3) All femur fractures. Many of these will require prolonged traction, special casting, or surgery. (4) Most fractures of both bones of the lower leg in adults. In addition, there are several specific fractures in children and adults that should be treated only by an orthopedic surgeon (Table 2–3).

PATHOLOGIC FRACTURES

Pathologic fractures develop because of some abnormal local condition that causes the bone to become weakened. The most common causes are tumors that metastasize to bone. Other causes are infection, cystic lesions of bone, and Paget's disease. With the increase in the survival rate of cancer victims, there has also been an increase in the incidence of pathologic features. In order to maintain the highest possible level of function in patients, aggressive management of these fractures is frequently indicated.

The treatment is usually surgical (Fig 2–17).

TABLE 2–3.

Common Fractures and Their Complications

Fracture	Complication
In Children	
Supracondylar fracture of the humerus	Volkmann's contracture, malunion
Lateral condylar fracture of the humerus	Nonunion, cubitus valgus, late ulnar nerve paralysis
Epiphyseal fractures III, IV, V	Growth disturbance
Radial neck and head fracture	Growth disturbance
In Adults	
Fracture of both bones of the forearm or displaced single forearm bone	Malunion, nonunion, restricted forearm rotation
Displaced malleolar or bimalleolar fracture	Nonunion, traumatic arthritis
Supracondylar, intercondylar fracture of the humerus	Traumatic arthritis, joint stiffness
Displaced olecranon fracture	Nonunion
Displaced radial head fracture	Traumatic arthritis, joint stiffness

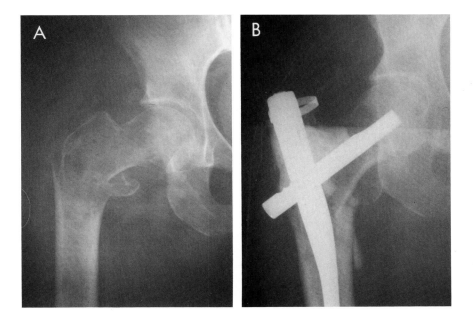

FIG 2–17.
A, pathologic fracture of the femur due to metastatic breast cancer. **B,** following open reduction and internal fixation, pain-free ambulation was possible.

Operative procedures are especially indicated in the lower extremities in order to encourage ambulatory activities. Although radiation therapy may relieve the pain, it can actually impede fracture healing. By stabilizing the fracture surgically, immediate use of the extremity is frequently pos-sible. This is accomplished by curetting the tu-mor, filling the resultant cavity with methyl-methacrylate cement, and adding the appropriate internal fixation device. The procedure is often performed on a prophylactic basis.

THE BATTERED CHILD

This term refers to a young child who is the vic-tim of physical abuse inflicted by a person usu-ally responsible for the child's care. As a general rule, these children tend to be young, under 4 years of age.

The diagnosis is often difficult. The history is usually suggestive. The parents are often evasive, or the cause of injury seems implausible. The parents are frequently quite young and seem poorly adjusted. A history of previous injuries should make the physician suspicious. Multiple bruises or signs of other soft tissue trauma may be present. The child may seem malnourished or in poor general health.

The injuries may be visceral, cranial, or mus-culoskeletal. The characteristic musculoskeletal lesions are (1) multiple bony lesions, frequently epiphyseal fractures, in various stages of healing and (2) excessive periosteal reaction indicative of recent trauma with or without fracture (Fig 2–18).

A complete skeletal survey is indicated in the workup. A bone scan may also be helpful to de-lineate other fractures. An attempt should also be

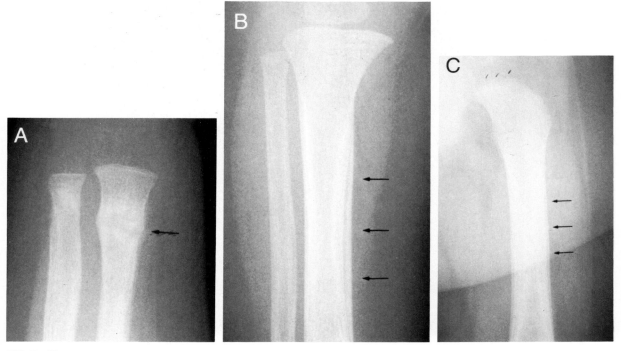

FIG 2–18.
Roentgenograms of a battered child. The child had multiple rib fractures as well as a fractured forearm **(A).** Note the periosteal reaction in the lower extremities **(B** and **C).**

made to rule out other possible causes of multiple fractures, especially osteogenesis imperfecta.

The treatment of the fractures is no different from that described in the sections on fractures of specific bones. In addition, it is the responsibility of the physician who suspects this condition to report it to the appropriate social service agency in order to protect the child from further mistreatment.

FATIGUE FRACTURES

Fatigue or stress fractures are incomplete fractures that occur as the result of prolonged, repetitive strains. They may occur in any weight-bearing bone but are most common in the metatarsal ("march" fracture), neck of the femur, calcaneus, tibia, and fibula. Unconditioned athletes are prone to this injury. It is also common in military personnel who are subjected to long hikes or marching in their physical training program.

Clinically, a history of unusual stress with subsequent pain over a bone is common. Local tenderness and swelling over the affected bone are usually present.

The roentgenogram is usually normal early in the disorder, although a bone scan would be positive. If this condition is suspected, treatment is instituted, and roentgenograms are repeated at 2-week intervals (Fig 2–19). A healing stress line is usually seen in 2 to 4 weeks. Exuberant periosteal bone formation may even simulate malig-

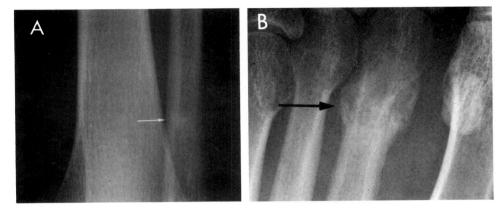

FIG 2–19.
A, fatigue fracture of the lower portion of the fibula with a sclerotic transverse line. **B,** "march" fracture of the second metatarsal neck with abundant callus.

nancy. Stress fractures in *cancellous* bone usually produce only a sclerotic transverse line without periosteal reaction. In *cortical* bone, however, there is generally considerable formation of periosteal new bone.

Treatment consists of protecting the bone from stress. Elimination of the offending activity is usually curative, although crutches are occasionally necessary. Gradual resumption of normal activity is allowed after the pain and tenderness subside.

ELECTRICAL STIMULATION OF BONE HEALING

In the early 1950s it was demonstrated that when bone is placed under stress, it exhibits a separation of charge. The side of the bone under compression becomes electronegative, and the side under tension becomes electropositive, thus creating an electrical potential. This is known as the piezoelectric effect. As a result of the findings, researchers began studying the effects of electricity on bone and cartilage. It was found that delivery of the proper amount of voltage and current by electrodes can stimulate osteogenesis.

A number of bone-stimulating devices are now available: (1) a semi-invasive percutaneous cathode system, (2) an invasive implant system, and (3) a noninvasive external inductive coupling device. These devices are used in conjunction with traditional fracture management (good reduction, adequate immbolization). At this time, they are only used in cases of delayed union or nonunion. The "success" rate varies from 60% to 75%. The indications for the use of these devices remain to be clearly defined.

BIBLIOGRAPHY

Bassett CA: The development and application of pulsed electromagnetic fields (PEMFs) for ununited fractures and arthrodeses. *Orthop Clin North Am* 1984; 15:61.

Blount WP; *Fractures in Children.* Baltimore, Williams & Wilkins, 1955.
Charnley J: *The Closed Treatment of Common Fractures,* ed 3. Edinburgh, Churchill Livingstone, 1970.

Compere EL, Banks SW, Compere CL: *Pictorial Handbook of Fracture Treatment,* ed 5. Chicago, Year Book Medical Publishers Inc, 1963.

Connolly JF: *Fracture Complications.* Chicago, Year Book Medical Publishers Inc, 1988.

Flatt AE: *The Care of Minor Hand Injuries,* ed 3. St. Louis, CV Mosby Co, 1972.

Gitelis S, et al: The role of prophylactic surgery in the management of metastatic hip disease. *Orthopedics* 1982; 5:1004.

Harrington KD, et al: The use of methylmethacrylate as an adjunct in the internal fixation of malignant neoplastic fractures. *J Bone Joint Surg [Am]* 1972; 54:1665.

Holmes CM: Intravenous regional analgesia: A useful method of producing analgesia of the limbs. *Lancet* 1963; 1:245.

Howard PW, Makin GS: Lower limb fractures with associated vascular injury. *J Bone Joint Surg [Br]* 1990; 72:116.

Hunter JM, Cowen NJ: Fifth metacarpal fractures in a compensation clinic population: A report on 133 cases. *J Bone Joint Surg [Am]* 1970; 52:1159.

Lavine LS, Grodzinsky AJ: Current concepts review: Electrical stimulation of repair of bone. *J Bone Joint Surg [Am]* 1987; 69:626.

Marcove RC, Yang DJ: Survival times after treatment of pathologic fractures. *Cancer* 1967; 20:2154.

McLaughlin HL: *Trauma.* Philadelphia, WB Saunders Co, 1959.

Pool C: Colles' fracture. *J Bone Joint Surg [Br]* 1973; 55:540.

Rang M: *Children's Fractures,* ed 2. Philadelphia, JB Lippincott, 1983.

Rockwood CA, Green DP: *Fractures in Adults,* ed 2. Philadelphia, JB Lippincott, 1984.

Ryan JR, Rowe DE, Salciccioli GG: Prophylactic internal fixation of the femur in neoplastic lesions. *J Bone Joint Surg [Am]* 1976; 58:1071.

Silverman FN: The roentgen manifestations of unrecognized skeletal trauma in infants. *AJR* 1953; 69:413.

CHAPTER 3

The Cervical Spine

The cervical spine is exceeded only by the lumbar spine in the number of patients affected by conditions causing pain or dysfunction. These disorders vary from those that are annoying to those that may be functionally disabling. The diagnosis and treatment of these disorders are a major part of orthopedics.

ANATOMY

Seven cervical vertebrae make up the bony elements of the cervical spine. A typical cervical vertebra is similar to other vertebrae in that it is composed of a body and a neural arch (Fig 3–1). The neural arch is composed of two pedicles that form the sides and two laminae that meet in the midline to form the roof. Projecting dorsally where the laminae meet is the spinous process, and projecting laterally from the junction of the pedicle and lamina is a transverse process on each side. Two articular processes, the superior and inferior, project upward and downward, respectively, from the junction of the pedicle and laminae on each side and articulate with similar processes on adjacent vertebrae to form the zygoapophyseal or facet joints.

The first two cervical vertebrae are atypical in that C1, the atlas, has no body (Fig 3–2). Its body is attached to C2, the axis, and forms the dens, or odontoid process. This arrangement allows for most of the rotation in the cervical spine. Strong ligaments bind C1 to C2, the most important of which is the transverse ligament. The seventh cervical vertebra, vertebra prominens, is also somewhat atypical in that it has a long spinous process that is easily palpable beneath the skin.

Several major ligaments stabilize the cervical spine (Fig 3–3). The anterior and posterior longitudinal ligaments are applied to the respective surfaces of the vertebral bodies. Where the posterior longitudinal ligament crosses the disc, it tends to be somewhat weak laterally, thus forming a point where disc herniation may occur. Some gliding motion is allowed to occur between vertebrae by relatively weak capsular ligaments that bind together each articular joint. The ligamentum flavum, or yellow ligament, is situated between adjacent laminae, and in the cervical spine, extremely strong ligaments—the nuchal ligament and interspinous ligaments—provide posterior support.

The vertebrae are separated from each other

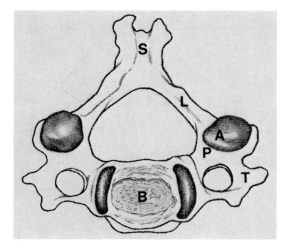

FIG 3–1.
A typical cervical vertebra: *S* = spinous process; *L* = lamina; *A* = articular facet; *P* = pedicle; *T* = transverse process; *B* = body.

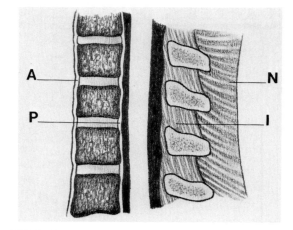

FIG 3–3.
Ligaments of the cervical spine: *A* = anterior longitudinal ligament; *P* = posterior longitudinal ligament; *N* = nuchal ligament; *I* = interspinous ligament.

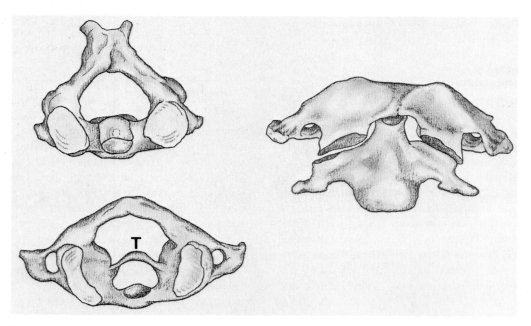

FIG 3–2.
The axis *(top),* atlas *(bottom),* and transverse ligament *(T). Right,* the articulation of the atlas and the axis.

by the intervertebral discs, which constitute approximately one fourth of the length of the vertebral column. Each disc is composed of an inner nucleus pulposus, which is mainly gelatinous, and an outer layer, the anulus fibrosis, which is mainly fibrous. The discs function to distribute stress over a wide area of the vertebrae, to absorb shock, and to allow mobility. The nucleus pulposus has a very high water content in early life, but with age this tends to diminish. With this loss of water, abnormal pressures begin to be exerted on the anulus, which leads to pathologic changes in adjacent structures.

Eight pairs of nerve roots arise from the cervical spinal cord. Each nerve exits above the vertebra of the same number. Thus, the sixth nerve root exits at the C5–C6 disc space. Each nerve except the first two pairs leaves the spinal column by passing through an intervertebral foramen (Fig 3–4). Each foramen has as its superior and inferior boundaries the pedicles of the adjacent vertebrae. Posterolaterally, it is bounded by the apophyseal joint and, anteromedially, by the so-called joint of Luschka. In the cervical spine,

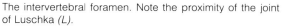
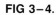

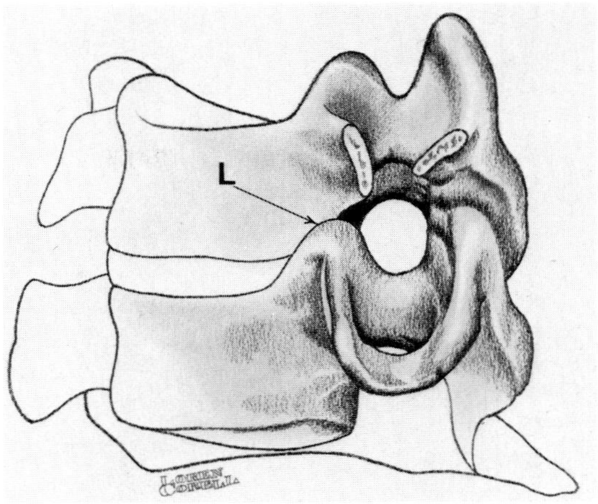

FIG 3–4.
The intervertebral foramen. Note the proximity of the joint of Luschka *(L)*.

this foramen is quite small and is almost entirely occupied by the nerve root. Thus, anything that compromises this space, such as disc degeneration with spur formation, will cause pressure on the nerve root.

EXAMINATION

Examination of the neck begins with observation of the posture of the head and neck in relation to the torso. Any decrease in the normal cervical lordosis is noted. The neck is gently palpated for tender areas, trigger points, and muscle spasm. The range of motion of the cervical spine is then measured and any movement that reproduces pain is noted. Flexion, extension, right and left bending, and right and left rotation are all recorded. A complete neurologic examination, including muscle strength testing, is always performed. The peripheral nerves are percussed for tenderness and tested for function. In addition, the shoulders and elbows are always carefully examined, particularly if there is any radiation of the pain or numbness and tingling.

ROENTGENOGRAPHIC ANATOMY

The examination of all neck disorders should include a standard roentgenographic evaluation. The roentgenographic features of the cervical spine are well visualized by the following: (1) anteroposterior view (Fig 3–5), (2) lateral views in flexion and extension, (3) oblique views in both directions to visualize the intervertebral foramen (Fig 3–6), and (4) an open-mouth odontoid view to visualize the odontoid process and the relationship between C1 and C2.

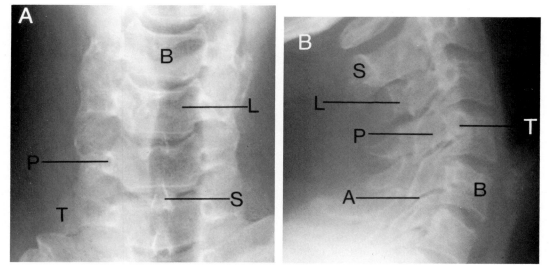

FIG 3−5.
Anteroposterior **(A)** and lateral **(B)** views of the cervical spine: *S* = spinous process; *T* = transverse process; *B* = body; *A* = articular (zygoapophyseal) facet joint; *P* = pedicle; *L* = lamina. Note the slight lordosis and even spacing of the vertebrae and discs.

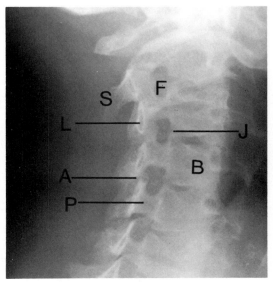

FIG 3−6.
Oblique view: *S* = spinous process; *F* = intervertebral foramen; *J* = joint of Luschka; *L* = lamina; *P* = pedicle; *A* = articular facet joint; *B* = body.

CERVICAL DISC SYNDROMES

More than 90% of disc lesions in the cervical spine occur at the C5 and C6 levels, those being the most mobile segments. As disc degeneration occurs, either gradually or following acute trauma, two types of lesions result that produce very similar symptoms. The first of these is the so-called *soft* disc protusion or nuclear herniation. With this lesion, a mass of nucleus pulposus begins to bulge outward, usually at the area of the greatest weakness in the anulus fibrosus (Fig 3–7). Complete extrusion of this disc material may even occur. This lesion is more common in the younger patient. With acute rupture of a cervical disc, immediate compression of the nerve root occurs and results in nerve root symptoms and radicular pain.

The second, more common lesion results from chronic disc degeneration with subsequent narrowing of the disc space and alterations in the surrounding structures. This is the so-called *hard* disc lesion, or cervical "spondylosis," and occurs primarily in the older age group. As narrowing and collapse of the disc proceeds, the vertebrae become more closely approximated, which leads

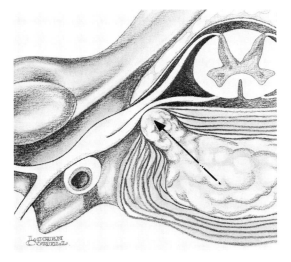

FIG 3–7.
Disk herniation *(arrow)* causing nerve root compression. Spur formation may occur in the same area.

to spur formation along the disc edges and at the joints of Luschka. Mild subluxation of the facet joint also occurs. All of these changes decrease the size of the intervertebral foramen, which results in pressure on the nerve root. Mild inflammation and swelling are usually present in conjunction with osteophyte formation, which further contributes to the narrowing of the foramen and nerve root compression. Large posterior osteophytes may also cause pressure on the anterior portion of the spinal cord and produce mixed symptoms of upper extremity nerve root pain and lower extremity weakness. This is commonly termed *cervical spondylosis with myelopathy.*

Clinical Features

Pain associated with cervical disc disease may develop either gradually or acutely. Patients often complain of a tightness or stiffness in the neck that is made worse with activity. Morning stiffness is common, and certain movements, especially extension, exacerbate the pain. Coughing, sneezing, and straining can accentuate the pain, which may radiate into the shoulder and arm and along the radial aspect of the forearm (Fig 3–8). Numbness and tingling are often noted in these same areas, and referred pain, which does not follow a dermatome pattern, is common along the medial border of the scapula. Headaches are not uncommon, and dysphagia has even been reported secondary to large anterior osteophytes.

Examination frequently reveals a decreased range of motion. Pain on hyperextension and local tenderness in the cervical spine are often observed. Trigger point tenderness is commonly noted in the area of referred pain in the interscapular region. Pressure against the top of the head may reproduce the pain in the arm (Fig 3–9). Some sensory changes are occasionally seen along the specific dermatome, but the sensory examination is frequently not very helpful. Motor weakness and reflex changes are frequently noted (Table 3–1).

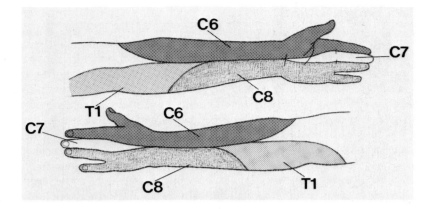

FIG 3–8.
Volar and dorsal dermatome pattern of the forearm and hand. Pain and paresthesias may radiate into these areas when the affected nerve root is compressed.

Spondylosis in the cervical spine may occasionally produce symptoms referable to the lower extremities (cervical spondylotic myelopathy). These symptoms occur as a result of pressure of posterior osteophytes on the anterior portion of the cervical spinal cord. The symptom complex appears as a combination of cervical *root* and *cord* symptoms. The patient may have a typical disc syndrome in the upper extremities, but in addition, gait difficulties, weakness, and spasticity may be present in the lower extremities. The lower extremity symptoms have a gradual onset at about 50 years of age and progress slowly.

Special Studies

In most cases, the diagnosis is clear without further testing. Neck, interscapular, and/or arm pain that is aggravated by neck motion is typical. Eventually, however, the following studies may be needed:

1. Plain roentgenograms are usually performed first and within the first few weeks. Anteroposterior (AP) and lateral views are sufficient. They are usually normal in soft disc rupture. With chronic degenerative disc disease, however, loss of the height of the disc space, anterior and posterior osteophyte formation, and

TABLE 3–1.
Clinical Features of Common Cervical Disc Syndromes

Disc	Pain	Sensory Change	Motor Weakness, Atrophy	Reflex Change
C4–5 (C5 root)	Base of neck, shoulder, anterolateral aspect of arm	Numbness in deltoid region	Deltoid, biceps	Biceps
C5–6 (C6 root)	Neck, shoulder, medial border of scapula, lateral aspect of arm, dorsum of forearm	Dorsolateral aspect of thumb and index finger	Biceps, extensor pollicis longus	Biceps, brachioradialis
C6–7 (C7 root)	Neck, shoulder, medial border of scapula, lateral aspect of arm, dorsum of forearm	Index, middle fingers, dorsum of hand	Triceps	Triceps

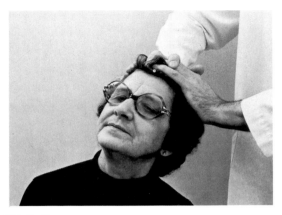

FIG 3–9.
Vertex compression test. Reproduction of neck and arm pain may be observed.

encroachment on the intervertebral foramen by osteophytes are noted on routine films (Fig 3–10).

2. Myelography, sometimes followed by computed tomography (CT), remains important for the evaluation of cervical radiculopathy. It is helpful in localizing the lesion but is not without some morbidity and is indicated only under two circumstances: (1) if surgical intervention is contemplated or (2) if other serious spinal abnormality is suspected. Loss of the normal root "sleeve" and indentation of the dural sac are often seen (Fig 3–11). Spinal fluid analysis performed at the time of myelography may show a slight increase in protein content.

3. Magnetic resonance imaging is also valuable in the assessment of the cervical spine and may eventually replace myelography. It is attractive partly because it is noninvasive and uses no ionizing radiation. It should be used selectively due to its continuing high cost. Many patients are excluded from this modality for various reasons: obesity, the presence of pacemakers, internal fixation devices, and claustrophobia among others (although newer models cause less claustrophobia). The examination time is also quite lengthy. Indications for its use are generally the same as those for myelography. Like myelography, it is usually indicated late in the disorder, after several weeks have passed without recovery.

CT scanning, while less expensive, is not as

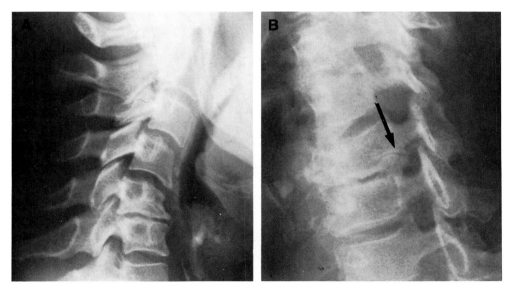

FIG 3–10.
Lateral **(A)** and oblique **(B)** roentgenograms showing degenerative disc disease at the C5–C6 level. Note the osteophyte formation and narrowing of the intervertebral foramen *(arrow)*.

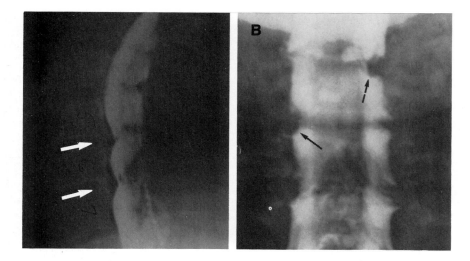

FIG 3–11.
Myelographic findings in cervical disc disease. Note the filling defects from osteophyte formation on the lateral view **(A)** and absence of the normal root sleeve *(arrows)* on the AP view **(B).**

helpful in evaluating *degenerative* disc disease in the cervical spine as it is in the assessment of *traumatic* conditions of the neck.

4. Electromyography and discography are also occasionally performed in the evaluation of cervical disc disease, but the diagnosis can usually be well established on the basis of the history, physical examination, and myelogram alone.

5. Thermography is mentioned only for com-

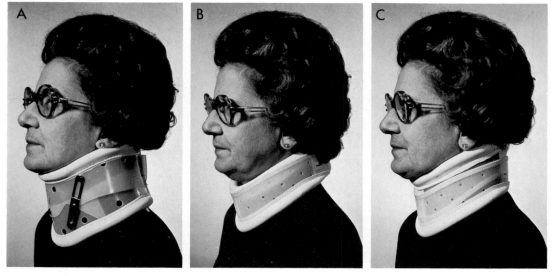

FIG 3–12.
Proper usage of the cervical collar. **A,** a collar too high places the neck in too much extension. **B,** a collar too short does not immobilize and allows too much flexion. **C,** proper height of the collar maintains the head in a slightly flexed or neutral position.

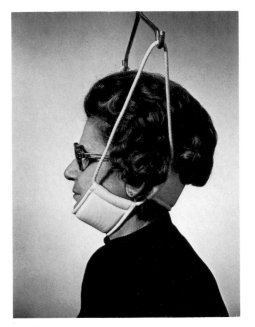

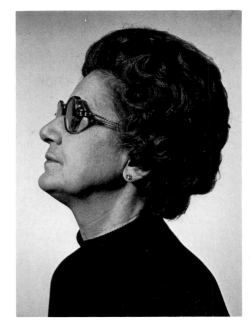

FIG 3–13.
Proper usage of cervical traction. The direction of pull should be neutral; 4 to 6 lb of weight should be used for 20 to 30 minutes. It should be repeated three to four times daily, depending on the response. The pressure should be equally distributed between the chin and the occiput.

FIG 3–15.
The hyperextended "spectator" attitude that often causes neck strain and aggravates disc disease. The head and neck should be maintained in a neutral position at all times. Positions that produce sharp angulation or rotation of the head, such as sleeping on the abdomen or resting on a couch with the armrest as a "pillow," should also be avoided.

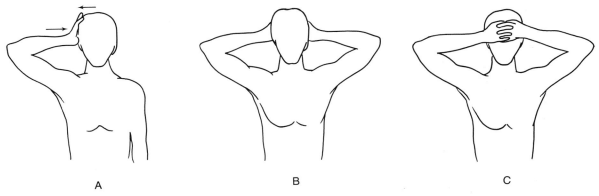

A   B   C

FIG 3–14.
Isometric neck exercises. The hand is placed against the side of the head slightly above the ear, and pressure is gradually increased while resisting with the neck muscles and keeping the head in the same position **(A).** The position is held 5 seconds, relaxed, and repeated five times. The exercise is performed on the other side and then from the back and front **(B and C).** The exercise should be performed three to four times daily.

pleteness. Its validity is uncertain, and it is not commonly used.

Note: Roentgenographic studies are not always conclusive. False-negative and false-positive results are fairly common. These studies should be performed only as an adjunct to, not instead of, a good history and clinical examination. When the results are uncertain, it is best to re-examine the patient. If the symptoms do not correlate well with the roentgenographic findings, it is best to continue to treat the symptoms and not the roentgenogram. Remember that "abnormal" roentgenographic findings in the spine are present in up to 35% of *asymptomatic* adults.

Treatment

1. Rest is the cornerstone of therapy for cervical disc disease. In acute disc protusion, it permits the healing of soft parts to occur. In chronic disc disease, it allows the inflammatory reaction to subside. Rest is accomplished by various means, but absolute bed rest is the most beneficial. Various soft collars that restrict motion and give support are also helpful (Fig 3–12).

2. Moist heat applied to the affected area will help relieve tenderness and muscle pain. Massage may also give temporary relief of the trigger point soft-tissue pain. Cervical traction, which may be used at home, is also beneficial (Fig 3–13). Formal physical therapy in the form of di-

TABLE 3–2.

Algorithm for Suspected Cervical Disk Syndrome

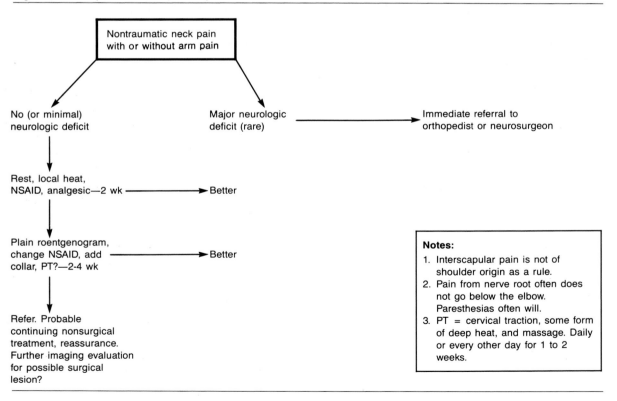

Notes:
1. Interscapular pain is not of shoulder origin as a rule.
2. Pain from nerve root often does not go below the elbow. Paresthesias often will.
3. PT = cervical traction, some form of deep heat, and massage. Daily or every other day for 1 to 2 weeks.

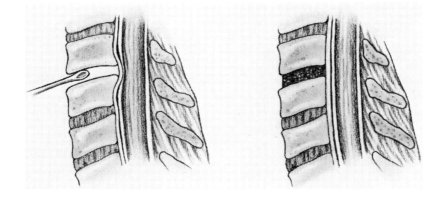

FIG 3–16.
Arthrodesis of the cervical spine. The disc is removed and replaced with a bone graft.

athermy or ultrasound, massage, and cervical traction may also provide temporary improvement. (Although most forms of physical therapy are of an unproven scientific value, some patients do respond to these treatments. Pain relief with physical therapy, however, seems short-lived, and any overall improvement usually parallels what would have probably occurred naturally.)

3. Aspirin given in adequate doses for analgesia and inflammation is probably the most effective of the anti-inflammatory drugs, but any of these medications may be used. Muscle "relaxers" are not effective. The problem is not caused by muscle tissue. The pain is simply referred to the surrounding soft parts. These medications probably are only effective via their tranquilizing effect. They may be helpful when given at night to allow the patient to rest. Narcotic analgesics are often necessary to control pain.

4. After the acute pain subsides, a program of gentle, graded isometric exercises is recommended (Fig 3–14). Recurrences are prevented by avoiding fatigue and poor postural habits, especially hyperextension (Fig 3–15). A pillow approximately 7.5 to 10 cm thick should be used for sleeping and should be placed under the neck rather than under the head. An overly thick pillow may place the head in too much flexion, while a thin one may allow too much extension to occur. Most patients may continue a reasonable daily work schedule unless the pain is particularly intense (Table 3–2).

Prognosis

Most patients will improve with time and, fewer than 5% will require surgery. Patience is important. The time period required for improvement varies considerably among patients. Several weeks may be needed before full recovery occurs. They may be advised, however, that there is generally no danger in waiting and continuing conservative treatment. Recurrences occur occasionally and are treated in the same manner.

Surgery is reserved for those patients in whom the pain and level of disability become intolerable or in whom a major neurologic deficit has developed. It is not as helpful for neck pain as for arm pain. The procedure consists of removal of the affected disc, usually followed by arthrodesis of the two adjacent vertebrae with a bone graft (Fig 3–16). Some soft disc protrusions are occasionally removed without fusion. The arm pain usually subsides immediately after surgery, and osteophytes that have formed in the foramen and adjacent structures are usually absorbed within 9 to 18 months.

CERVICAL SPRAIN

Most soft-tissue injuries of the cervical spine are the result of a hyperextension force. This is the nature of the injury most commonly sustained in a rear-end automobile collision. Rarely is there any osseous injury. Most of the force is absorbed by ligaments, muscles, and disc. Acute disc protrusion is not common, but disc injury is, and serial roentgenograms taken at later dates may show significant progressive degenerative changes.

All soft structures, including muscle, anterior longitudinal ligament, esophagus, and trachea, may be severely stretched. Dysphagia and hoarseness are sometimes seen shortly after the injury. Hemorrhage and edema may be present in the prevertebral area, and the sympathetic nerve chains, which are located near the vertebral bodies, are occasionally stretched. This may produce somewhat unusual symptoms such as nausea, tinnitus, blurred vision, and dizziness.

Chronic pain that continues for weeks or months is not uncommon. Degenerative changes may result from the injury at one or more levels in a previously normal cervical spine, and this may lead to significant disability. Similarly, patients with previously asymptomatic degenerative disc disease may develop their first symptoms of a cervical disc syndrome following a hyperextension injury.

Clinical Features

Frequently there are very few symptoms immediately following the injury. A few hours later, however, the patient begins to notice stiffness in the neck followed by pain and an inability to move the neck normally. The pain is generalized to the neck region and may radiate to the occiput along the path of the greater occipital nerve. Shoulder, arm, and interscapular pain may be noted, and there may even be pain in the anterior chest wall. Symptoms such as nausea, tinnitus, blurred vision, and occipital headaches are not uncommon.

Examination may reveal generalized tenderness in the anterior and posterior neck muscula-ture. Motion may be greatly limited, and extension of the spine is often quite painful. Mild torticollis may be present. The results of the neurologic examination are usually normal.

Special Studies

After the initial examination, if there is any reason to suspect a significant cervical spine injury, a full lateral roentgenogram of the cervical spine should be taken without moving the patient. This view should always include the body of the seventh cervical vertebra; if it does not, the vertebra is probably being obscured by the shoulder soft tissue shadow. In this case, the shoulders should be pulled down manually and the roentgenogram repeated. If a satisfactory view of C7 still

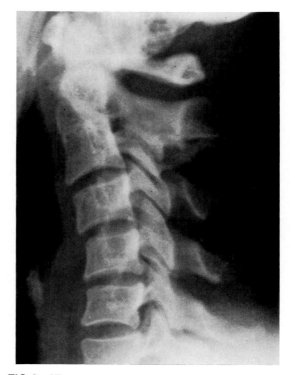

FIG 3–17.
Lateral roentgenogram showing reversal of the cervical lordosis.

has not been obtained, then a "swimmer's" view may be performed. If no significant injury is seen on this view, then the remainder of the cervical spine films are obtained.

Usually, results of the initial roentgenographic examination are normal, but with the passage of time, reversal of the normal cervical lordosis may be observed (Fig 3–17). This finding is often seen in patients with prolonged disability. Late degenerative changes may even occur. "Loss of the normal cervical lordosis," often quoted on early roentgenograms, is probably not significant.

Any degenerative changes present in the cervical spine at the time of the initial injury should also be noted for both medical and medicolegal purposes. Further roentgenographic studies are usually not indicated. CT and bone scanning may be helpful to rule out fracture, however.

Treatment

1. Rest is the most important treatment modality in acute cervical strain. It should be continuous and consist primarily of bed rest for the

TABLE 3–3.
Algorithm for Cervical Strain

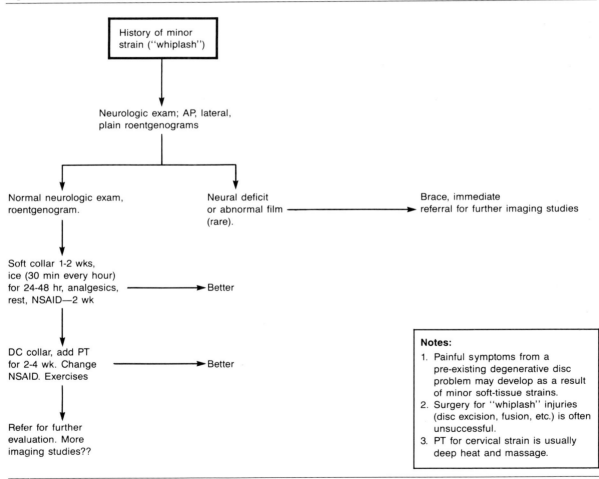

History of minor strain ("whiplash")

Neurologic exam; AP, lateral, plain roentgenograms

Normal neurologic exam, roentgenogram.

Neural deficit or abnormal film (rare). → Brace, immediate referral for further imaging studies

Soft collar 1-2 wks, ice (30 min every hour) for 24-48 hr, analgesics, rest, NSAID—2 wk → Better

DC collar, add PT for 2-4 wk. Change NSAID. Exercises → Better

Refer for further evaluation. More imaging studies??

Notes:
1. Painful symptoms from a pre-existing degenerative disc problem may develop as a result of minor soft-tissue strains.
2. Surgery for "whiplash" injuries (disc excision, fusion, etc.) is often unsuccessful.
3. PT for cervical strain is usually deep heat and massage.

first few days, especially if the injury is very painful. A soft cervical collar holding the neck in slight flexion is worn day and night for approximately 1 to 2 weeks, depending upon response.

2. Analgesics are given in amounts sufficient to relieve pain. Anti-inflammatory drugs given soon after the injury may be helpful, especially in the patient who has preexisting degenerative disc disease of the cervical spine.

3. Cold should be used initially. Heat should be avoided early after the injury because it may further increase swelling. It may be helpful later in the course of care. Cervical traction should also be avoided early in the treatment because it may stretch already stretched soft parts.

4. When the acute pain subsides, isometric and gentle range-of-motion exercises are started, and wearing of the collar is gradually discontinued. General measures including a proper pillow and the avoidance of stress should be instituted. If symptoms persist after 4 to 6 weeks, cervical traction and physical therapy may be beneficial. (Table 3–3).

Prognosis

Most patients will improve in 4 to 6 weeks if the initial treatment has been adequate. Less long-term disability and anxiety on the part of the patient will result if aggressive, conservative treatment is instituted, especially in the initial stage of the injury.

This disorder is well known for its chronicity, however, and frequently defies all attempts at cure. It is best, however, to continue with nonoperative management as long as possible. Surgery is rarely necessary, and the results are often unrewarding. Part of the reason for this is that it is often difficult to localize the exact source of the pain.

Eventually, some patients develop a "chronic pain syndrome." Daily exercise, resuming a normal life-style, and avoiding excessive *passive* treatment may help these individuals.

Tension Strain

Neck and upper dorsal pain may also result from tension and strain. The common clinical settings are those in which the individual is required to sit at a desk typing or studying for long periods of time. Positional strain, sometimes combined with tension and stress, often leads to muscular pain in the upper dorsal and cervical spine. The neck pain may radiate to the occiput.

The examination usually has negative results except for local tenderness and occasional limitation of neck movement. Treatment usually involves changes in work activities and work or study positions and taking frequent breaks from activities for gentle stretching exercises.

DISC CALCIFICATION

Calcification of the intervertebral disc is not uncommon. It frequently occurs in the dorsal spine of adults in the anulus fibrosus and is probably secondary to a degenerative process. Multiple disc calcifications also occur with ochronosis. Disc calcification is usually an incidental roentgenographic finding and generally does not produce symptoms.

In children, however, disc calcification occurs more commonly in the cervical spine, and in this age group it appears as a definite clinical entity with symptoms. The cause is unknown, but it may represent a nonspecific inflammatory reaction. It is probably not infectious in nature. In contrast to the adult, it is the nucleus pulposus that calcifies.

Clinical Features

The disorder has its onset at about the age of 7 years and usually begins with neck pain and stiff-

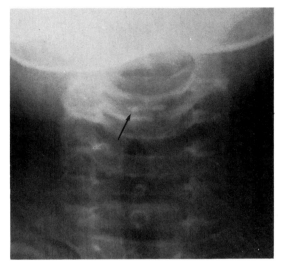

FIG 3–18.
Disk space calcification (arrow).

ness. Localized tenderness and a decrease in the range of motion of the cervical spine are usually present. A mild torticollis may be noted. There is usually an elevation of the temperature, sedimentation rate, and white blood cell (WBC) count.

Roentgenograms reveal the disease to primarily affect the lower discs in the cervical spine (Fig 3–18). Multiple discs may be affected, and the calcification usually begins to regress with the onset of symptoms.

Treatment

Treatment is conservative and consists of a soft collar, cervical traction, and analgesics as necessary. Antibiotics are not as a rule indicated. Patients usually become asymptomatic in 1 to 2 weeks without any sequelae.

TORTICOLLIS

Torticollis is a deformity of the neck that causes rotation and tilting of the head, usually in opposite directions. It may be present on a congenital basis or acquired as a result of trauma or disease.

Congenital Muscular Torticollis

This deformity is usually noted at birth and is much more common after breech deliveries. It results from a unilateral contracture of the sternocleidomastoid muscle. The cause is unknown, but fibrosis of the muscle occurs, possibly secondary to a vascular disturbance in the muscle. A "tumor" consisting of dense fibrous tissue is often found in the muscle shortly after birth. This mass gradually subsides over the ensuing weeks to leave a shortened and contracted sternocleidomastoid muscle. If untreated, secondary changes appear in the cervical vertebrae, and marked asymmetry of the face becomes apparent. These changes frequently persist in spite of later treatment.

Clinical Features

The diagnosis generally can be made shortly after birth. The "mass" is usually palpable, and the head is characteristically tilted toward the side of the mass and rotated in the opposite direction (Fig 3–19). Roentgenograms of the cervical spine are usually performed to rule out injury and congenital osseous disorders of the cervical spine.

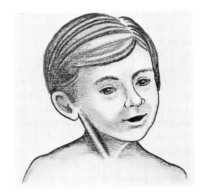

FIG 3–19.
Congenital muscular torticollis.

Treatment

Conservative treatment, if instituted early, will usually result in a cure. No improvement can be expected without treatment. In mild deformities, gentle stretching exercises carried out by the mother will usually correct the problem. The exercises should be repeated several times daily. The crib should be placed so that the child must turn toward the corrected position when someone enters the room.

Surgery is reserved for late cases or those who fail to respond to conservative treatment. The procedure consists of the release of the sternocleidomastoid muscle followed by traction or casting and exercises. The results are usually good.

Torticollis Secondary to Inflammation

Torticollis may be seen in the 5- to 10-year-old age group following an upper respiratory tract infection or cervical lymphadenitis. A few days after onset of the infection, spontaneous subluxation of the atlas or unilateral subluxation of C2 on C3 occurs. There may be a history of a minor neck injury. Typically, there is no sternocleidomastoid tightness or spasm; if any is present, it is on the long side of the neck rather than on the short side as seen in myositis and congenital muscular torticollis. Examination may reveal tenderness of the spinous process of C2 and an obvious tilting of the head. Treatment consists of cervical traction and warm, moist packs. The subluxation will usually improve, and a collar is worn afterward until all symptoms subside.

An inflammatory condition sometimes referred to as "myositis" often causes tenderness of the cervical musculature. The cause is unknown, but the disorder usually follows exposure to cold air or a draft. Clinically, there is tenderness in the musculature of the cervical spine, and the head is held toward the side of the tenderness. This entity is treated with rest, moist heat, and a soft collar until symptoms subside.

Spasmodic Torticollis

Spasmodic torticollis is a term that refers to a disease entity consisting of the spontaneous onset of painful contractions of various muscles about the cervical spine, including the sternocleidomastoid muscle. The cause is unknown, and the disease has a gradual onset in adulthood. "Spasms" may occur in the cervical musculature, and they may be bilateral. These spasms tend to hold the head toward the affected side and are uncontrollable.

These patients have strong psychoneurotic tendencies, and there is little likelihood of spontaneous recovery. The disease is usually resistant to ordinary conservative treatment and surgical treatment is sometimes required. This consists of sectioning the spinal accessory nerves and upper cervical rhizotomies. The surgical results are only fair.

Miscellaneous Causes of Torticollis

Spinal cord tumor, neuritis of the spinal accessory nerve, cervical spine anomalies, and rheumatoid arthritis will occasionally produce torticollis. Ocular disturbances may produce the same symptoms, and any child who has gradually increasing torticollis should have a complete eye examination. Fracture or unilateral rotatory subluxation may also cause torticollis and should always be ruled out by an adequate roentgenographic examination.

BIBLIOGRAPHY

Adson AW, Young HH, Ghormley RK: Spasmodic torticollis. *J Bone Joint Surg* 1946; 28:299.

Bohlman HH: Cervical spondylosis with moderate to severe myelopathy. *Spine* 1977; 2:151.

Canale ST, Griffin DW, Hubbard CN: Congenital muscular torticollis: a long-term follow-up. *J Bone Joint Surg [Am]* 1982; 64:810.

Clark E, Robinson PK: Cervical myelopathy: A

complication of cervical spondylosis. *Brain* 1856; 79:483.

Coventry MB, Harris LE: Congenital muscular torticollis in infancy. *J Bone Joint Surg [Am]* 1959; 41:815.

Deans GT, et al: Neck sprain: A major cause of disability following car accidents. *Injury* 1987; 18:10.

DePalma AF, Rothman RH: *The Intervertebral Disc.* Philadelphia, WB Saunders Co, 1970.

Dubousset J: Torticollis in children caused by congenital anomalies of the atlas. *J Bone Joint Surg [Am]* 1986; 68:178.

Eyring EJ, Peterson CA, Bjornson DR: Intervertebral-disc calcification in childhood: A distinct clinical syndrome. *J Bone Joint Surg [Am]* 1964; 46:1432.

Ferke RD, et al: Muscular torticollis: A modified surgical approach. *J Bone Joint Surg [Am]* 1983; 65:894.

Hohl M: Soft tissue injuries of the neck in automobile accidents. *J Bone Joint Surg [Am]* 1974; 56:1675.

Miller GM, Forbes GS, Onofrio BM: Magnetic resonance imaging of the spine. *Mayo Clin Proc* 1989; 64:986.

Norris SH, Watt I: The prognosis of neck injuries resulting from rear-end vehicle collisions. *J Bone Joint Surg [Br]* 1983; 65:608.

Pennie BH, Agambar LJ: Whiplash injuries. *J Bone Joint Surg [Br]* 1990; 72:277.

Robinson RA: The results of anterior interbody fusion. *J Bone Joint Surg [Am]* 1962; 44:1569.

Robinson RA, Smith GW: Anterolateral cervical disc syndrome. *Bull Johns Hopkins Hosp* 1955; 96:223.

Robinson RA, et al: Cervical spondylotic myelopathy: Etiology and treatment concepts. *Spine* 1977; 2:89.

Ruge D, Wiltse LL: *Spinal Disorders: Diagnosis and Treatment.* Philadelphia, Lea & Febiger, 1977.

Scoville WB: Types of cervical disc lesion and their surgical approaches. *JAMA* 1966; 196:105.

Sherman WD, et al: Calcified cervical intervertebral discs in children. *Spine* 1976; 1:55.

Sonnabend DH, Taylor TKF, Chapman GK: Intervertebral disc calcification syndromes in children. *J Bone Joint Surg [Br]* 1982; 64:25.

Tachdjian MO: *Pediatric Orthopedics.* Philadelphia, WB Saunders Co, 1972.

Tamura T: Cranial symptoms after cervical injuries: Aetiology and treatment of Barre-Lieou syndrome. *J Bone Joint Surg [Br]* 1989; 71:283.

CHAPTER 4

The Cervicobrachial Region

Affections of the brachial plexus are usually the result of either compression or injury. The resultant symptoms and signs are often confusing, but these disorders should always be considered in the differential diagnosis of neuropathies of the upper extremity.

ANATOMY

The brachial plexus is formed by the anterior rami of the last four cervical and first thoracic nerves (Fig 4–1). In general, the upper portion of the plexus innervates the shoulder abductors and external rotators and the elbow flexors. It also provides sensation to the shoulder and radial side of the arm. The lower portion of the plexus primarily innervates the forearm and hand muscles and provides sensation to the ulnar side of the arm, forearm, and hand. The first thoracic ramus also communicates with the first thoracic ganglion, through which sympathetic fibers are carried to the face from the spinal cord.

Thus, involvement of the lower portion of the plexus by disease or injury may produce Horner's syndrome (ptosis, miosis, enophthalmos, and anhidrosis).

The plexus passes distally between the middle and anterior scalene muscles, which attach to the first rib (Fig 4–2). Beneath the clavicle, it is joined by the subclavian artery. The subclavian vein passes anterior to the scalenus anticus muscle. Artery, vein, and plexus then enter the axilla beneath the pectoralis minor muscle, with the lower trunk of the plexus (C8, T1) lying on the first rib.

THORACIC OUTLET SYNDROMES

Thoracic outlet syndrome is a term given to four different syndromes that have in common neurovascular compression at the base of the neck. These syndromes are referred to as the cervical rib syndrome, the scalenus anticus syndrome, the costoclavicular syndrome, and the hyperabduction syndrome. These disorders all have very similar clinical features and it is often impossible

to differentiate among them on this basis alone. The symptoms and signs are related to the degree of involvement of each of the various structures at the level of the first rib. Primary neural involvement may lead to pain and numbness. Arterial involvement usually causes the extremity to feel "asleep." This symptom may have a glove type of distribution and is occasionally associated

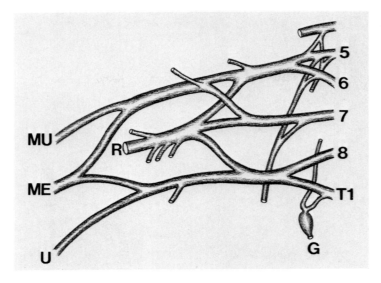

FIG 4–1.
The brachial plexus. Five rami normally combine to form three trunks, which divide to form three cords. The lower trunk *(C8, T1)* lies on the first rib and is most commonly involved in thoracic outlet syndromes. The posterior cord continues as the radial nerve *(R)*. The medial cord contributes half of the median nerve and continues as the ulnar nerve *(U)*. The lateral cord continues as the musculocutaneous *(MU)* nerve after contributing the other half of the median nerve *(ME)*. G = ganglion.

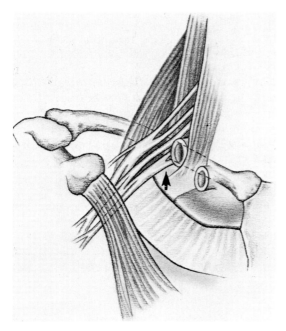

FIG 4–2.
Anatomy of the cervicobrachial region. Note that the lower portion of the trunk of the brachial plexus lies on the first rib *(arrow)*.

with paresis. Venous involvement may produce swelling.

Cervical Rib Syndrome

The cervical rib usually arises from the seventh cervical vertebra and is the most common cause of neurovascular compression at the base of the neck (Fig 4–3). The condition may be bilateral. The rib or its fibrous extension narrows the interval between the anterior and middle scalene muscles and produces a higher barrier that the neurovascular structures must arch over on their way into the arm. In older patients or those with muscular weakness, the shoulder may also sag more than normal, which further increases the tension on the neurovascular structures. The compression is also increased by carrying a heavy object in the hand.

The lowest components (C8, T1) of the plexus are most commonly involved because of their position against the rib. The symptoms therefore tend to be most noticeable in the hand and inner aspect of the forearm. Pain and paresthesias are

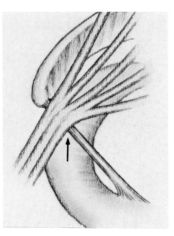

FIG 4–3.
Compression caused by a cervical rib *(arrow).*

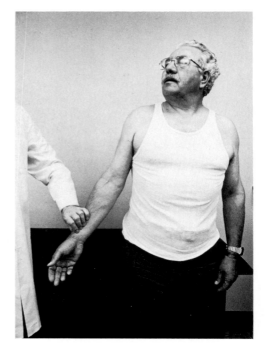

FIG 4–4.
Adson's test.

frequently produced along the distribution of the ulnar nerve. Weakness, numbness, and clumsiness in use of the hand are common complaints. Coldness, Raynaud's phenomenon, or even gangrene may be the initial symptom.

Clinically, the cervical rib may be palpable, and the brachial plexus is often tender. Weakness and atrophy of the muscles supplied by the lower trunk (interosseous, hypothenar muscles) are occasionally seen. Sensation may be diminished over the ulnar aspect of the forearm, arm, and the ulnar 1½ fingers. Swelling, coldness, cyanosis, trophic skin changes, and other signs of circulatory insufficiency are occasionally observed.

Adson's test may be positive (Fig 4–4). This test takes advantage of the fact that by tensing the scalene muscles the interval between them is decreased and any existing compression is increased. The test is performed by having the patient breathe deeply, extend the neck, and turn the chin toward the affected side. When the test is positive, a decrease in the radial pulse is noted. If the test is negative, it is repeated with the chin turned to the opposite side. Although a positive test is highly suggestive of compression in the interscalene region, it is sometimes positive in the normal population and is not neces-

sarily diagnostic of cervical rib or scalenus anticus syndrome.

Roentgenographic examination reveals an extra rib extending from the transverse process of the seventh cervical vertebra (Fig 4–5). The rib may be fully developed or rudimentary, and it is often bilateral. Its presence does not necessarily imply that it is symptomatic, however, because it may be present in asymptomatic individuals.

Nerve conduction studies are not very useful in the diagnosis of any of the thoracic outlet syndromes. Noninvasive vascular studies are occasionally helpful if diminished pulsations and reproduction of the neurologic and/or vascular symptoms occur during one of the various maneuvers.

Scalenus Anticus Syndrome

In the absence of a cervical rib, compression can still occur between the middle and anterior

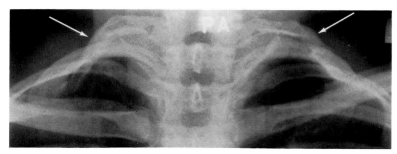

FIG 4−5.
Bilateral cervical ribs *(arrows)*.

scalene muscles. This may be due to abnormal scalene muscle insertions or the presence of additional muscle slips in the interscalene interval (Fig 4−6). The clinical findings are the same as those produced by a cervical rib.

Costoclavicular Syndrome

The space between the clavicle and the first rib may be narrowed by downward and backward pressure on the shoulders for a prolonged period of time. Abnormalities of the clavicle, such as malunion or nonunion following fracture, may contribute to the narrowing.

The syndrome is occasionally seen in individ-

uals who are required to carry heavy packs on their shoulders. Intermittent numbness and pain in the hand and arm are the most common symptoms. They may be reproduced by the costoclavicular maneuver (Fig 4−7). In this test, the shoulders are drawn downward and backward, and any change in the radial pulse or reproduction of symptoms is noted.

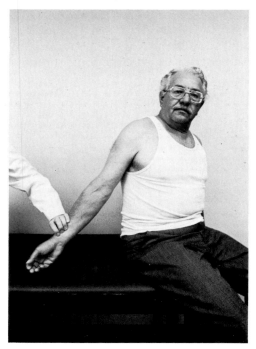

FIG 4−7.
The costoclavicular maneuver. The radial pulse may be diminished in many normal individuals.

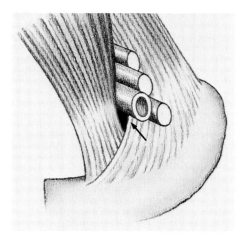

FIG 4−6.
Abnormal scalene muscle insertions that may cause compression at the cervicobrachial region *(arrow)*.

Hyperabduction Syndrome

Neurovascular symptoms may also follow prolonged assumption of the position of shoulder hyperabduction. This position is often assumed during sleep and in certain occupations such as overhead painting. The neurovascular structures are compressed as they pass under the coracoid process and pectoralis minor muscle with the arm in hyperabduction (Fig 4–8). Numbness and paresthesias are common, but the pain tends to be less severe than that seen in the other compression syndromes. Wright's test (diminution of pulse or reproduction of symptoms on hyperabduction of the arm) may be positive (Fig 4–9).

Treatment

The initial treatment is conservative in all thoracic outlet syndromes except those with vascular complications. Symptomatic relief may be obtained by resting the elbow of the affected side on the arm of the chair, thereby elevating the shoulder. A sling may serve the same purpose. Physical therapy in the form of moist heat, ultrasound, and pendulum exercises may also be helpful (Chapter 5). Specific strengthening exercises for the shoulder girdle muscles are begun (Fig 4–10). Faulty posture should be cor-

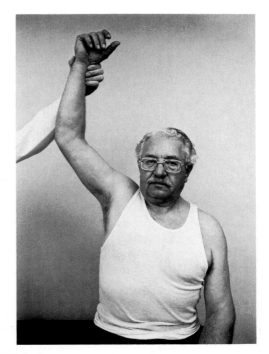

FIG 4–9.
Wright's test.

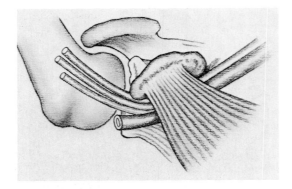

FIG 4–8.
Hyperabduction of the upper extremity that may produce neurovascular compression.

rected, and positions that aggravate the condition are avoided. For the hyperabduction syndrome, avoidance of the hyperabducted position is usually the only treatment necessary. A gauze strip tied to the wrist and attached to the foot of the bed to prevent hyperabduction at night may be temporarily necessary for those patients whose symptoms occur primarily at night.

Operative treatment is considered when conservative measures fail to obtain significant relief after 4 to 6 months. Removal of the first dorsal and cervical ribs combined with release of any abnormal scalene muscle insertions is recommended for the cervical rib and scalenus anticus syndromes. First-rib removal is also recommended for the costoclavicular syndrome, except when abnormalities of the clavicle are the primary causative factor. In this case, excision of the outer clavicle may be recommended. Clavicular

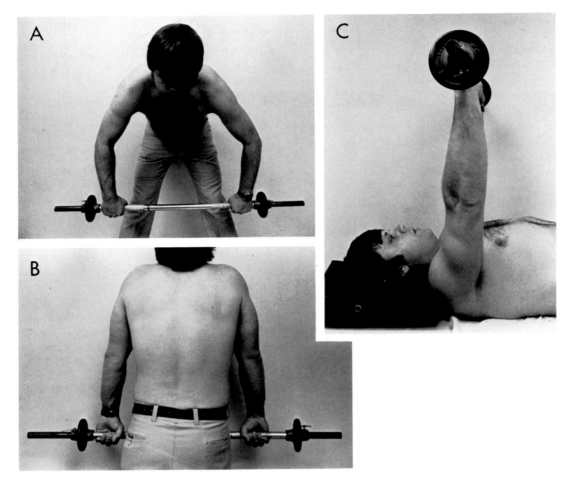

FIG 4–10.
Shoulder exercises for thoracic outlet syndrome. **A** and **B,** the trapezius is strengthened by raising and drawing the shoulders backward to bring the scapulae upward and together. **C,** to strengthen the serrati, the weight is pushed upward so that the shoulders are lifted off the table.

excision, however, is cosmetically more deforming than first-rib resection and is usually reserved for unusual cases. For those cases of hyperabduction syndrome that fail to respond to conservative treatment, first-rib resection, sometimes combined with release of the pectoralis minor muscle, is usually the treatment of choice. These procedures are all combined with vascular repair when indicated.

Note: Although these disorders are discussed at some length, they are probably quite uncommon. The standard physical tests (Adson's, etc.) are of somewhat limited value, and there are no good special studies that can be used to confirm the diagnosis in most cases. The results from surgery are also quite variable. These disorders should rank very low on any differential diagnosis of arm pain.

BIRTH PALSY

Paralysis of the upper extremity at birth usually follows a difficult and prolonged delivery. The upper plexus is usually injured by lateral flexion of the neck against either a fixed head or a fixed shoulder, and the lower plexus is damaged by an injury that forces the arm upward. The damage may vary from simple stretching to complete avulsion of nerve roots.

Clinically, the involved extremity is noted to remain motionless at the side with the elbow extended. The Moro reflex is also absent on the affected side. There may be swelling above the clavicle due to hemorrhage. Tenderness to palpation is often present from a traumatic neuritis. Fractures of the clavicle or upper portion of the humerus may be present and cause a "pseudoparalysis." They should always be ruled out in cases of birth palsy. Horner's syndrome may be observed if the injury involves the thoracic root.

Recovery may occur within a few days or may take 3 to 6 months. No improvement can be expected after the age of 2 years. In older patients, underdevelopment of the entire upper extremity is frequently seen, and the humerus is often markedly shortened. Contractures and disuse atrophy are also observed. Unawareness of the extremity, despite satisfactory motor and sensory recovery, may also be noted in late cases.

Three types of paralysis are seen, depending on the area of the injury: Erb-Duchenne or upper-arm paralysis, whole-arm paralysis, and Klumpke's or lower-arm paralysis.

Erb-Duchenne Paralysis

This is the most common type of obstetric paralysis. Damage to the upper roots (C5 and C6) leads to paralysis of the deltoid muscle, the external rotators of the shoulder, the elbow flexors, and the supinators of the fore-arm. Residual weakness of these muscles leads to the characteristic "waiter's-tip" position in which the arm is held adducted and internally rotated and the forearm is pronated (Fig 4–11). Wrist and finger function are usually normal.

Whole-Arm Paralysis

The limb is often completely flaccid and without motor function in this uncommon type of birth palsy. The hand tends to be dry and atrophic, and extensive sensory loss is often present.

Klumpke's Paralysis

In Klumpke's paralysis, the lower cervical and first thoracic roots are involved. This is the least common of the birth palsies. The finger and

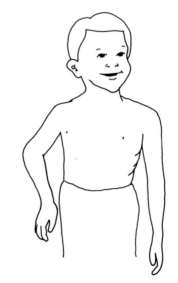

FIG 4–11.
The "waiter's-tip" position. Following partial upper arm paralysis, the upper extremity is frequently shortened and slightly smaller, and the palm often faces backward at rest.

wrist flexors are denervated along with the intrinsic muscles. A clawhand deformity often results. Horner's syndrome may also be present. Sensory loss involves the affected dermatomes of the lower plexus. The upper part of the arm is frequently uninvolved.

Treatment and Prognosis

Treatment is designed to prevent fixed soft tissue contractures from developing so that any muscles that regain function will have a flexible joint on which to act. Gentle, repetitive, meticulous range-of-motion exercises to the shoulder and elbow are instituted as soon as the tenderness disappears (usually about 2 weeks). Supportive splints for the wrist and fingers are helpful when used in conjunction with but not instead of a good exercise program. The "Statue of Liberty" splint or cast is not recommended because it may lead to overimmobilization and abduction contractures.

Reconstructive surgery is often beneficial for late deformities. Muscle transfers and osteotomies are utilized to restore motor function and correct malposition.

The overall prognosis for Erb's palsy is relatively good when compared with that for Klumpke's and whole-arm paralysis. Over 50% to 80% of upper-arm paralyses show fair to good recovery of arm function. Only about one in ten patients, however, will have complete return of normal use of the extremity.

BRACHIAL PLEXUS INJURIES

Injuries of the brachial plexus are uncommon and frequently severe. They are usually caused by motorcycle accidents. Traction and compression of the plexus may both occur anywhere along its course.

The diagnosis is sometimes delayed because the patient often has other serious injuries, frequently to the head and chest. Eventually, it is noted that the arm is completely paralyzed and hangs loosely from the shoulder. It may be completely anesthetic except for a small area on the inner aspect of the upper portion of the arm that is innervated by T2. Severe pain is common. If the site of injury is close to the spinal cord, Horner's syndrome may be present. This usually implies a poor prognosis.

The initial treatment is always conservative for the first several weeks. Range-of-motion exercises are begun to prevent joint stiffness. During this time, the patient is observed for spontaneous recovery. If this occurs, the prognosis is often favorable. If it does not occur, the patient should be evaluated to determine whether a reparable lesion is present. Myelography and electromyography can be helpful in this regard. If the myelogram shows the presence of several traction meningoceles or dye pockets, this indicates that the nerve roots have been avulsed from the cord. This suggests that the injury is probably complete and not reparable and that the prognosis is poor. This status is also suggested by the absence of any appropriate electromyographic activity.

If results of the myelogram are normal and there is some potential for recovery suggested, early surgery with microscopic assistance may be beneficial. Neurolysis and nerve repair may then be performed. Some improvement can be expected following the surgery.

Patients with irreversible lesions are faced with a difficult decision. Their extremity is now anesthetic, flail, and often painful and frequently gets in their way during normal activities. Amputation above the elbow is usually recommended about 1 year after the injury. A prosthesis may be tried, but these are frequently discarded. Amputation should not be expected to relieve pain, however. Most patients are able to adapt to being one-handed.

BIBLIOGRAPHY

Aston JW: Brachial plexus palsy. *Orthopedics* 1979; 2:594.

Britt LP: Nonoperative treatment of thoracic outlet syndrome symptoms. *Clin Orthop* 1967; 51:45.

Burge P, Rushworth G, Watson N: Patterns of injury to the terminal branches of the brachial plexus: The place for early exploration. *J Bone Joint Surg [Br]* 1985; 67:630.

Derkash RS, et al: The results of first rib resection in thoracic outlet syndrome. *Orthopedics* 1981; 4:1025.

Dunkerton MC: Posterior dislocation of the shoulder associated with obstetric brachial palsy. *J Bone Joint Surg [Br]* 1989; 71:764.

Eng GD: Brachial plexus palsy in newborn infants. *Pediatrics* 1971; 48:18.

Ferguson AB Jr: *Orthopaedic Surgery in Infancy and Childhood,* ed 3. Baltimore, Williams & Wilkins, 1968.

Grant JCB: *A Method of Anatomy,* ed 6. Baltimore, Williams & Wilkins, 1958.

Hardy AE: Birth injuries of the brachial plexus: Incidence and prognosis. *J Bone Joint Surg [Br]* 1981; 63:98.

Jackson ST, Hoffer MM, Parish N: Brachial plexus palsy in the newborn. *J Bone Joint Surg [Am]* 1989; 70:1217.

Nichols HM: Anatomic structures of the thoracic outlet. *Clin Orthop* 1967; 51:17.

Omer GE Jr, Spinner M: *Management of Peripheral Nerve Problems.* Philadelphia, WB Saunders Co, 1980.

Ransford AO, Hughes SPF: Complete brachial plexus injuries: A ten-year follow-up of twenty cases *J Bone Joint Surg [Br]* 1977; 59:417.

Rorabeck CH, Harris WR: Factors affecting the prognosis of brachial plexus injuries. *J Bone Joint Surg [Br]* 1981; 63:404.

Sedal L: The results of surgical repair of brachial plexus injuries. *J Bone Joint Surg [Br]* 1982; 64:54.

Tachdjian MO: *Pediatric Orthopedics.* Philadelphia, WB Saunders Co, 1972.

Telford ED, Mottershead S: Pressure at the cervicobrachial junction: An operative and anatomical study. *J Bone Joint Surg [Br]* 1948; 30:249.

Travlos J, Goldberg I, Boome RS: Brachial plexus lesions associated with dislocated shoulders. *J Bone Joint Surg [Br]* 1990; 72:68.

Wickstrom J: Birth injuries of the brachial plexus: Treatment of defects of the shoulder. *Clin Orthop* 1962; 23:187.

CHAPTER 5

The Shoulder

The shoulder is a complex series of joints that provide an extraordinary range of motion. This extreme mobility is accomplished at the expense of some stability, however. This lack of stability, combined with its relatively exposed position, makes it vulnerable to injury and degenerative processes.

ANATOMY

The shoulder is composed of three bones: the scapula, the clavicle, and the humerus. The scapula is a thin bone that articulates widely and closely with the posterior chest wall. It also articulates with the humerus by way of a small, shallow glenoid cavity and with the clavicle at the acromion process. The clavicle and scapula are suspended from the cervical and thoracic vertebrae by the trapezium, levator scapulae, and rhomboid muscles.

Four articulations constitute the shoulder joint: the glenohumeral, scapulothoracic, acromioclavicular, and sternoclavicular joints. The stability of these joints is provided by a series of ligaments and muscles (Fig 5–1).

Motion of the arm results from the coordinated efforts of several muscles. With the initiation of shoulder motion, the scapula is first stabilized. The muscles of the rotator (musculotendinous) cuff then steady the humeral head in the glenoid cavity and cause it to descend (Fig 5–2). Elevation of the arm results from a combination of scapulothoracic and glenohumeral joint movements. One third of total shoulder abduction is provided by forward and lateral movement of the scapula. The remaining two thirds occurs at the glenohumeral joint through progressively increasing activity of the deltoid and supraspinatus muscles. Thus, even in the complete absence of glenohumeral motion, scapulothoracic movement can still abduct the arm approximately 60 to 70 degrees.

The muscles of the rotator cuff (supraspinatus, teres minor, infraspinatus, and subscapularis) are separated from the overlying "coracoacromial arch" by two bursae, the subdeltoid and the subcoracoid (Fig 5–3). These bursae frequently communicate and are affected by lesions of the musculotendinous cuff, acromioclavicular joint, and adjacent structures. They are frequently referred to as the subacromial bursa. Primary diseases of this bursa are rare, although secondary involvement is quite common.

55

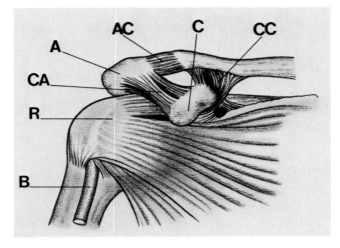

FIG 5–1.
Bones and ligaments of the shoulder: *R* = rotator cuff; *B* = long head of the biceps; *AC* = acromioclavicular joint capsule; *CC* = coracoclavicular ligaments; *A* = acromion; *C* = coracoid process; *CA* = coracoacromial ligaments.

EXAMINATION

The examination is performed with both shoulders widely exposed (Fig 5–4). The general contour of the shoulder is noted, as well as any atrophy or swelling. The shoulder is thoroughly palpated, and any areas of tenderness are determined. These are frequently located over the acromioclavicular joint and the rotator cuff.

Active and passive ranges of motion are tested and compared with those of the opposite arm. The examiner should determine whether the scapula and humerus move together or independently. Any crepitus during the examination is also noted. Active motion is measured in abduc-

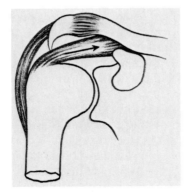

FIG 5–2.
Abduction of the shoulder. By stabilizing the humeral head in the glenoid *(arrow)*, the superior portion of the rotator cuff prevents it from being forced into the acromion by the deltoid muscle.

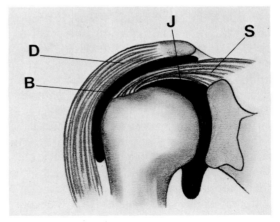

FIG 5–3.
The subacromial bursa *(B)* is shown between the deltoid *(D)* and supraspinatus *(S)* muscles. Deep to the rotator cuff is the glenohumeral joint cavity *(J)*.

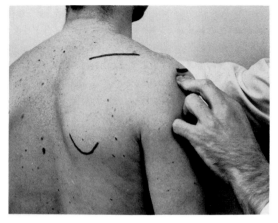

FIG 5–4.
Superficial landmarks of the shoulder. The spine of the scapula lies at the level of the third dorsal vertebra. The inferior angle lies at the level of the seventh rib and eighth dorsal vertebra. The rotator cuff is palpated just distal to the acromion process.

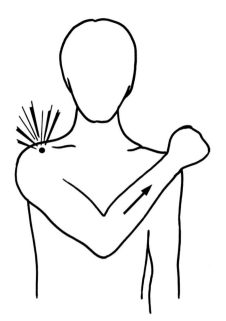

FIG 5–5.
Testing for acromioclavicular pain by having the patient touch behind the opposite shoulder *(arrow)*. Local AC tenderness may also be present.

tion, forward flexion, and extension. External and internal rotation can be measured by instructing the patient to reach behind the head and then backward behind the shoulder blades. Involvement of the acromioclavicular joint is tested by directing the patient to adduct the arm across the front of the chest and touch the opposite shoulder (Fig 5–5). Pain with this test suggests acromioclavicular or sternoclavicular disease. The strength of the shoulder, especially at 90 degrees of abduction, is tested and compared with the opposite arm.

ROENTGENOGRAPHIC ANATOMY

The shoulder is routinely examined by anteroposterior views with the arm rotated externally and internally (Fig 5–6). A lateral view may be obtained by utilizing a transaxillary or transthoracic exposure.

DISORDERS OF THE ROTATOR CUFF

The tendons of the rotator cuff muscles fuse together near their insertions into the tuberosities of the humerus to form a musculotendinous cuff. With advancing age and repeated trauma these tendons, especially the supraspinatus, undergo degeneration. This is most severe near the tendon insertion. Secondary changes in the form of thickening and chronic inflammation frequently develop in the overlying bursa. It is agreed by many authors that the rotator cuff is the source of the majority of all shoulder pain.

A great deal of difficulty is encountered in di-

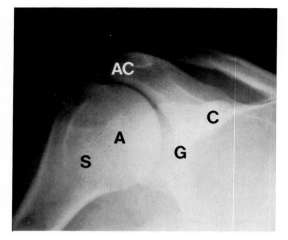

FIG 5–6.
Roentgenographic anatomy of the shoulder: *S* = surgical neck of the humerus; *A* = anatomic neck of the humerus; *T* = greater tuberosity; *C* = coracoid process; *AC* = acromion process; *G* = glenoid fossa.

agnosing nonarticular soft-tissue lesions of the shoulder. Tendinitis, bursitis, complete and incomplete rotator cuff ruptures, calcific deposits, and other lesions are all capable of producing similar signs and symptoms. A variety of terms have developed to describe these diseases: supraspinatus syndrome, chronic impingement syndrome, painful arc syndrome, and internal derangement of the subacromial joint. The treatment for all of these lesions tends to be similar except for that of complete rupture of the capsular rotator muscles, which causes loss of motor function. Surgical repair is frequently necessary for this lesion.

Chronic Strains and Tendinitis

At any age, a chronic strain of the musculotendinous unit may develop. Small tears of the rotator cuff may even be produced in the young athlete or laborer from repetitive use. Scarring and thickening of the involved area of tendon occurs with secondary irritation of the overlying bursa. Thickening of all of these tissues decreases the distance between the cuff and the overlying cora-

coacromial arch. Pain and crepitus may be noted when motions of the arm squeeze and pinch these tissues between the humerus and the overlying arch.

Clinical Features

The major clinical manifestations are pain, tenderness, muscle spasm, and occasionally, atrophy. The patient is frequently unable to lie on the affected shoulder and may feel a locking sensation with certain motions, especially abduction. The pain is often referred to the deltoid region. When abducting the shoulder, the patient will often automatically turn the palm up, thereby externally rotating the shoulder, a maneuver that gives the rotator cuff more room beneath the coracoacromial arch.

Maximum tenderness is usually noted over the supraspinatus insertion because this is the most common area of involvement. The acromioclavicular joint may also be tender due to degenerative changes. There is usually little loss of muscle power. The pain and crepitus are most severe in the arc of motion between 60 and 120 degrees of abduction. This is where the traumatized soft tissues are maximally compressed between the tuberosity and the overlying arch. The roentgenogram is usually normal, but some sclerosis may be present in the tuberosity secondary to long-standing local inflammation.

Treatment

1. Relief of pain and restoration of function are the therapeutic goals. The most important part of the treatment program is rest. This allows the inflammatory process to subside, relieves pain, and restores function. Rest should not be complete, however, because stiffness is prone to develop in the shoulder joint, especially in the older patient. Rest may be accomplished by simply avoiding excessive use of the arm, but occasionally, a sling is needed temporarily. The patient should avoid all "overhead" work, that is, work performed at a level higher than shoulder height.

2. Anti-inflammatory medication is usually helpful.

3. Moist heat is applied several times each day.

4. Local steroid injections often relieve pain and swelling but should be used with caution, especially in the young patient: 1 to 2 mL of steroid mixed with equal amounts of lidocaine is injected, under sterile conditions, into the subdeltoid bursa (Fig 5–7). The injection may be repeated two to three times every 2 weeks.

5. Physical therapy in the form of diathermy, ultrasound, or phonophoresis is occasionally beneficial. (Phonophoresis is ultrasound with cortisone cream. Theoretically, the ultrasound "drives" the cortisone into the affected area.)

6. Function is restored by an exercise program directed at preserving muscle tone and preventing stiffness (Fig 5–8). Pendulum exercises are begun early but are performed only within the limits of pain. As pain subsides, the exercises are increased, and further range-of-motion exercises are added. Swimming is an excellent means of restoring shoulder strength and motion. Work habits and other activities that cause compression and pinching of the inflamed tissue should be avoided. A sling may be worn initially between the exercises in order to rest

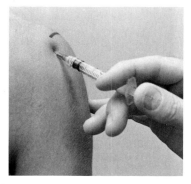

FIG 5–7.
Injection of the rotator cuff and bursa. A slightly posterior approach is best. The needle is angled slightly upward and placed in the sulcus between the head of the humerus and the acromion (marked). It should be able to be inserted completely, and the fluid should flow easily.

the shoulder, but it is gradually discontinued as the exercises are increased.

Improvement is usually seen within 3 to 5 weeks. If it is not, a more serious cuff lesion such as a rupture should be suspected. Surgery is reserved for those cases that fail to respond to conservative treatment, and it consists of partial excision of the acromion, release of obstructing soft tissue, and repair of any rotator cuff tears.

Ruptures of the Rotator Cuff

Ruptures of the rotator cuff result from continued deterioration and degeneration (Fig 5–9). The tear may be partial or complete. Ruptures are uncommon before the age of 40 years, but may occur in the young athlete secondary to a sudden forceful motion of the shoulder.

Clinical Features

A history is frequently obtained of a fall on the outstretched hand or an attempt at lifting a heavy object. A snap may be felt in the shoulder, and acute pain begins immediately after the injury. The pain may become progressively worse for the next few hours and the patient will note an inability to abduct or flex the shoulder, depending on the area of the tear. The pain is often referred down the deltoid muscle.

If the rupture is partial, the clinical findings are similar to those seen in chronic tendinitis. Even with complete rupture, the shoulder may have a full range of motion because of continued function of the other rotator muscles. Usually, however, with both partial and complete ruptures, there is significant weakness in abduction or flexion. The weakness is usually most severe in abduction because the muscle most commonly torn is the supraspinatus. If the tear is more anterior into the subscapularis, forward flexion will be weak. It may be impossible to actively abduct the arm more than 45 to 50 degrees, after which further abduction is obtained by scapulothoracic motion. A painful "catch" may be noted on passive motion between 50 and 100

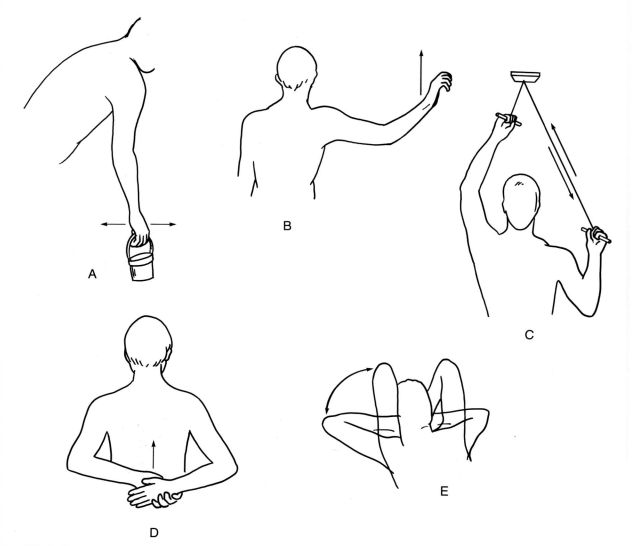

FIG 5–8.
Shoulder exercises. **A,** pendulum exercises. **B,** wall-climbing exercise. **C,** pulley exercises. The normal arm assists in the elevation of the stiffened arm. **D,** exercise for restoring internal rotation. **E,** exercise for restoring external rotation. Each exercise should be performed hourly or at least four times a day. Applying moist heat before the exercise may be helpful. In addition, activities that aggravate the pain, such as overhead work, should be avoided. For sitting work, a chair that supports the arms and shoulders should be used, and the patient should sit as close to the working surface as possible.

degrees, where compression of the swollen tissues between the tuberosity and the overlying arch occurs. Tenderness at the site of the tear is a common finding, and with complete ruptures a defect in the cuff may be palpated through the

deltoid muscle. Passive range of motion is frequently normal in the pain-free shoulder.

Atrophy of the cuff muscles is frequently present, and the "drop-arm" test may be positive. In this test, the arm is passively abducted to 90

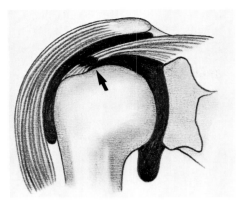

FIG 5–9.
Rupture of the rotator cuff *(arrow).*

degrees and then released. If abduction is able to be maintained, slight downward pressure is applied to the forearm, and the strength of the affected shoulder is compared with the normal shoulder. If pain is severe during the examination, it can be relieved by lidocaine infiltration of the tender area and the strength measured again. Inability to maintain shoulder abduction with this test is suggestive of a rotator cuff tear.

Special Studies

In patients who have shoulder pain clearly of shoulder origin, it may be difficult to differentiate tendinitis from partial or complete rotator cuff tears on a clinical basis. Roentgenographic evaluation may be of assistance:

1. Plain films should be obtained within the first few weeks of symptoms although they may not be necessary on the first visit. They are often indicated simply because of the nonspecific nature of rotator cuff symptoms and to rule out other obvious causes of shoulder pain. The examination may reveal chronic changes in the tuberosity of the humerus or calcific deposits (Fig 5–10). Degenerative arthritis may also be present in the acromioclavicular or glenohumeral joint.

2. Arthrography of the shoulder may help distinguish between complete and incomplete tears (Fig 5–11). Its main drawback is its invasive nature. It should probably only be performed if there has been serious discussion regarding surgery.

3. Ultrasonography is gaining some popularity

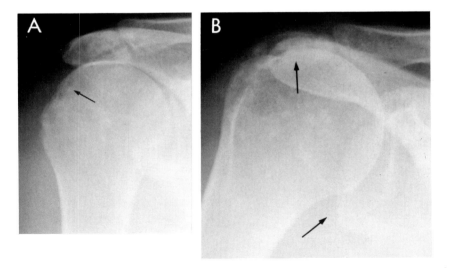

FIG 5–10.
A, cystic changes and sclerosis *(arrow)* frequently seen in the humeral head in chronic rotator cuff disorders. **B,** proximal migration of the humeral head is occasionally seen in rotator cuff tears *(arrows).* This occurs because the cuff can no longer stabilize the head in the glenoid. The deltoid, acting alone in abduction, pulls the head proximally.

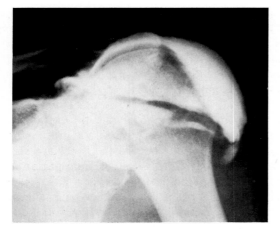

FIG 5–11.
Arthrography of the shoulder reveals dye leakage through the rotator cuff into the subacromial bursa; this indicates a complete rupture.

in the evaluation of the rotator cuff. It is safe and noninvasive, and its accuracy approaches 90% in some centers. It is most accurate in large and moderately large tears.

4. Magnetic resonance imaging (MRI) may eventually play a major role in diagnosing rotator cuff disease.

Treatment

Partial tears usually respond well to the conservative treatment program outlined for chronic tendinitis. Occasionally, it is necessary to surgically repair the rupture and remove any impinging structures beneath the coracoacromial arch.

Complete tears should also be repaired if they are sufficiently disabling. Frequently, however, there is very little loss of function and minimal pain. In these patients, especially if they are relatively inactive, operative intervention is probably not justified.

Calcific Deposits in the Rotator Cuff

Calcium deposits in the rotator cuff tendon are frequently associated with pain and stiffness in the shoulder. These deposits result from degenerative changes in the same area where ruptures

take place and are most frequently found in the supraspinatus tendon. Many of them remain small and deep in the tendon and, consequently, do not irritate the overlying bursa. Others slowly increase in size until they contact the bursa and produce an inflammatory reaction and swelling of the bursa. Impingement of these swollen tissues on the overlying coracoacromial arch may increase the inflammation and pain. Intermittent mechanical locking of the shoulder may even occur.

Clinical Features

The onset of symptoms may be gradual or acute. The pain is characteristically severe and accentuated by the slightest motion. Night pain and an inability to sleep on the shoulder are common complaints. The pain may radiate to the deltoid and even down the arm and forearm. It may subside suddenly when the milky deposit ruptures into the overlying bursa.

Examination in the acute stage reveals markedly limited motion and exquisite tenderness over the bursa and calcific deposit. There may be pronounced spasm of the rotator cuff muscles.

The symptoms and signs in chronic cases are less pronounced. Shoulder motion is frequently normal, and muscle spasm is absent. Symptoms of intermittent impingement and tenderness of the rotator cuff are usually present, however.

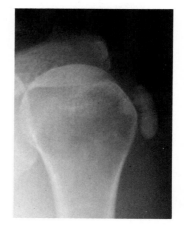

FIG 5–12.
Large calcific deposit in the rotator cuff.

Roentgenographic examination in internal and external rotation will usually reveal the deposit (Fig 5–12). If the deposit is anterior in the subscapularis muscle or posterior, a transaxillary view may be necessary to demonstrate it.

Treatment

Treatment is directed at relief of the inflammation and tension under the bursa from the swollen calcific mass. An injection of 2 mL of steroid mixed with equal amounts of lidocaine will often give dramatic relief. If the deposit appears soft, fluffy, and irregular on roentgenographic examination, aspiration and needling of the deposit may also be indicated. If the deposit is dense, round, and well circumscribed, however, this procedure is less helpful.

Aspiration and needling are performed under local anesthesia. A syringe with an 18-gauge needle is partially filled with lidocaine or saline and inserted directly into the deposit. Multiple areas are then injected and aspirated. A fine, flaky material may be withdrawn. The aspiration and needling are repeated over several areas until all accessible material is withdrawn. A second large needle placed in the calcific mass can be used for aspiration while the first needle is used for injection. At the end of the procedure, 2 mL of steroid is left in the bursa.

Analgesics and sedatives are given as necessary. Continuous warm, moist packs are applied to the shoulder. Diathermy and ultrasound may also be beneficial. The arm is allowed to hang in a sling until the acute pain subsides, and pendulum exercises are then initiated within the limits of pain. Motion progresses as tolerated.

Surgical excision of the calcific deposit is reserved for cases that fail to respond to conservative treatment. The results are usually excellent.

DISORDERS OF THE BICEPS TENDON

Tenosynovitis

Tenosynovitis of the long head of the biceps is a common cause of shoulder pain in adults over 40 years old. It may also occur in the young athlete from repeated strains, such as those caused by the throwing motion. The basic lesion is an inflammation in the tendon and its sheath in the bicipital groove. The disorders may be primary or secondary to disease of the overlying rotator cuff.

Clinical Features

The most common symptom is pain over the anterolateral aspect of the shoulder that may be referred down the anterior aspect of the arm. Muscle spasm and limitation of motion are frequently present. The most constant physical finding is tenderness to palpation over the bicipital groove. Active and passive shoulder motions are often restricted because of pain. Maneuvers that stretch the biceps tendon or cause it to glide in the groove may reproduce the pain. Forceful exter-

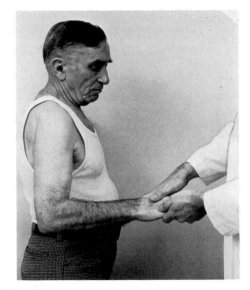

FIG 5–13.
Yergason's test. The forearm is supinated against resistance. Pain in the region of the bicipital groove is suggestive of bicipital tenosynovitis.

nal rotation with abduction or backward flexion of the extremity is often painful. Supination against resistance with the elbow flexed is also frequently uncomfortable (Fig 5–13). The roentgenograms are usually normal.

Treatment

In the acute stage, treatment consists of rest, moist heat, and gentle range-of-motion exercises. All motions that stretch the biceps tendon should be avoided. A sling may be used temporarily. Local steroid injections into the tendon sheath are frequently beneficial, and anti-inflammatory drugs are given as necessary.

The majority of cases respond well to conservative treatment. Surgery is recommended for those cases that fail to improve. Anchoring the tendon in the bicipital groove to prevent its motion will relieve the pain. The results are usually excellent.

Rupture of the Biceps Tendon

The biceps tendon may rupture as a result of advanced degeneration from chronic tendinitis. The rupture is usually complete and may follow a forceful contraction of the biceps muscle.

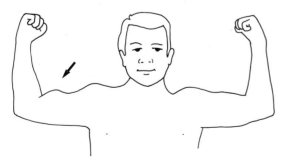

FIG 5–14.
Rupture of the long head of the biceps. A localized bulge *(arrow)* that is more prominent when the elbow is flexed against resistance is present in the distal part of the biceps.

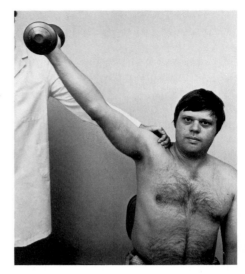

FIG 5–15.
Test for a subluxing biceps tendon. With a weight in the hand, the arm is elevated and externally rotated. As the arm is slowly adducted from this position, a snap may be heard or felt in the bicipital groove.

Clinical Features

The onset is usually sudden. A sharp snap may be felt by the patient, followed by pain and weakness of the arm. The diagnosis is easily made by the observation of an abnormally large mass in the arm that represents the retracted muscle belly of the long head of the biceps (Fig 5–14). There may be some loss of elbow flexion power.

Treatment

No treatment is necessary in many cases. There is only minimal loss of function and usually little pain associated with this condition. In the young patient, however, surgical repair of the rupture is often indicated.

Subluxing Biceps Tendon

The biceps tendon may occasionally dislocate from the bicipital groove. The usual cause is a tear in the overlying subscapularis tendon as the result of degenerative changes, but the condition may result from a congenitally shallow groove. The disorder may also occur in the young patient on forceful external rotation and abduction of the shoulder. Recurrences are frequent and may be reproducible by the patient (Fig 5–15). Tenosynovitis frequently develops and leads to pain and stiffness.

The only cure for this lesion is anchoring the tendon in the bicipital groove surgically. The results are uniformly good.

FROZEN SHOULDER (ADHESIVE CAPSULITIS)

Frozen shoulder is a disorder characterized by the insidious onset of pain and restriction of motion. The disease tends to be chronic, and full recovery may take several months. The cause is unknown, but bicipital tenosynovitis, rotator cuff tendinitis, and reflex sympathetic dystrophy have all been blamed.

Clinical Features

The onset is usually gradual and begins in the fifth decade. The disorder frequently develops during a period of inactivity in the use of the extremity or following a relatively minor injury to the shoulder. Pain is a constant symptom but frequently does not occur until much of the shoulder motion has already been lost. It is usually well localized in the region of the rotator cuff and may radiate down the deltoid and anterior aspect of the arm. It frequently interferes with sleep, especially when the patient attempts to lie on the affected shoulder.

Examination reveals an apprehensive patient who holds the arm protectively at the side. Spasm of the scapular muscles and trapezius is often present, and varying degrees of deltoid and spinatus atrophy may be noted. Generalized tenderness is present around the rotator cuff and biceps tendon. Shoulder motion is usually restricted to varying degrees, depending on the stage of the disease. The signs of reflex sympathetic dystrophy are often present in the involved extremity (edema of the hand, coolness, and discoloration).

Roentgenograms should always be performed. Although their findings are usually normal, a missed *posterior shoulder dislocation* should always be ruled out.

The course of the disease is variable. Some patients recover relatively early in the disorder, but in many cases the condition is progressive over several months. In these patients, shoulder motion gradually decreases and the pain subsides. As soon as the pain diminishes, the shoulder begins to regain its motion. Recovery is slow, and complete recovery in less than 6 months is rare. Most patients will eventually regain full motion of their shoulder, however.

Treatment

The most important facet of treatment is prevention. Every attempt should be made to maintain motion in the shoulder during those periods of time when the patient may be inactive due to disease or injury. Once the disease process has begun, treatment is directed at the relief of pain. Bed rest, moist heat, sedation, and analgesics are prescribed as necessary. A local injection of a steroid/lidocaine mixture into the rotator cuff may also prove beneficial. Pendulum and overhead pulley exercises are begun as soon as possible and initially are performed on an hourly basis.

Most patients will eventually respond to a well-supervised program of physical therapy. Those patients who fail to respond may benefit from careful manipulation of the shoulder under general anesthesia followed by aggressive range-of-motion exercises. Repeated cervical sympathetic blocks may also be indicated in those patients who have a significant sympathetic component to their symptoms. Surgical intervention is rarely necessary.

SNAPPING SCAPULA

Snapping scapula is an uncommon disorder in which an audible grating sound occurs with motion of the scapulothoracic joint. Normally, the serratus anterior and subscapularis muscles cushion the scapula from the underlying rib cage. The scapula is poorly protected at its medial border and at its superior and inferior angles, however. Abnormal angulations at these locations may cause pain and snapping sensations. Tumors of the scapula or ribs, bursae between these bones, and poor posture with sagging of the shoulder joint are other causes of crepitus in this area. Often, no cause is found.

Clinical Features
The onset is usually gradual, but the process is frequently precipitated by a traumatic event. The snapping is often palpable and painful. The origin of these noises can frequently be well localized by the patient to a specific area in the scapulothoracic articulation.

Roentgenograms of the scapula, including oblique views, are obtained to discover such lesions as exostoses and tumors when they are present (Fig 5–16).

Treatment
If the roentgenograms are normal, physical therapy, rest, and local steroid injections will often relieve the pain. Correction of poor posture is also frequently beneficial. If the snapping is secondary to tumor or exostosis and the pain and disability are sufficient to justify surgery, the involved area of the scapula is removed surgically.

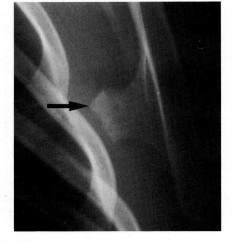

FIG 5–16.
Osteochondroma *(arrow)* of the inner wall of the scapula.

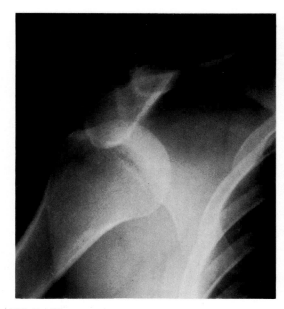

FIG 5–17.
Anterior dislocation of the shoulder.

GLENOHUMERAL DISLOCATION

Dislocations of the shoulder are most commonly anterior in direction and usually result from a fall on the externally rotated, abducted arm (Fig 5–17). This force levers the humerus out of the glenoid cavity into its anterior position.

Posterior dislocations are less common and may result from a force directed against the internally rotated arm. Many posterior dislocations occur at the time of a seizure in patients with convulsive disorders. Occasionally, some individuals can reproduce a posterior dislocation voluntarily and use this maneuver to attract attention.

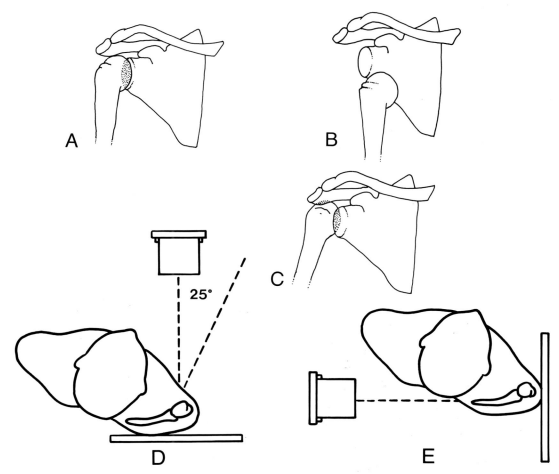

FIG 5–18.
A, the "normal" AP roentgenographic anatomy of the glenohumeral joint. There is normally a 50% elliptical overlap or "half moon" of increased density where the humeral head overlaps the posterior glenoid rim. The anterior edge of the glenoid should parallel the medial border of the humeral head, and the distance between these two lines should not exceed 6 mm. **B,** anterior dislocation, which is usually not a problem in diagnosis. **C,** posterior dislocation. Up to 50% of these are missed initially. The humeral head barely overlaps the glenoid and may be higher or lower than normal. The greater tuberosity is usually internally rotated, and the area of overlap is abnormal. **D,** the "true" AP view of the glenohumeral joint is taken 25 degrees toward the midline. **E,** a true lateral (the scapular "Y") view may be taken at a right angle to this film. (The "Y" is formed at the glenoid fossa where the bases of the coracoid and spine of the scapula join the distally projecting body.)

Clinical Features

The diagnosis is usually not difficult. Clinically, the acromion is much more prominent than normal, and there is an absence of the normal fullness of the humeral head beneath the deltoid and acromion process. Little movement of the shoulder is possible without severe pain. With anterior dislocations, the arm is held externally rotated, the anterior shoulder is full, and internal rotation is painful. In posterior dislocations, the arm is held in internal rotation, with the forearm resting on the abdomen. The anterior portion of the shoulder is flat, and external rotation is painful. The integrity of the neurovascular structures of the arm should always be assessed, especially the axillary nerve. Numbness in the middle of the deltoid may be present.

Roentgenographic evaluation is mandatory, but interpretation is sometimes difficult with posterior dislocations (Fig 5–18). A "true" antero-posterior (AP) view of the shoulder may be helpful, and a lateral view of the glenohumeral joint is essential. A variety of lateral views may be performed (trans-scapular "Y", transthoracic, tranaxillary). Perhaps the easiest to perform and interpret is the transaxillary (Fig 5–19).

Treatment and Prognosis

Shoulder dislocations are usually reducible without general anesthesia if good muscular relaxation can be obtained. Intravenous sedation or analgesia is often helpful. Gentle, straight traction on the arm is usually sufficient to reduce both the anterior and posterior dislocation (Fig 5–20). If straight traction does not reduce the dislocation, Stimson's method may be used for the anterior dislocation. The patient is placed in a prone position with the affected arm hanging over the side of the table. A 5- to 10-kg weight is tied to the wrist for traction. As the shoulder muscles re-

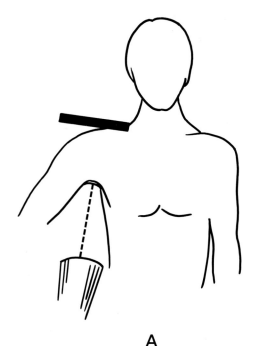
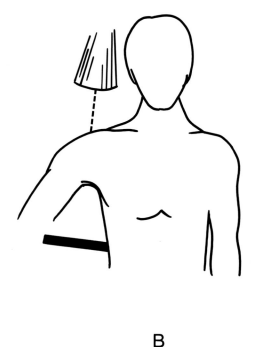

A   **B**

FIG 5–19.
A and **B,** Transaxillary lateral views of the glenohumeral joint. Even with a fracture or dislocation, the arm can be gently abducted enough to obtain a view from below or above. It may be done standing or supine.

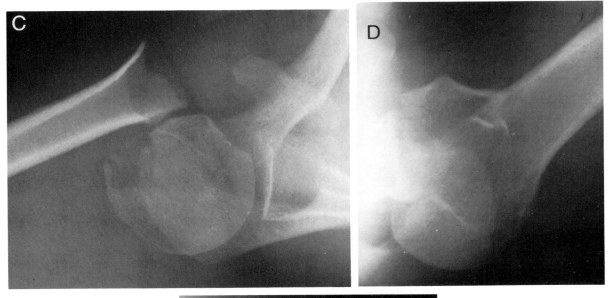

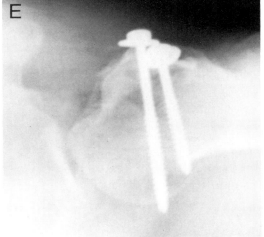

FIG 5–19 (cont'd.).
C, the roentgenographic appearance. Also present is a displaced fracture of the surgical neck of the humerus, but the humeral head is properly positioned in the glenoid. **D,** a posterior fracture-dislocation. **E,** the injury in **D** is reduced and internally fixed.

lax, spontaneous reduction frequently occurs. If the shoulder remains dislocated, reduction with the patient under a general anesthetic is usually necessary. Open reduction is rarely required.

Primary dislocations in either direction in patients under the age of 30 years have a high rate of recurrence. These recurrences frequently take place with little or no trauma and often can be reduced by the patient. In order to prevent recurrences and allow for proper healing of the anterior shoulder joint capsule after the initial anterior dislocation, strict immobilization for 4 weeks

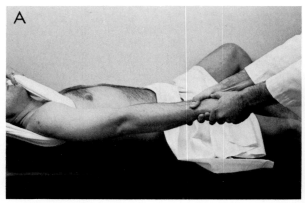

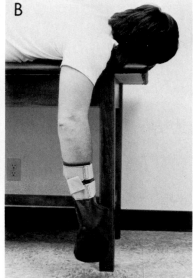

FIG 5–20.
Reduction of shoulder dislocation. **A,** straight traction is applied to the wrist with countertraction to the axilla. If straight traction fails, try pulling upward. **B,** Stimson's method for anterior dislocations. Kocher's maneuver is usually not necessary.

is necessary following the acute dislocation. A shoulder immobilizer is satisfactory treatment of the anterior dislocation, but the patient must not be allowed to externally rotate the arm (Fig 5–21). The posterior dislocation should be immobilized with the arm in external rotation and abduction. This may necessitate the use of an abduction splint. An exercise program may be beneficial (Fig 5–22). Recurrent dislocations in either direction usually require corrective surgery. The most common procedures used are those that restrict rotation or reinforce the weakened shoulder joint capsule.

Primary dislocations in patients over the age of 40 years are not generally complicated by recurrence but frequently result in shoulder joint stiffness. In this age group, light immobilization with a sling for 1 to 2 weeks is all the treatment that is necessary, and active motion is then encouraged in order to prevent stiffness.

Occasionally, an old anterior dislocation is seen in the elderly patient. The length of time the shoulder has been dislocated may be impossible to determine. Closed reduction may be attempted, but if the injury is over 2 to 3 weeks old, enough soft-tissue healing will probably

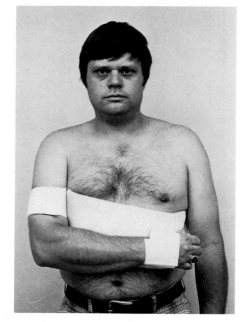

FIG 5–21.
Shoulder immobilizer. Sometimes a simple sling is more comfortable. It should be worn beneath a knit shirt to keep the arm against the body.

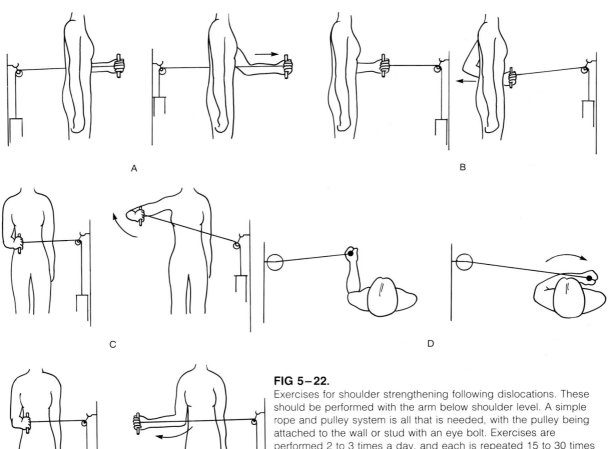

A

B

C

D

FIG 5–22.
Exercises for shoulder strengthening following dislocations. These should be performed with the arm below shoulder level. A simple rope and pulley system is all that is needed, with the pulley being attached to the wall or stud with an eye bolt. Exercises are performed 2 to 3 times a day, and each is repeated 15 to 30 times beginning with a 2-kg weight and progressing to 10 kg. **A,** flexion; **B** extension; **C,** abduction; **D,** internal rotation; and **E,** external rotation.

E

have occurred to make the procedure unsuccessful. If it fails, accepting the disability and working to improve motion may be the most logical treatment in this age group.

ACROMIOCLAVICULAR DISLOCATION

Acromioclavicular dislocations and separations occur as the result of a fall on the shoulder or from a direct blow to the top of the shoulder. They are classified as complete or incomplete. A complete dislocation is present when both the acromioclavicular and coracoclavicular ligaments are disrupted (Fig 5–23). Incomplete separations are those in which only the acromioclavicular joint ligaments are disrupted.

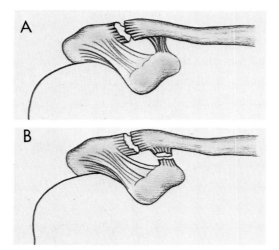

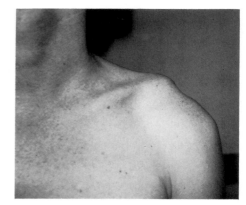

FIG 5–24.
Clinical deformity with acromioclavicular dislocation.

FIG 5–23.
A, incomplete dislocation of the acromioclavicular joint. The coracoclavicular ligaments are intact. **B,** complete dislocation.

ening between the coracoid process and the clavicle will be present on the affected side (Fig 5–25).

Clinical Features

These injuries are characterized by tenderness and swelling over the acromioclavicular joint. The outer clavicle is usually elevated in both complete and incomplete dislocations (Fig 5–24). Downward traction on the arm may increase the deformity.

Complete dislocations may be differentiated from incomplete dislocations by an AP roentgenogram taken while the patient has a 10-kg weight hanging from both arms. If complete rupture of the coracoclavicular ligaments has occurred, wid-

Treatment

Reduction of the incomplete separation by manual pressure is usually easy, but maintenance of the reduction is frequently difficult. Strapping between the elbow and clavicle may maintain the reduction, but usually no treatment is necessary for these injuries. A sling is used for a few days to minimize the pain, and active shoulder motion is begun as tolerated. The outer end of the clavicle may remain prominent, but this is usually painless and does not interfere with function. If it does, the tip of the clavicle may be surgically re-

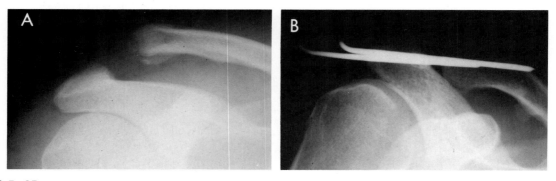

FIG 5–25.
A, complete acromioclavicular dislocation. **B,** the postoperative appearance. The pins are removed in 7 to 8 weeks.

moved at a later date. Complete acromioclavicular dislocations sometimes require surgical intervention with reduction of the dislocation and repair of the ruptured ligaments.

STERNOCLAVICULAR DISLOCATION

Sternoclavicular dislocations are uncommon injuries that occur as the result of a fall on the shoulder. The anterior dislocation is more common. The rare posterior dislocation may cause pressure on the anterior structures of the neck and lead to dyspnea and vascular compression that may require immediate reduction.

The injury usually produces a tender, visible prominence at the sternoclavicular joint. Some discomfort with shoulder motion is usually present.

This is an area that is difficult to visualize roentgenographically. A view angled upward including the uninjured side may give some information.

Anterior dislocations are reduced by traction and manipulation, but the reduction is frequently difficult to maintain. Recurrence after the reduction is common, but except for minor cosmetic deformity, no function is lost. Surgical intervention, therefore, is rarely justified in the acute case. If post-traumatic arthritis occurs, surgical excision of the medial 1 to 2 cm of clavicle will usually relieve the symptoms.

Spontaneous anterior sternoclavicular (SC) dislocation may occasionally occur without any clear history of trauma. The patient may present with a relatively painless "mass," the enlargement being the sternal end of the clavicle. This is most commonly seen in the older adult. Reassurance is usually the only treatment, following routine examination and plain films.

In the child, an *epiphyseal fracture* can also occur in this area, sometimes causing confusion with an SC dislocation. Reduction may be able to be obtained by manipulation but is difficult to maintain. Fortunately, some remodeling occurs and will diminish the size of the fracture lump. Surgery would be required to keep the fracture reduced, but an unsightly scar usually results. As with SC dislocations, only nonsurgical management is needed.

DEGENERATIVE ARTHRITIS

Degenerative arthritis of the glenohumeral joint is relatively uncommon. It is usually the end stage of chronic rheumatoid arthritis or long-standing chronic rotator cuff disease (Fig 5–26). It may also be the result of recurrent shoulder dislocations or severe fractures of the shoulder joint. Chronic pain and limited shoulder motion are common, and crepitus is frequently present.

Treatment is usually directed at providing symptomatic relief by injections and anti-inflammatory medication. These often provide only temporary relief, and many have to be repeated at frequent intervals. The surgical options are fusion, resection of the humeral head, and total joint replacement, although the latter two have had inconsistent results.

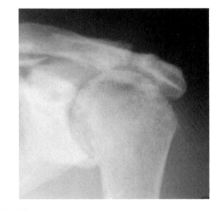

FIG 5–26.
Osteoarthritis of the glenohumeral joint.

FRACTURES OF THE SHOULDER REGION

Fracture of the Clavicle

The clavicle is the only rigid bony connection between the shoulder and the chest, and it functions to hold the shoulder upward and backward. It may be injured by a fall on the outstretched hand (Fig 5–27).

Reduction is obtained by manipulating both shoulders upward, outward, and backward in order to reestablish the length of the clavicle (Fig 5–28). Infiltration of the fracture site with a local anesthetic will usually eliminate the pain. The reduction is maintained by a figure-of-8 dressing for 4 to 5 weeks in the child and 5 to 6 weeks in the adult. The addition of a sling may be helpful. A prominence at the fracture site will often persist in the adult, but it usually disappears in the child a few months after remodeling of the bone has occurred. If undue pressure on the axillary vessels and nerves occurs during use of the dressing, pressure can be relieved by allowing the patient to lie down and temporarily abduct the shoulders. Open reduction is never

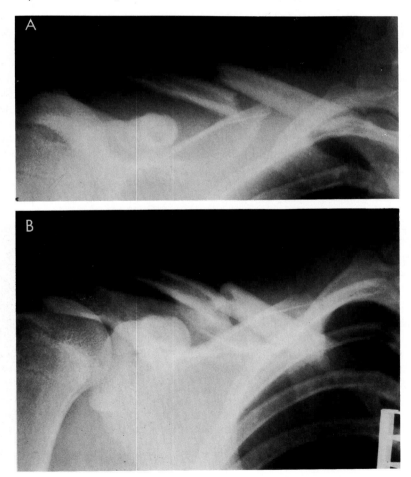

FIG 5–27.
A, fracture of the clavicle with overriding. **B,** the length has been restored by manipulation.

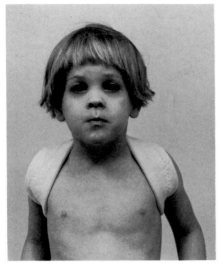

FIG 5–28.
After restoring the length to the clavicle, the fracture is immobilized by a figure-of-8 dressing. The dressing should remain snug and may have to be tightened.

indicated in the child and only rarely in the adult.

Fractures of the Scapula

Fractures of the scapula usually result from a direct blow or fall (Fig 5–29). Fractures that do not involve the articular surface of the glenoid cavity require little treatment. A sling or shoulder immobilizer may be used for 1 to 2 weeks until the pain subsides. Gentle motion of the shoulder is encouraged as soon as possible, and the results are usually excellent. The rare fracture that in-

volves the shoulder articulation may require more extensive surgical treatment.

Fractures of the Upper Portion of the Humerus

Undisplaced or impacted fractures of the surgical neck of the humerus are common in elderly patients (Fig 5–30). Slight degrees of malalignment should be accepted in this age group.

Treatment consists of a dressing that immobilizes the arm and forearm to the chest and abdomen. This is continued for approximately 2 weeks and is followed by a sling for 2 more weeks. Pendulum exercises are performed in the sling. All immobilization is discontinued after 4 weeks. A hanging cast should not be used in these fractures because it may disimpact the bony fragments. The disability in this injury results not from the fracture itself, which usually heals readily, but from the secondary stiffness that develops in the shoulder, especially in elderly patients. It is not uncommon for some permanent loss of abduction to result from this injury, and full range of motion may take several months to return.

Displaced fractures of the surgical neck may

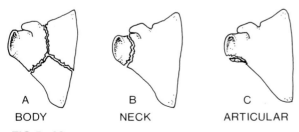

FIG 5–29.
Various fractures of the scapula.

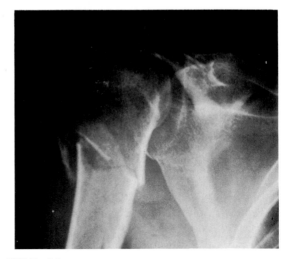

FIG 5–30.
Fracture of the surgical neck of the humerus.

require manipulative reduction and a hanging long arm cast. If closed methods fail, open reduction is occasionally indicated.

Fractures of the tuberosities of the upper humerus may occur from a fall or in association with a shoulder dislocation (Fig 5–31). Undisplaced fractures require only a sling for 7 to 10 days, followed by early range-of-motion exercises. Fractures that are displaced over 5 to 10 mm frequently require open reduction and internal fixation. If this is not performed, a bony impingement to abduction may result.

Fractures of the Shaft of the Humerus

Fractures of the shaft of the humerus usually heal well with nonoperative treatment. The function of the radial nerve should always be evaluated because it may be injured in its course around the humeral shaft.

Manipulative reduction under local anesthesia may be required, but distraction of the fracture fragments should be avoided. With the patient sitting on a stool and leaning forward, the weight of the arm will frequently reduce the fracture (Fig 5–32). The wrist is supported to overcome apprehension, but the elbow should hang free.

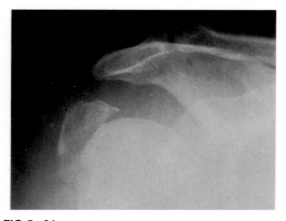

FIG 5–31.
Displaced fracture of the greater tuberosity of the humerus.

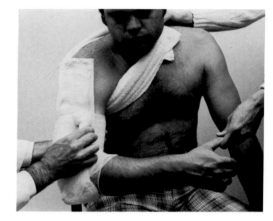

FIG 5–32.
Fracture of the humerus reduced by downward traction and countertraction. A "sugar-tong" or "U"-shaped splint is then applied and wrapped with gauze or elastic bandage. The splint begins in the axilla and ends over the shoulder. It may have to be tightened at intervals. A collar and cuff are added.

Gentle traction and countertraction are applied, and the fracture fragments are manipulated to correct any angulation. End-to-end apposition is tested by upward pressure on the elbow. If no "telescoping" of the fracture fragments occurs, apposition is usually secure. The fracture is immobilized by the application of a "U"-shaped plaster splint. Additional fixation may be obtained by strapping the humerus to the chest wall. After 4 to 6 weeks, gentle motion is encouraged. Healing is usually complete by 8 to 10 weeks (Fig 5–33).

Inferior Subluxation of the Humeral Head

Inferior displacement of the head of the humerus may occur in a number of situations including: (1) following fractures about the shoulder area (Fig 5–34), (2) as a result of local neurogenic impairment such as brachial neuritis, and (3) following strokes or other central nervous system (CNS) disorders.

The most common cause is "hypotonicity,"

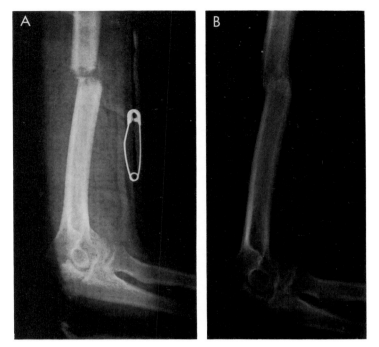

FIG 5–33.
A, transverse fracture of the humerus immobilized in a "U"-shaped splint. **B,** the end result.

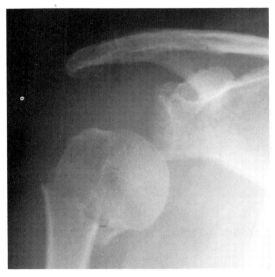

FIG 5–34.
Inferior "subluxation" of the humeral head.

which may develop in conjunction with fractures of the upper aspect of the humerus or dislocations of the glenohumeral joint. When the musculoskeletal injury heals, muscle tone usually returns to normal, and the abnormal increase in acromiohumeral distance disappears. Simple strengthening and range-of-motion exercises after the injury has healed are the only necessary treatment.

If the subluxation is atraumatic, electromyography may be needed to determine whether a neurogenic disorder has developed.

MEDICAL CAUSES OF SHOULDER PAIN

Shoulder pain may develop not only from primary disease of the neck and shoulder but also by referral from disorders of thoracic or abdominal origin. Care should be taken not to always assume the patient's description of shoulder pain to be "arthritis." Visceral disorders must be borne in mind, especially when other causes of the pain are not apparent.

Abdominal Causes

It is well known that pain may be referred to the shoulder via the phrenic nerve. This pain may refer to any part of the shoulder but is most commonly on top of the shoulder, in the supraspinous fossa, or over the acromion or clavicle, that is, in the region of distribution of the cutaneous branches of the fourth cervical nerve. Lesions affecting a certain portion of the diaphragm may cause pain over the corresponding part of the shoulder on the same side of the body. In general, pain on top of both shoulders indicates a median diaphragmatic irritation. When the diaphragm is irritated by a neighboring lesion such as blood from a ruptured spleen, tenderness may even be elicited by pressure on the corresponding phrenic nerve in the neck.

When a gastric or intestinal ulcer perforates, the escaping fluid may impinge on the lower surface of the diaphragm. This may irritate the terminations of the phrenic nerve on one or both sides and can be the cause of pain on top of one or both shoulders. Pain felt on top of both shoulders at the onset of the attack suggests that the perforation has occurred in the anterior portion of the stomach and is causing irritation of the median portion of the diaphragm. In the case of pyloric duodenal ulcer, the shoulder pain is usually felt in the right supraspinous fossa or on the corresponding side.

Referred shoulder pain may also develop in cases of subphrenic abscess, diaphragmatic pleurisy, acute pancreatitis, gallstones, ruptured spleen, and appendicitis with peritonitis. It may be the only signal with a liver abscess that is threatening to perforate the diaphragm. Pelvic inflammatory disease with perihepatic inflammation (so-called Fitz-Hugh-Curtis syndrome) is also an occasional cause of shoulder pain.

In addition, a history of shoulder pain should be sought in all patients who have had serious abdominal trauma. Injury to solid viscera such as liver, spleen, pancreas, and kidney may result in hemorrhage, which in turn may cause diaphragmatic irritation and shoulder pain.

Note: In summary, while most shoulder pain is musculoskeletal in origin, it behooves the clinician to keep a high index of suspician for abdominal causes of the pain. This is especially true if the pain is not aggravated by neck or shoulder movement and the patient has a history of gastrointestinal symptoms. In these cases, further studies and referral to a gastroenterologist may be indicated.

Thoracic Causes

While most disorders of intrathoracic origin will cause chest pain, shoulder discomfort is not uncommon and may be the main presenting complaint. Diseases of *cardiac* origin (pericarditis, etc.) commonly cause left arm and shoulder pain. Cardiac pain may also be referred to the neck, lower jaw, and interscapular area. The pain associated with ischemic disease is usually exertional but may occur at rest and cause more confusion. Clinically, there is usually no tenderness or aggravation of the pain by neck or shoulder motion.

Pulmonary diseases (carcinoma, pneumonia, abscess, etc.) may also result in shoulder pain. Of special interest are tumors of the superior sulcus of the lung (Pancoast). This tumor produces a syndrome by virtue of its growth in the thoracic inlet. This region is bounded roughly by the first rib, the first costal cartilage, the manubrium, and the body of T1. The apex of the lung occupies most of the area. The superior pulmonary sulcus is a groove in the lung tissue made by the subclavian artery as it crosses the apex of the lung, and because the majority of apical lung tumors occur in relation to this sulcus, they are often called superior sulcus tumors. The structures in this area are the internal jugular and subclavian veins; the vagus, phrenic, and recurrent laryngeal nerves; the subclavian and common carotid arteries; the eighth cervical and first thoracic nerves; and the stellate ganglion and sympathetic chain. Any of these structures may be involved, and therefore the symptoms may be variable and complex. Pain is the most common initial complaint. Its distribution is often wide and unusual, frequently being present throughout the shoulder, scapular or infrascapular area, upper anterior portion of the chest, arm, neck, and axilla. Other components of this syndrome include Horner's syndrome, weakness and sensory disturbances on the involved side (possibly due to involvement of the lower portion of the brachial plexus), supraclavicular fullness, venous distension, and edema of the extremity. A superior sulcus tumor should always be kept in mind in patients with neck or shoulder pain, especially if there is a history of cigarette smoking. Shoulder roentgenograms may reveal the lesion, but usually a more complete roentgenographic examination is needed (Fig 5–35).

Other diseases of thoracic origin that may cause shoulder pain are disorders of the mediastinum, aorta, and esophagus. The pain of hiatus hernia, in particular, can radiate to the top of both shoulders and down the arms.

Miscellaneous Causes

Malignant tumor, either primary, locally spread, or metastatic from a distant origin, may also be the cause of shoulder pain. The diagnosis may be obvious in the patient with a known history of malignancy. The major sources are tumors of thyroid, prostate, breast, lung, and kidney and Hodgkin's disease. The most common primary tumor that metastasizes to bone is multiple myeloma. The shoulder is less commonly involved than the ribs, spine, and pelvis. Pathologic fractures may occur but are uncommon in the upper extremity. Plain roentgenograms may be normal because over 50% bone destruction is needed before destructive changes become apparent. Bone scanning is usually helpful, but myeloma and some aggressive sarcomas may destroy bone so fast that repair cannot occur, thereby resulting in a false-negative study.

Paget's disease may also cause localized bone pain. As a result of periosteal bone formation impinging on cranial and spinal nerves, impairment of nerve function may even occur. Most patients with Paget's disease have minimal or no symptoms. The onset of increased pain in an area of Paget's disease should suggest sarcomatous degeneration.

Shoulder-hand syndrome, a form of reflex neurovascular dystrophy, is a poorly understood disorder (see Chapter 18). The disease is probably caused by reflex sympathetic stimulation analogous to that proposed for causalgia. The patients are usually above the age of 50 years and often have had a recent acute illness, frequently a myocardial infarction, cerebrovascular accident (CVA), pulmonary disorder or minor musculoskeletal trauma. The patient develops pain, stiffness in the shoulder, and swelling and vasomotor phenomena in the involved extremity. There is a marked variability in the intensity of the pain,

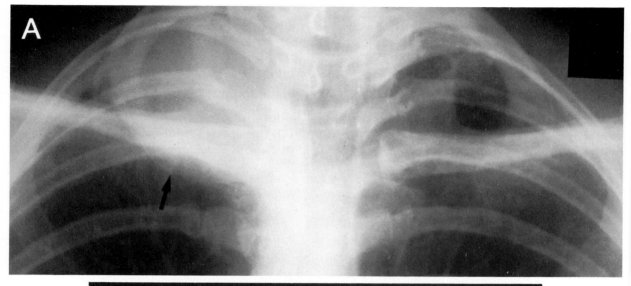

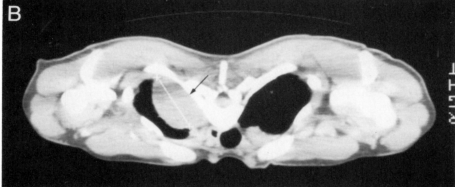

FIG 5–35.
Pancoast tumor *(arrows).* **A,** plain film. **B,** computed tomographic (CT) appearance.

duration of acute symptoms, and extent of dystrophic change. A frequent complication is frozen shoulder. Treatment is nonspecific and includes (1) an active exercise program facilitated by analgesics; (2) physical therapy; (3) a trial of a corticosteroid (prednisone, 10 to 20 mg/day) for a short time; and (4) stellate ganglion blocks if all other forms of medical management are unsuccessful. The condition will usually resolve on its own in the course of several months.

Herpes zoster ("shingles") is an acute viral infection that produces an inflammatory reaction in

a segmental nerve. Initially, fever with unilateral pain and paresthesias may be present. In a few days, an erythematous rash appears that becomes vesicular. Early, before the rash develops, its symptoms may be confused with other painful disorders.

Brachial neuritis is an unusual disorder of unknown cause that can also be confused with other causes of shoulder pain or weakness. Many terms have been used to describe this syndrome: shoulder-girdle syndrome of Parsonage and Turner, acute brachial radiculitis, neuralgic amy-

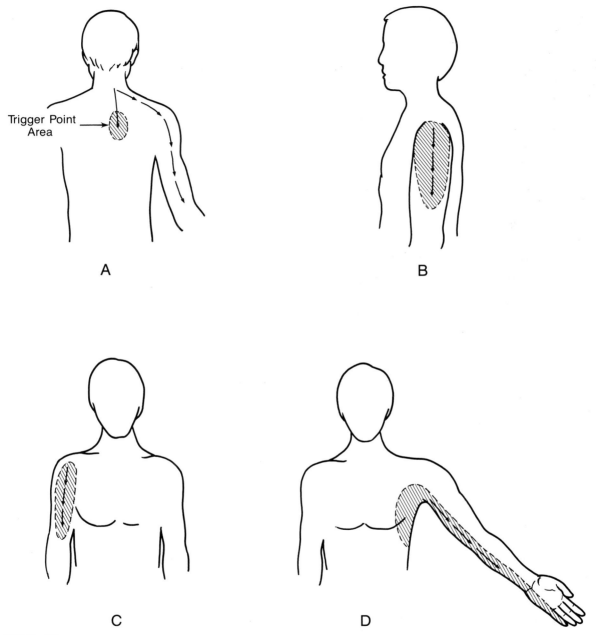

FIG 5–36.
General pain distribution of common neck and arm disorders. **A,** cervical disc syndrome. **B,** rotator cuff syndrome. **C,** bicipital tendinitis. **D,** disorders involving the lower portion of the brachial plexus (Pancoast tumor, thoracic outlet syndrome). When the shoulder pain has a visceral origin, the patient sometimes recognizes it as "deep" and perhaps not arising in the exact region where it is felt.

otrophy, and brachial plexus neuropathy. The cause is unknown, but a viral or allergic reaction is suspected. It is characterized by acute severe pain, usually in the shoulder but frequently in the arm and neck. The pain is often worse at night. Shoulder weakness follows the pain, usually within a month and sometimes as soon as a day. The pain is typically of short duration. The deltoid, rotator cuff, biceps, and triceps are commonly involved, and electromyography usually demonstrates changes of neurogenic atrophy. The prognosis is usually good, although recovery may take 2 to 3 years. Treatment is symptomatic.

Carpal tunnel syndrome (see Chapter 7) is a common cause of shoulder pain. While the predominant symptoms occur in the hand, they are frequently accompanied by arm and shoulder pain. Carpal tunnel syndrome and cervical disc syndrome with radiculopathy occasionally occur at the same time and involve the same extremity.

DIFFERENTIAL DIAGNOSIS (TABLE 5–1)

TABLE 5–1.

Differential Diagnosis of Common Causes of Neck and/or Arm Pain*

Disorder	Most Common Pain Location or Radiation	Findings Present	Findings Absent
Cervical disc syndrome	Posterior neck, usually unilateral, intrascapular and trapezius pain. May radiate down one shoulder (if nerve root pressure), lateral arm, dorsoradial forearm to thumb, index, or long finger (see Fig 5–36)	Pain aggravated by neck movement. Weak biceps or triceps. Paresthesias in forearm, hand. Trigger point in interscapular area	Symptoms not aggravated by shoulder motion. Usually no radicular symptoms on ulnar aspect of arm or hand
Rotator cuff syndrome	Acromion down to deltoid insertion. (often worse at night)	Painful shoulder motion especially abduction, external rotation. Mild limitation of shoulder motion. Crepitus. Tender rotator cuff. Mild weakness	No interscapular pain or pain with neck motion. No paresthesias. Usually no symptoms below elbow
Bicipital tendinitis	Bicipital groove down anterior arm	Tender bicipital groove, pain on shoulder extension. Positive Yergason's test	No symptoms below elbow, no pain with neck motion, no neurologic symptoms
Pancoast tumor	Variable symptoms. Shoulder, plexus pain into arm	Supraclavicular tenderness. Horner's syndrome? Palpable mass. Pain with shoulder motion	Pain not increased with neck movement
Thoracic outlet syndrome	Shoulder, medial arm, forearm, and hand symptoms (C8, T1)	Ulnar (medial) paresthesias; signs of vascular compression?	No neck findings. Full, painfree shoulder motion

*NOTES: (1) Symptoms of *cervical strain* are usually bilateral and involve the neck and occiput. The symptoms are often diffuse, and the areas of soft-tissue tenderness frequently change. (2) *Acromioclavicular arthritis* has localized acromioclavicular pain and tenderness. (3) *Glenohumeral arthritis* presents with generalized shoulder pain and considerable loss of shoulder movement. (4) *Carpal tunnel syndrome* may cause shoulder aching, but the symptoms are mainly in the hand and forearm.

TABLE 5–2.
Algorithm for Rotator Cuff Inflammation

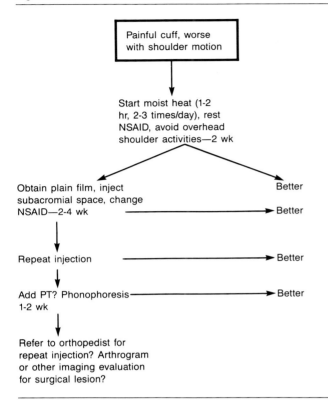

Notes:
1. Night pain is common with cuff tendinitis.
2. No trauma—always consider METS.
3. Bone scans are often abnormal in tendinitis and reflect the local increased bone circulation caused by the adjacent soft-tissue inflammation.

This situation is called the "double-crush" syndrome. Under this circumstance then, there may be two causes of shoulder pain, neither of which has its origin in the shoulder itself.

BIBLIOGRAPHY

Andersen K, Jensen PO, Lauritzen J: Treatment of clavicular fractures: Figure-of-eight bandages versus a simple sling. *Acta Orthop Scand* 1987; 57:71.

Arendt EA: Multidirectional shoulder instability. *Orthopedics* 1988; 11:113.

Bacevich BB: Paralytic brachial neuritis. A case report. *J Bone Joint Surg [Am]* 1976; 58:262.

Bannister GC, et al: The management of acute acromioclavicular dislocation. *J Bone Joint Surg [Br]* 1989; 71:848.

Bateman JE: The diagnosis and treatment of ruptures of the rotator cuff. *Surg Clin North Am* 1963; 43:1523.

Baxter MP, Wiley JJ: Fractures of the proximal humeral epiphysis. Their influence on humeral growth. *J Bone Joint Surg [Br]* 1986; 68:570.

Bergenudd H, et al: Shoulder pain in middle age: A study of prevalence and relation to occupational work load and psychosocial factors. *Clin Orthop* 1988; 231:234.

Buckerfield CT, Castle ME: Acute traumatic retrosternal dislocation of the clavicle. *J Bone Joint Surg [Am]* 1984; 66:379.

Bush LH: The torn shoulder capsule. *J Bone Joint Surg [Am]* 1975; 57:256

Cofield RH: Rotator cuff disease of the shoulder. *J Bone Joint Surg [Am]* 1985; 67:974.

Cope Z: *The Early Diagnosis of the Acute Abdomen,* ed 12. Oxford, England, Oxford University Press, 1963.

Crass JR, Craig EV: Noninvasive imaging of the rotator cuff. *Orthopedics* 1988; 11:57.

DeDeuxchaisnes CN, Krone SM: Paget's disease of bone: Clinical and metabolic observation. *Medicine (Baltimore)* 1964; 43:233.

DePalma AF: *Surgery of the Shoulder,* ed 2. Philadelphia, JB Lippincott, 1973.

Dillin L, Hoaglund FT, Scheck M: Brachial neuritis. *J Bone Joint Surg [Am]* 1985; 67:878.

Fery A, Sommelet S: Dislocation of the sternoclavicular joint: A review of 49 cases. *Int Orthop* 1988; 12:187.

Fronek J, et al: Posterior subluxation of the glenohumeral joint. *J Bone Joint Surg [Am]* 1989; 71:205.

Gerber C, Garz R: Clinical assessment of instability of the shoulder. *J Bone Joint Surg [Br]* 1984; 66:551.

Gore DR, et al: Shoulder-muscle strength and range of motion following surgical repair of full-thickness rotator-cuff tears. *J Bone Joint Surg [Am]* 1986; 68:266.

Goss TP: Anterior glenohumeral instability. *Orthopedics* 1988; 11:87.

Grant JCB: *A Method of Anatomy,* ed 6. Baltimore, Williams & Wilkins, 1958.

Hammond G: Complete acromionectomy in the treatment of chronic tendinitis of the shoulder. *J Bone Joint Surg [Am]* 1971; 53:173.

Hawkins RJ, McCormack RG: Posterior shoulder instability. *Orthopedics* 1988; 11:101.

Howell SM, et al: Normal and abnormal mechanics of the glenohumeral joint in the horizontal plane. *J Bone Joint Surg [Am]* 1988; 70:227.

Jupiter JB, Leffert RD: Non-union of the clavicle. Associated complications and surgical management. *J Bone Joint Surg [Am]* 1987; 69:753.

Kessel L, Watson M: The painful arc syndrome: Clinical classification as a guide to management. *J Bone Joint Surg [Br]* 1977; 59:166.

Kozin F, et al: The reflex sympathetic dystrophy syndrome: I. Clinical and histologic studies: Evidence for bilaterality, response to corticosteroids, and articular involvement. *Am J Med* 1976; 60:321.

Laskin RS, Schreiber S: Inferior subluxation of the humeral head: The drooping shoulder. *Radiology* 1971; 98:585.

McLaughlin HL: The "frozen" shoulder. *Clin Orthop* 1961; 20:126.

Moseley HF: *Ruptures of the Rotator Cuff.* Springfield, Ill, Charles C Thomas Publisher, 1952.

Neer CS: Anterior acromioplasty for the chronic impingement syndrome in the shoulder. *J Bone Joint Surg [Am]* 1972; 54:41.

Neer CS, Craig EV, Fukuda H: Cuff-tear arthropathy. *J Bone Joint Surg [Am]* 1983; 65:1232.

Parker RD, et al: Frozen shoulder. *Orthopedics* 1989; 12:869.

Parsons TA: The snapping scapula and subscapular exostosis. *J Bone Joint Surg [Br]* 1973; 55:345.

Percy EC, Birbragen D, Pitt MJ: Snapping scapula: A review of the literature and presentation of 14 patients. *Can J Surg* 1988; 31:248.

Quigley TB: The nonoperative treatment of symptomatic calcareous deposits in the shoulder. *Surg Clin North Am* 1963; 43:1495.

Rockwood CA, Odor JM: Spontaneous atraumatic anterior subluxation of the sternoclavicular joint. *J Bone Joint Surg [Am]* 1989; 71:1280.

Rowe CR, Zarins B, Ciullo JV: Recurrent anterior dislocation of the shoulder after surgical repair: Apparent causes of failure and treatment. *J Bone Joint Surg [Am]* 1984; 66:159.

Samelson RL, Prieto V: Dislocation arthropathy of the shoulder. *J Bone Joint Surg [Am]* 1983; 65:456.

Silferskiold JP, Straehley DJ, Jones WW: Roentgenographic evaluation of suspected shoulder dislocation: A prospective study comparing the axillary view and the scapular "Y" view. *Orthopedics* 1990; 13:63.

Spengler DW, Kirsh MM, Kaufer H: Orthopedic aspects and early diagnosis of superior sulcus tumor of lung (Pancoast). *J Bone Joint Surg [Am]* 1973; 55:1645.

Steinbrocher O: The painful shoulder, in Hollander JL, McCarty D Jr (eds): *Arthritis and Allied Conditions,* ed 8. Philadelphia, Lea & Febiger, 1972.

Taft TN, Wilson FC, Oglesby JW: Dislocation of the

acromioclavicular joint: An end-result study. *J Bone Joint Surg [Am]* 1987; 69:1045.

Tsairis P, Dyck PJ, Mulder DW: Natural history of brachial plexus neuropathy. *Arch Neurol* 1972; 27:109.

Watson M: Major ruptures of the rotator cuff: The results of surgical repairs in 89 patients. *J Bone Joint Surg [Br]* 1985; 67:618.

Young TB, Wallace WA: Conservative treatment of fractures and fracture-dislocations of the upper end of the humerus. *J Bone Joint Surg [Br]* 1985; 67:373.

CHAPTER 6

The Elbow

The elbow is a strong hinge joint that allows flexion and rotation of the forearm. It also provides the bony origin for most of the extrinsic muscles of the wrist and hand. It is frequently affected by inflammatory and traumatic conditions that seriously alter its function.

ANATOMY

The elbow joint is formed by the articulation between the humerus and the radius and ulna (Fig 6–1). The humerus widens distally to form the lateral and medial condyles. The capitellum of the lateral condyle articulates with the radial head, and the trochlea articulates with the ulna. The head of the radius also articulates with the lateral aspect of the ulna and is held in position by the orbicular ligament. Medial and lateral collateral ligaments provide additional stability.

Adjacent to each condyle are the epicondyles, which are the bony attachments for many forearm muscles. The flexor-pronator muscle group takes its origin from a common tendon that attaches to the medial epicondyle, and the extensor-supinator group arises in a similar manner from the lateral epicondyle. Posteriorly, the triceps attaches to the olecranon; anteriorly, the biceps and brachialis attach to the radius and ulna, respectively.

Three major nerves cross the elbow joint on their way into the forearm. The median nerve passes deep in the antecubital fossa medial to the biceps and brachialis, and the radial nerve passes lateral to them. The ulnar nerve reaches the forearm by coursing posteriorly in a groove between the medial epicondyle and the olecranon process, where it is easily palpated. It is also vulnerable to injury in this superficial location.

EXAMINATION

The tip of the olecranon process and the epicondyles form useful bony landmarks (Fig 6–2). When the elbow is fully extended and viewed from behind, these points form a straight, transverse line. With the elbow flexed, they form an isosceles triangle. Just distal to the lateral epi-

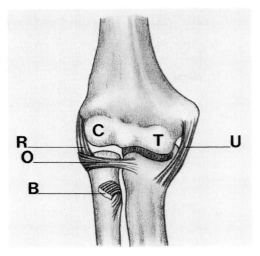

FIG 6-1.
Bony and ligamentous anatomy of the elbow: *R* = radial collateral ligament; *O* = orbicular ligament; *B* = biceps insertion; *U* = ulnar collateral ligament; *C* = capitellum; *T* = trochlea.

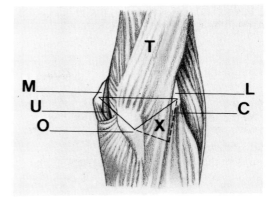

FIG 6-2.
The flexed elbow from behind: *T* = triceps; *M* = medial epicondyle; *U* = ulnar nerve; *L* = lateral epicondyle; *C* = common extensor tendon; *X* = the posterolateral triangle. The isosceles triangle between the epicondyles and the olecranon *(O)* is altered in most fractures and dislocations of the elbow except the supracondylar fracture, where all three points move together.

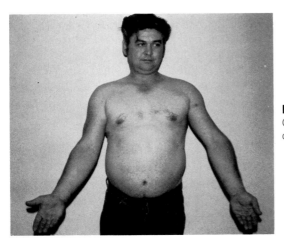

FIG 6-3.
Gunstock deformity (cubitus varus) of the left elbow with reversal of the carrying angle due to an old fracture with malunion.

condyle lies the radial head. These two points, along with the olecranon process, form another triangle on the posterolateral aspect of the joint. This triangle is occupied by the anconeus muscle. This area usually bulges when the joint is distended by fluid and is an excellent site for joint aspiration.

With the forearm in the supinated position, an angle is formed with the arm at the elbow joint. This is referred to as the "carrying angle" and normally measures 15 to 20 degrees (Fig 6-3). Alterations in this angle may occur following injury or infection, especially in the young, and may lead to cubitus valgus or varus.

ROENTGENOGRAPHIC ANATOMY

The roentgenographic features of the elbow are well visualized by standard anteroposterior and 90-degree flexion lateral views (Fig 6–4). Comparison views of the opposite elbow should be obtained whenever necessary.

TENNIS ELBOW

Tennis elbow, or epicondylitis, is one of a large group of musculoskeletal disorders commonly termed "overuse syndromes." It is an inflammatory condition characterized by pain at the origin of the flexor muscles at the medial epicondyle or the extensor muscles at the lateral epicondyle. The cause is unknown, but minor tears in the tendinous attachments of these muscles are often present. The disorder is common in those individuals whose activities require repeated use of the extensor or flexor mechanism of the forearm. The lateral side is more commonly involved.

Clinical Features

The onset is usually gradual. A dull ache appears over the affected epicondyle that is worsened with use of the involved muscles. Activities that require rotation and grasping, such as opening a jar, increase the pain. The pain often radiates into the forearm. Extension or flexion of the hand against resistance will reproduce the pain at the affected epicondyle. The point of maximum tenderness can usually be well localized by digital pressure applied to the epicondyle. The roentgenograms are usually normal.

Treatment

Treatment is similar to that for other "musculotendinous overuse syndromes." The most important aspect of treatment is rest, and this can frequently be obtained merely by avoiding the offending activity. The inflammation may be further decreased by the application of moist heat or ultrasound. Aspirin, eight to ten tablets per day, is given as necessary. Local infiltration of the affected area with 1 to 2 mL of a steroid/lidocaine mixture will often give permanent relief. The injection is placed in the area of maximum local tenderness and may be repeated at weekly intervals for 2 or 3 weeks. A special tennis elbow dressing may also be effective. If these modalities are not effective, the elbow and wrist should be

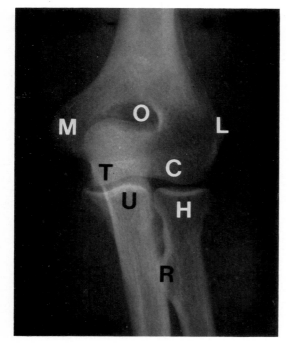

FIG 6–4.
Roentgenographic anatomy of the elbow: M = medial epicondyle; O = olecranon fossa; L = lateral epicondyle; T = trochlea; C = capitellum; U = coronoid process of the ulna; H = radial head; R = radial tuberosity. Regardless of the position of the elbow, the long axis of the radius always passes through the capitellum.

immobilized in a long arm cast. The cast is applied so that the wrist is immobilized in a position that maintains relaxation of the affected muscles. For the more common lateral epicondylitis, the cast is applied with the elbow flexed 90 degrees, the forearm supinated, and the wrist slightly dorsiflexed.

The disease is usually self-limited, but symptoms may persist for several months before full recovery occurs. Conservative treatment is effective in most cases. Surgery is reserved for resistant cases and usually consists of resection of the injured portion of the tendon and repair.

OSTEOCHONDRITIS DISSECANS

Osteochondritis dissecans is a condition in which a portion of subchondral bone undergoes avascular necrosis. This segment of bone, with its overlying articular cartilage, may partially or completely separate from the adjacent bone and even extrude into the joint to form a loose body. The disorder is most commonly seen in the knee joint, but a similar condition also occurs in the elbow, ankle, and hip joints. The cause is unknown, but it is probably traumatic in origin.

Clinical Features
In the elbow, the disorder is most common during adolescence, and males are usually affected. The onset of symptoms is gradual, and a history of trauma may be elicited. The patient will fre-

quently complain of a dull, aching pain that is often associated with stiffness. Occasionally, episodes of locking will occur if the fragment has become extruded into the joint. The physical findings consist of limitation of motion, local tenderness, and joint effusion. Roentgenographically, the capitellum is the most common site of involvement (Fig 6–5).

Treatment
The treatment in early cases consists of rest. This may be accomplished by the use of a sling or a cast. All throwing activities are discontinued. Surgery is indicated for removal of any loose bodies. The prognosis is usually good, although some residual stiffness may occur.

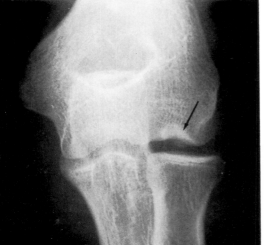

FIG 6–5.
Osteochondritis dissecans of the elbow. Sclerosis, rarefaction, and a small loose body are present (arrow).

PULLED ELBOW

Pulled elbow, or "nursemaid's elbow," is a term that is used to describe a disorder in which the head of the radius becomes subluxed beneath the orbicular ligament (Fig 6–6). This occurs as a result of longitudinal traction on the hand with the elbow extended and the forearm in a pronated position. A common situation in which this occurs is when a child is lifted up by the wrist or hand.

Clinical Features

The disorder is most common between the ages of 1 and 3 years and is rare after the age of 6. Clinically, an audible snap may be heard when the radial head subluxes. The arm is then held motionless at the side in slight flexion and pronation. The radial head is tender. Roentgenographic findings are usually normal.

Treatment

Reduction is easily accomplished by supinating and flexing the forearm while applying manual pressure over the radial head (Fig 6–7). A palpable click can be noted as reduction occurs, and the pain is immediately relieved. Reduction sometimes occurs in the radiology department when the technician places the forearm and the elbow in the flexed and supinated position in order to obtain a lateral view of the elbow. After reduction, a sling is worn for 5 to 7 days. Recurrences occasionally take place and are treated in a similar manner.

OLECRANON BURSITIS

The olecranon bursa overlies the olecranon process and is extremely vulnerable to direct trauma and repeated irritation. After an acute traumatic episode, a tender, painful swelling may develop over the tip of the olecranon (Fig 6–8). The bursa sac fills with blood or clear fluid. At this stage, aspiration of the fluid with application of a compression dressing and ice may prevent reformation of the fluid and recurrence. Many acute lesions will spontaneously subside, however.

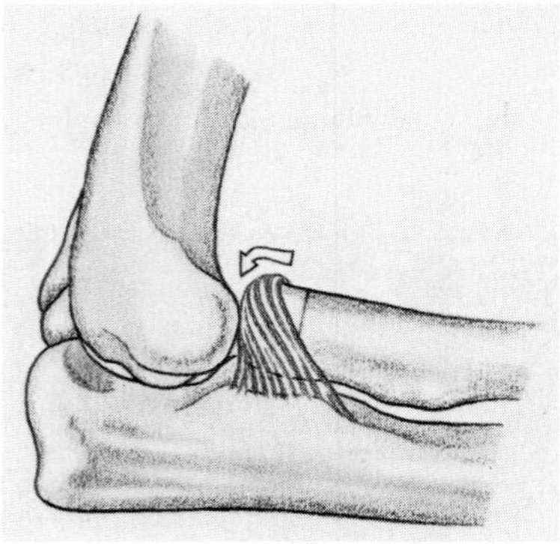

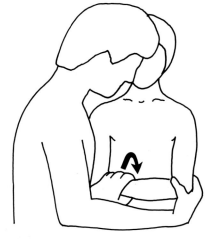

FIG 6–6.
The radial head is pulled beneath the orbicular ligament.

FIG 6–7.
Reduction of a "pulled elbow."

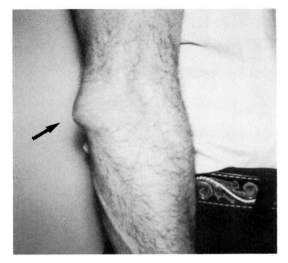

FIG 6–8.
Chronic olecranon bursitis *(arrow)*.

With repetitive trauma, a chronic inflammatory reaction occurs that results in the formation of a thickened, rubbery bursa. This bursa is usually not painful, in contrast to the swelling that occurs after an acute injury. Palpation may reveal multiple, small, hard nodules that feel like loose bodies. These usually are not chips of bone but instead represent villous thickenings of the bursa. Aspiration of the bursa may be attempted but will often fail at this stage. Incision is not recommended, for a chronic draining infection is often the end result. If the bursa is chronically painful, excision is recommended.

Occasionally, the bursa is the site of an acute infection that sometimes follows trauma. The treatment is the same as that for any other infection and consists of antibiotics, moist heat, and splinting, with incision and drainage when necessary.

DISTAL RUPTURE OF THE BICEPS TENDON

The distal end of the biceps tendon may rupture as the result of degenerative changes near its insertion into the radial tuberosity. The distal end of the biceps tendon undergoes the same attritional changes as those that occur in the long head at the shoulder. Sudden, forceful flexion of the elbow against resistance may then cause it to rupture at its insertion into the radius.

A painful snap is felt at the elbow and is followed by swelling and tenderness. Flexion of the elbow and supination of the forearm are weakened. The overlying deep fascia of the antecubital fossa may remain intact, thus preventing a significant loss of elbow flexion power. On flexion of the elbow, the belly of the biceps retracts, to produce a bulbous swelling in the upper arm similar to that seen with proximal rupture of the long head.

Surgical repair of the ruptured tendon is usually indicated if a significant amount of motor power is lost. If the strength is satisfactory, surgical repair then becomes elective.

DISLOCATION OF THE ELBOW

Dislocation of the elbow is a common injury and is usually posterior in direction (Fig 6–9). It is generally the result of a fall on the outstretched hand with the elbow extended. Examination will reveal obvious deformity that must be differentiated from a supracondylar fracture. Avulsion fractures of the medial epicondyle and fractures of the radial head occasionally occur that may require surgical intervention.

Reduction is performed as soon as possible. It can usually be accomplished by gentle, steady traction on the wrist with countertraction on the shoulder (Fig 6–10). A general anesthetic is usually unnecessary. Extension of the elbow to un-

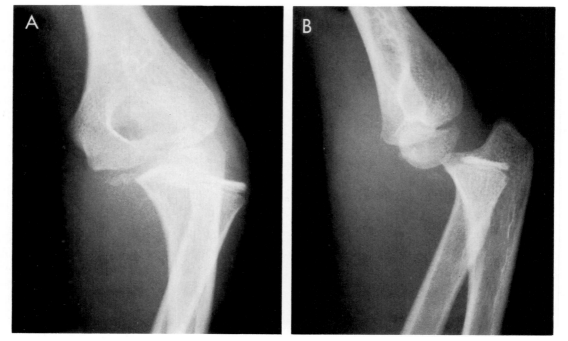

FIG 6–9.
Posterior dislocation of the elbow. It should be noted that a line drawn through the center of the radius no longer passes through the capitellum.

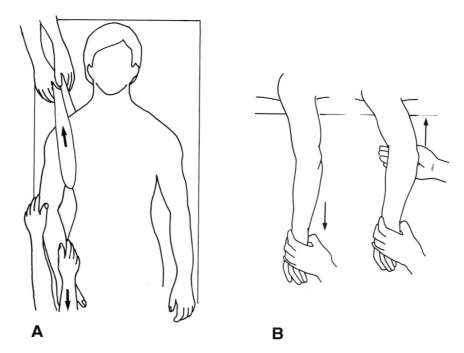

FIG 6–10.
A, reduction of an elbow dislocation by straight traction. **B,** Parvin's method. With the patient prone, gentle downward traction is applied to the wrist. A few minutes later, the arm is gently lifted upward, often reducing the dislocation.

lock the olecranon may be necessary. After reduction, the elbow is immobilized in a molded posterior plaster splint for 3 weeks in a position of 90 degrees of flexion to allow ligamentous and capsular healing. Gentle range-of-motion exercises are then instituted after removal of the splint. Temporary stiffness is common, and full recovery of elbow motion may take several months. Motion should never be forced. The patient should be allowed to progress as tolerated. Forced passive motion only encourages more swelling, which leads to more stiffness. Some residual restriction of motion is not uncommon, but it is usually of such a minor degree that it does not interfere with function.

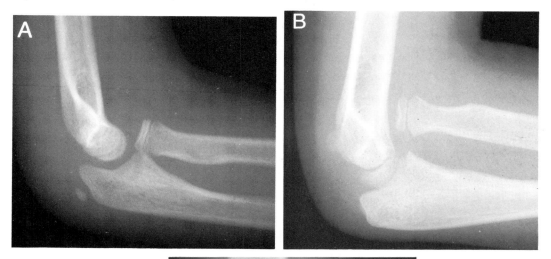

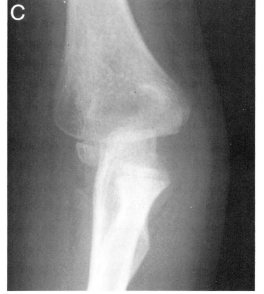

FIG 6–11.
Anterior radial head dislocation. **A,** lateral view showing subtle anterior dislocation. **B,** a more obvious dislocation. **C,** anteroposterior view.

DISLOCATION OF THE RADIAL HEAD IN CHILDREN

This is an uncommon disorder that is usually traumatic but may occasionally be congenital or developmental in nature. Most of the traumatic cases dislocate anteriorly (Fig 6–11). The mechanism of injury is usually a fall on the outstretched pronated arm, and the injury is frequently missed. Some cases may be associated with a "bent" ulna suggesting a Monteggia type of injury.

Congenital dislocations are usually posterior and are frequently bilateral. They may be associated with other congenital anomalies such as Ehlers-Danlos syndrome. *Developmental* dislocations are usually the result of cerebral palsy or neurologic injury and are commonly posterolateral. These two types of radial head dislocations usually have no pain and little functional impairment. No treatment is required.

Traumatic dislocations, however, need early reduction to prevent stiffness and pain. Old neglected dislocations may benefit from surgery.

Recognition is important. Remember, a line drawn through the long axis of the radius should always pass through the capitellum in any view.

FRACTURES OF THE ELBOW REGION

Fractures of the Head and Neck of the Radius

Fractures of the radial head and neck result from a fall on the outstretched hand with the elbow extended (Fig 6–12). All are characterized by tenderness over the radial head, local swelling, and pain on rotation or flexion of the forearm.

Undisplaced or minimally displaced fractures in adults and children are treated conservatively. If the swelling is extremely painful, the joint may be aspirated through the posterolateral triangle. A light posterior plaster splint and sling are applied with the elbow flexed 90 degrees. The splint is removed in 1 to 2 weeks, and early motion is encouraged. The sling is continued for another 1 to 2 weeks.

Displaced or comminuted fractures in adults are usually treated by early (24 to 48 hours) excision of the entire radial head. Otherwise, permanent restriction of joint motion and traumatic arthritis may result. Early removal is especially indicated in grossly comminuted and displaced fractures because the fracture fragments may act as a nidus for soft tissue calcification in the anterior elbow region, and myositis ossificans may result (Fig 6–13).

Children's fractures with less than 15 to 30 de-

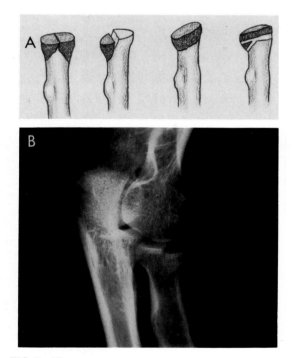

FIG 6–12.
A, various types of fractures of the radial head or neck that may be treated nonsurgically. **B,** typical head fracture in which full, pain-free motion was restored following conservative treatment.

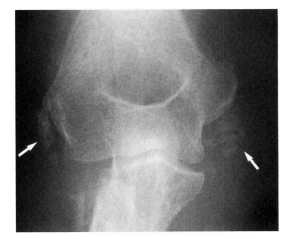

FIG 6–13.
Roentgenogram of the elbow following a comminuted radial head fracture shows multiple areas of ossification (myositis ossificans) in the adjacent soft tissue *(arrows)*.

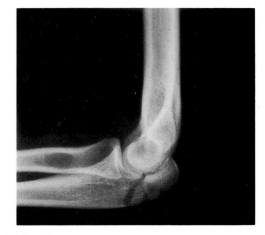

FIG 6–14.
Fracture of the olecranon.

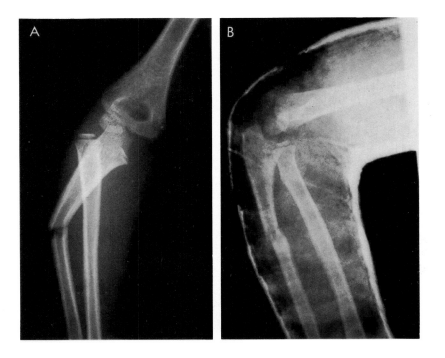

FIG 6–15.
A, Monteggia's fracture-dislocation of the elbow. Note the angulation of the ulna. Also, a line drawn through the shaft of the radius no longer passes through the capitellum. **B,** after reduction it is always important to obtain a roentgenogram of the joint above and below any fracture.

grees of angulation are treated as undisplaced fractures. Displaced fractures, or fractures that are angulated greater than 15 to 30 degrees, are treated by closed or open reduction. The radial head is never removed in the growing child, however, because removal of the epiphysis will result in unequal growth of the forearm bones.

Regardless of the method of treatment, some loss of extension of the elbow is not uncommon. However, little functional impairment usually results.

Fractures of the Olecranon

Fractures of the olecranon usually result from falls on the tip of the elbow (Fig 6–14). They are either displaced or undisplaced. The extensor mechanism is intact in undisplaced fractures, and further displacement is unlikely. The undisplaced fracture is easily treated with a molded posterior plaster splint for 2 weeks, followed by a sling and gradually increasing range-of-motion exercises.

Displaced fractures usually require open reduction and internal fixation in order to restore the bony alignment and repair the triceps insertion.

Monteggia's Fracture-Dislocation

This injury consists of a fracture of the proximal third of the ulna and a dislocation of the radial head (Fig 6–15). Closed treatment may suffice in the child, but open reduction with internal fixation is frequently necessary in the adult.

Occasionally, especially in children, the fracture of the ulna may not be obvious, or the ulna fracture may be greenstick in nature and the radial head dislocation overlooked. **Remember:** always obtain roentgenograms of the joint *above* and *below* any fracture.

BIBLIOGRAPHY

Ackerman G, Jupiter JB: Nonunion of fractures of the distal end of the humerus. *J Bone Joint Surg [Am]* 1988; 70:57.

Adams JE: Bone injuries in very young athletes. *Clin Orthop* 1968; 58:129.

Baker BE, Bierwagen D: Rupture of the distal tendon of the biceps brachii: Operative versus non-operative treatment. *J Bone Joint Surg [Am]* 1985; 67:414.

Blount WP: *Fractures in Children.* Baltimore, Williams & Wilkins, 1955.

Boyd HB, McLeod AC: Tennis elbow. *J Bone Joint Surg [Am]* 1973; 55:1183.

Broberg MA, Morrey BF: Results of delayed excision of the radial head after fracture. *J Bone Joint Surg [Am]* 1986; 68:669.

Dobbie RP: Avulsion of the lower biceps brachii tendon: Analysis of 51 previously unreported cases. *Am J Surg* 1941; 51:662.

Garden RS: Tennis elbow. *J Bone Joint Surg [Br]* 1961; 43:100.

Goldberg I, et al: Late results of excision of the radial head for an isolated closed fracture. *J Bone Joint Surg [Am]* 1986; 68:675.

Hudson DA, DeBeer JD: Isolated traumatic dislocation of the radial head in children. *J Bone Joint Surg [Br]* 1986; 68:378.

Letts M, Locht R, Wiens J: Monteggia fracture-dislocations in children. *J Bone Joint Surg [Br]* 1985; 67:724.

Lloyd-Roberts GC, Bucknell TM: Anterior dislocation of the radial head in children. Aetiology, natural history and management. *J Bone Joint Surg [Br]* 1977; 59:402.

March HC: Osteochondritis of the capitellum (Panner's disease). *AJR* 1944; 51:682.

Mehlhoff TL, et al: Simple dislocation of the elbow in the adult: Results after closed treatment. *J Bone Joint Surg [Br]* 1988; 70:244.

O'Donoghue DH: *Treatment of Injuries to Athletes,* ed 3. Philadelphia, WB Saunders Co, 1976.

Pirone AM, Krajbich JE: Management of displaced extension-type supracondylar fractures of the humerus in children. *J Bone Joint Surg [Am]* 1988; 70:641.

Reckling FW: Unstable fracture-dislocations of the forearm (Monteggia and Galeazzi lesions). *J Bone Joint Surg [Am]* 1982; 64:857.

Roberts N, Hughes R: Osteochondritis dissecans of the elbow joint. *J Bone Joint Surg [Br]* 1950; 32:348.

Salter RB: *Disorders and Injuries of the Musculo skeletal System.* Baltimore, Williams & Wilkins, 1970.

Tullos HS, King JW: Lesions of the pitching arm in adolescents. *JAMA* 1972; 220:264.

Woodward A, Bianco A: Osteochondritis dissecans of elbow, ankle, and hip: A comparison survey. *Clin Orthop* 1980; 148:245.

CHAPTER 7

The Forearm, Wrist, and Hand

The importance of the wrist and hand is evidenced by the fact that the rest of the upper extremity functions primarily to place the hand in a position where it can operate most effectively. Treatment of the wide variety of disorders that occur in the hand requires an understanding of the complicated anatomy and functional physiology.

ANATOMY

Skin, Fascia, and Nail

The skin on the dorsum of the hand is loose and overlies a subcutaneous space through which pass many veins and most of the lymph vessels of the hand. This abundance of lymph vessels accounts for the dorsal lymphedema that commonly occurs secondary to infection in the palm or fingers.

The palmar skin, however, is firmly attached to the underlying palmar aponeurosis, which is continuous with the palmaris longus tendon (Fig 7–1). This thick fascia sends extensions into the fingers and serves to protect the important deeper structures of the hand. It may become nodular and shortened in Dupuytren's contracture.

The nail of each finger originates close to the distal interphalangeal joint and is surrounded on the sides and at the base by thick folds of tissue, the paronychium, and the eponychium, respectively. It covers a rich capillary bed that may be tested to determine the circulation of the extremity. The nail should be retained, whenever possible, in fingertip injuries.

Blood Supply

Most of the blood supply to the hand enters on the palmar aspect through the radial and ulnar arteries. Each of these arteries terminates in a superficial and a deep branch. The superficial branches join to form the superficial palmar arch, which is located at the level of the base of the first web space. The deep palmar arch, which is located 1 cm proximal to the superficial arch, is formed by the junction of the deep branches. The arches are so named because of their position relative to the flexor tendons. Many branches and anastomoses from these arches provide the blood supply to the fingers and hand. In the fingers, digital vessels lie just ventral to the flexor skin crease of the interphalangeal joints (Fig 7–2).

Muscles of the Hand

Motions of the wrist and fingers are controlled by groups of muscles that are classified as either intrinsic or extrinsic. Intrinsic muscles arise within the hand and are responsible for the deli-

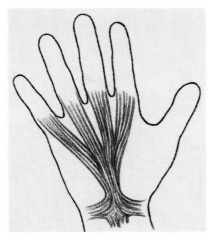

FIG 7-1.
The palmar aponeurosis.

cate movements of the fingers. Extrinsic muscles are those that take origin within the forearm.

Extrinsic Muscles

Motion at the wrist is accomplished by the various wrist flexors and extensors. In addition to providing wrist motion, these muscles stabilize the wrist in slight dorsiflexion, a position that allows maximum function of the extrinsic flexors.

Nine finger flexors and the median nerve pass

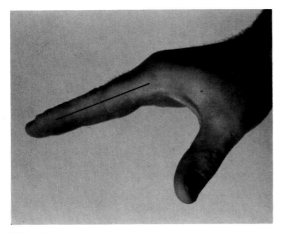

FIG 7-2.
The neurovascular bundle is situated just ventral to the flexor skin crease.

into the hand through the carpal tunnel beneath the transverse carpal ligament (Fig 7-3). Five deep flexors pass to the distal phalanx of each finger and thumb, and four superficial flexors pass to the middle phalanx of each finger. Each of these finger flexors can be tested individually (Fig 7-4).

The finger flexors pass beneath a series of ligaments between the distal palmar crease and the distal interphalangeal joint. These annular ligaments, or "pulleys," prevent the tendon from bowstringing. Tendon repair in this area called "no-man's-land" is often unrewarding because of adhesions that form between the lacerated tendon ends and these ligaments.

The extensor tendons pass dorsally over each finger and thumb and insert into the phalanges. They extend the proximal phalanges and assist the intrinsic muscles in interphalangeal joint extension. The thumb extensors are easily palpated at the anatomic "snuffbox."

Intrinsic Muscles

The thenar (median nerve) and hypothenar (ulnar) muscles act primarily to position the thumb and small finger for the purpose of pinching. The

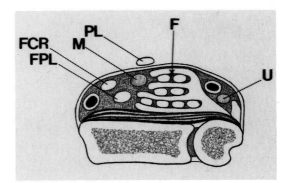

FIG 7-3.
Structures proximal to the wrist joint. The ulnar nerve *(U)* and artery continue distally through the ulnar tunnel of Guyon. The nine finger flexors *(F, FPL)* and median nerve *(M)* pass through the carpal tunnel beneath the transverse carpal ligament. Note the superficial location of the median nerve and the sublimis to the long and ring fingers. *FCR* = flexor carpi radialis; *PL* = palmaris longus.

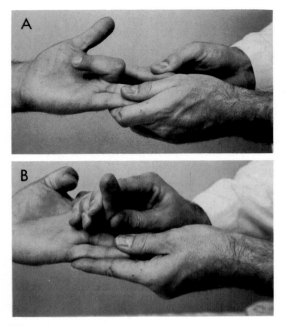

FIG 7–4.
A, the sublimis is functioning if the proximal interphalangeal joint can be flexed while the adjacent fingers are held extended. **B,** the profundus is functioning if the distal interphalangeal joint can be flexed while the rest of the finger is stabilized.

rest of the intrinsic muscles (interossei and lumbricals) insert into the proximal phalanges and extensor hoods and assist in flexion of the metacarpophalangeal joints and extension of the interphalangeal joints.

Nerve Supply

The ulnar nerve provides the motor supply to all of the intrinsic muscles of the hand except the two radial lumbricals and the thenar muscles. It also provides sensation to the entire ulnar 1½ fingers (Fig 7–5). Its function is easily evaluated by testing finger abduction and palpating the belly of the first dorsal interosseous muscle (Fig 7–6).

The thenar muscles and the two radial lumbricals are supplied by the median nerve, which also supplies sensation to the palmar aspect of the radical 3½ fingers as well as the tips of these

FIG 7–5.
Dorsal **(A)** and palmar **(B)** sensation of the hand: *R* = radial nerve; *U* = ulnar nerve; *M* = median nerve.

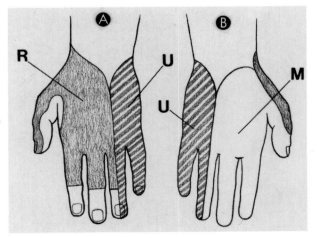

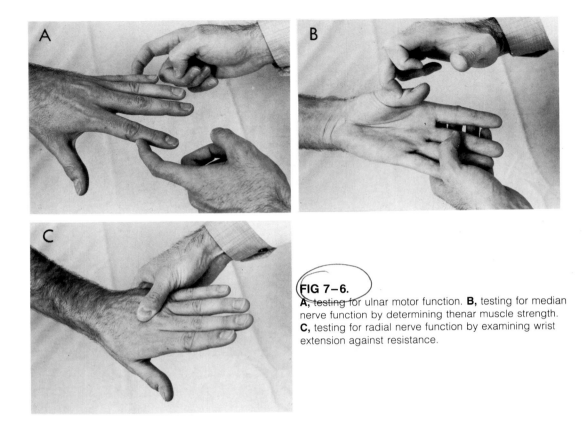

FIG 7–6.
A, testing for ulnar motor function. **B,** testing for median nerve function by determining thenar muscle strength. **C,** testing for radial nerve function by examining wrist extension against resistance.

fingers on their dorsal aspect. Its function is evaluated by testing opposition of the thumb to each finger and observing the thenar muscles for contractions.

The radial nerve has no intrinsic muscle supply but does provide sensation to the dorsum of the hand over the radial 3½ fingers. It supplies motor function to the extrinsic wrist and finger extensors.

Bones and Ligaments

The carpal bones contribute to the mobility of the hand by allowing flexion, extension, and radial and ulnar deviation to occur. The carpal bones are eight in number and are arranged into a distal and proximal row. Strong ligaments bind them together, one of the strongest being the transverse carpal ligament. At the metacarpophalangeal and interphalangeal joints, strong collateral ligaments provide mediolateral stability.

ROENTGENOGRAPHIC ANATOMY

The 27 bones of the hand are visualized by anteroposterior, lateral, and oblique roentgenograms when appropriate (Fig 7–7).

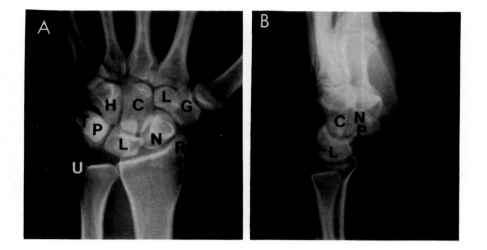

FIG 7–7.
Roentgenographic anatomy of the wrist: *H* = hamate with its prominent hook; *C* = capitate; *L* = lesser multangular (trapezoid); *G* = greater multangular (trapezium); *T* = triquetrum; *P* = pisiform; *L* = lunate; *N* = navicular (scaphoid); *U* = ulnar styloid; *R* = radial styloid. On the lateral view, note that the capitate, lunate, and distal portion of the radius are in a direct line.

CARPAL TUNNEL SYNDROME

Carpal tunnel syndrome, or compression of the median nerve at the wrist, is a common entity. It usually occurs as the result of compression of the nerve between the transverse carpal ligament and the flexor tendons with their enlarged synovium. Often, no cause is found, but the disorder is seen in association with hypothyroidism, rheumatoid and gouty arthritis, and aberrant or anomalous muscles in the wrist. A deficiency in vitamin B_6 has even been postulated. It is sometimes seen following fractures of the wrist and is not uncommon in the third trimester of pregnancy. (**Note:** When it does occur late in pregnancy, the symptoms tend to subside after delivery. Thus, treatment is strictly symptomatic, and surgery is generally not recommended in these cases.) The syndrome is bilateral in up to 50% of cases and may occur in the workplace as a result of repetitive hand activities. Sometimes, a combination of neck and hand pain occurs, especially in patients who suffer from degenerative cervical disc disease. This is termed the "double-crush syndrome" lesion and results from nerve com-

pression at two separate levels, the neck and the wrist. The suggestion is that proximal compression may decrease the ability of the nerve to tolerate a second, more distal compression.

Clinical Features
The onset is usually spontaneous, with gradually increasing night pain being common. The night pain is frequently the reason the patient seeks medical attention and occurs because of a slight increase in swelling at the wrist with inactivity or perhaps as a result of wrist flexion at night. The pain may radiate into the forearm, arm, and even the shoulder. Numbness and tingling occur along the median nerve distribution, but the sensory impairment rarely involves all 3½ fingers supplied by the median nerve. Often, only the long and index fingers are involved. A sense of weakness and clumsiness in the use of the hand is common. All of these symptoms may be precipitated by various manual activities such as typing or painting. They frequently subside after shaking and moving the hand or allowing it to hang

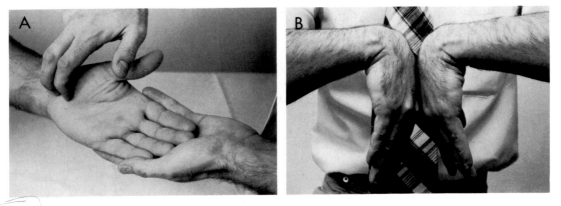

FIG 7–8.
A, Tinel's sign. Percussion of the median nerve at the carpal tunnel may reproduce the pain and tingling along the median nerve distribution. **B,** Phalen's test. The symptoms may also be reproduced after 1 minute of acute wrist flexion against resistance.

downward. The patient often describes "poor circulation" and "stiffness," but the hand is usually warm, and the motion is full. These symptoms are usually due to the numbness.

Physical examination may reveal some sensory disturbance along the median nerve. Tinel's sign and Phalen's test are often positive (Fig 7–8). Atrophy of the thenar muscles is seen in cases of long-standing duration.

Roentgenograms of the wrist are helpful in ruling out local bony abnormality. Nerve conduction studies may be of benefit but are frequently unnecessary in classic cases. Delayed electrical conduction across the wrist is usually present. Electromyography is generally unnecessary.

Treatment

1. Eliminate the cause. If repetitive trauma is a factor, cessation of that trauma may serve to alleviate the symptoms in some cases. Patients should avoid the extremes of wrist positions.

2. Anti-inflammatory medication for any tenosynovitis.

3. Splinting. Occupational ("job-specific") splints or braces or night splints may be helpful (Fig 7–9).

4. Injection of the carpal canal (avoiding the median nerve!) will occasionally provide some

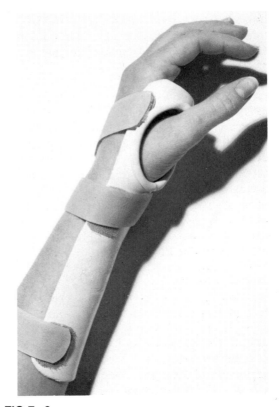

FIG 7–9.
Polypropylene occupational wrist splint.

relief. It can be harmful if improperly done. Inject on the ulnar side of the palmaris longus tendon.

Prognosis

Resolution of symptoms occurs fairly commonly with medical management. If symptoms warrant or motor weakness is developing, surgical re-lease of the transverse carpal ligament is indicated. This is usually followed by prompt and permanent relief of pain. Improvement of sensory and motor function may take several weeks or months, with motor function returning last. No disability results from sectioning the transverse ligament, and the surgical results are uniformly good.

ULNAR TUNNEL SYNDROME

Pain along the ulnar border of the hand secondary to compression of the ulnar nerve in its "tunnel" at the wrist is much less common than median nerve compression. It may result from pressure on the nerve by soft-tissue tumors, ganglia, constricting bands or muscles, or thrombosis of the ulnar artery. The symptoms and signs are similar to those found with carpal tunnel syndrome except that they are ulnar nerve in distribution. They are also similar to cubital tunnel syndrome except that the forearm is not affected and sensation to the dorsum of the hand and dorsal ulnar 1½ fingers is intact because the dorsal sensory branch of the ulnar nerve passes to the back of the hand proximal to the ulnar tunnel at the wrist.

The treatment is the same as that for carpal tunnel syndrome, and surgical release of the ulnar tunnel is usually necessary.

GANGLION

The ganglion cyst is the most common soft-tissue mass in the hand. It is always found adjacent to a joint or tendon sheath and may occur in any area of the body. The cause is unknown, but the cyst contains a mucinous material and usually has a stalk that can be traced to a tendon sheath or joint. Ganglion cysts are occasionally seen in children but frequently subside spontaneously in this age group in 2 to 3 years.

Clinical Features

A history of trauma is often elicited. Local pain and a feeling of weakness may be experienced by the patient. The mass may change in size, and this change is usually related to the level of activity of the patient. Ganglia are most common on the dorsum of the wrist. They are more prominent with the wrist flexed and are usually freely movable (Fig 7–10).

An "occult" ganglion may be the source of local dorsal wrist pain. Clinically, they are difficult to detect because they are deep to the extensor tendons. Special roentgenographic studies may be needed to determine its presence.

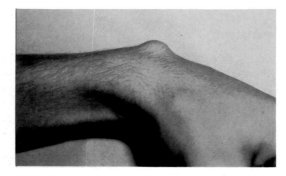

FIG 7–10.
Ganglion cyst.

Treatment

A cure may be effected by aspirating or puncturing the cyst in multiple areas and injecting it with a steroid compound. A compression dressing is then applied for 48 to 72 hours.

If symptoms persist, excision of the cyst may be indicated, although most patients tolerate the appearance and occasional minor discomfort.

The surgical procedure involves total removal of the cyst, its stalk, and a small portion of the adjacent joint capsule or tendon sheath. Methylene blue injected into the cyst may help localize the stalk. Recurrences are not uncommon, but the rate should be under 5% if the cyst is adequately removed.

DEGENERATIVE ARTHRITIS

Although osteoarthritis of the wrist and hand is much less common than in the lower extremities, it is sometimes more disabling. The most common area of involvement is the trapeziometacarpal or "base joint" of the thumb (Fig 7–11). Involvement at the base joint of the thumb is particularly bothersome because of the tremendous mobility required by this joint in daily use. Many other areas may also be affected, especially following fractures. When the distal interphalangeal (DIP) joints become involved with arthritis, persistent nodular swellings called *Heberden's nodes* may develop. Similar lesions at the proximal interphalangeal (PIP) joints are termed *Bouchard's nodes*. Occasionally, *mucous cysts* also develop at these interphalangeal (IP) joints.

Treatment

Treatment is similar to arthritis elsewhere. Antiinflammatory medication, intermittent splinting, moist heat, and occasional local cortisone injections are usually successful in temporarily relieving symptoms. Arthroplasty and arthrodesis are occasionally necessary.

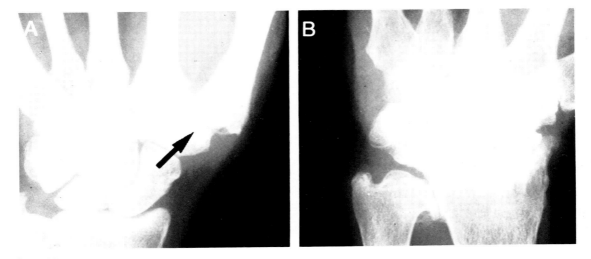

FIG 7–11.
A, osteoarthritis *(arrow)* of the carpometacarpal joint (CMJ) of the thumb. **B,** generalized osteoarthritis of the wrist.

DUPUYTREN'S CONTRACTURE

Dupuytren's contracture is a disease of the palmar fascia in which progressive contractures of the fascia occur and lead to a flexion deformity of the distal portion of the palm and fingers. The cause is unknown, but it is often hereditary and bilateral. It is more common in males and may be associated with fibrous contractures elsewhere in the body, especially in the plantar fascia of the foot. Pathologically, the contracture consists of proliferating vascular fibrous tissue that later develops into mature collagen.

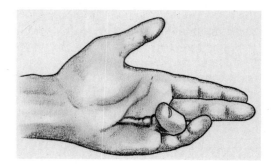

FIG 7–12.
Dupuytren's contracture. A flexion deformity of the finger is present, with nodular thickening of the fascia to the ring finger.

Clinical Features

The disorder is asymptomatic. Deformity and interference with the use of the hand by the flexed, contracted fingers are the most common complaints. The process usually begins on the ulnar side of the hand, often starting at the ring finger. An isolated nodule may appear in this area that eventually hardens and disappears. The overlying skin becomes adherent to the fascia, and a strong fibrous cord develops that extends into the finger (Fig 7–12). In the later stages of the disorder, the cord begins to contract and pull the finger into flexion. Multiple fingers may be affected.

Treatment

The treatment is often surgical. Fasciectomy is indicated as soon as joint contracture occurs. If performed early, complete restoration of extension can be anticipated. Nodules without contracture usually require no treatment.

STENOSING TENOSYNOVITIS

Tenosynovitis is a common condition that results from repetitive overuse or direct trauma. The resultant inflammation and irritation hinder the normal gliding motion of the tendon. Several distinct syndromes can be described, depending on the site of involvement. Many of them occur in the hand and some are associated with rheumatoid arthritis. They are common in the workplace.

de Quervain's Disease

Tenosynovitis frequently occurs in the first dorsal extensor compartment of the wrist (Fig 7–13). The extensor pollicis brevis and abductor pollicis longus occupy this compartment and are involved where they cross over the radial styloid.

Clinical Features

Pain and tenderness are usually present at the first dorsal compartment, and crepitus with motion of the tendon may be noted. The pain may radiate up the forearm and down into the thumb. Active and passive motion of the thumb aggravates the pain, and local thickening of the tendon sheath is frequently present. Characteristically, pain is reproduced by passive stretching of the affected thumb tendons (Finkelstein's test).

Treatment

Treatment in mild cases includes salicylates, immobilization, avoidance of the offending activity, and steroid injections into the tendon sheath. Moist heat is applied as necessary.

The symptoms usually subside with conserva-

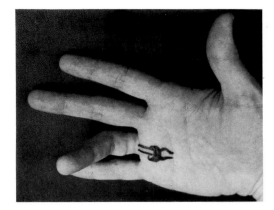

FIG 7-14.
Trigger finger. As the finger is extended, the nodular thickening of the tendon prohibits smooth passage of the tendon beneath the annular ligament. The finger may even lock in slight flexion.

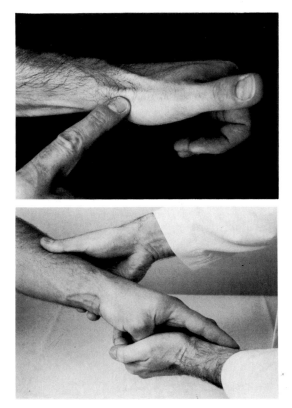
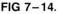

FIG 7-13.
Top, the first dorsal extensor compartment. *Bottom,* Finkelstein's test. Pain is reproduced in the first dorsal compartment by passively flexing the thumb and adducting the wrist.

tive treatment, but if they persist, surgical release of the tendon sheath is indicated.

Trigger Finger

If swelling of the flexor tendon and sheath occur, passage of the tendon through the constricted sheath may be difficult (Fig 7-14). This may result in snapping or "triggering" of the affected finger at the metacarpophalangeal joint as the swollen, nodular tendon passes through the constricted sheath. The symptoms are frequently worse after rest and improve with active use of the finger. The triggering effect itself is seen distal to the affected area, and the finger may even lock completely. A congenital form is occasionally seen in the thumb of children. Examination usually reveals tenderness, swelling, and a firm mass at the proximal flexor pulley.

The treatment is the same as that for de Quervain's disease. Surgical release is frequently necessary, but many cases, especially those that occur in children, recover spontaneously.

Extensor Carpi Radialis Tenosynovitis

Pain and tenderness affecting the radial wrist extensors are occasionally seen in heavy laborers. The symptoms, signs, and treatment are similar to those in de Quervain's disease.

REPETITIVE MOTION SYNDROME

This is one of several terms given to a controversial and increasingly common condition in which pain develops in the forearm and hand in the course of normal work activities in the workplace. Among other names used are cumulative trauma disorder and repetitive strain injury. A similar chronic pain syndrome may be seen in the neck and shoulder area as well as the lower part of the back. The disorder has been the subject of much media attention and has even set labor against management in many large industries. It has also been the source of a great deal of litigation, mainly directed at workers' compensation carriers.

Some of the reasons why it is so controversial are the following: (1) it is not known whether the condition is really an "injury" and is therefore compensable under law; (2) it is not known whether the syndrome is simply discomfort or whether any actual harm or damage ever results; (3) frequently, there is an absence or paucity of objective physical findings to support any clear working diagnosis or explanation for the pain; and (4) there is considerable controversy surrounding a number of epidemiologic studies based on data gathered from the workplace.

Clinical Features

Typically, pain in the forearms following the activity occurs. The pain may not even be improved by rest or restricted activities. The syndrome sometimes presents with symptoms consistent with one or more disorders known to cause upper extremity pain. Thus, some patients may present with symptoms compatible with tenosynovitis while others may suggest occupational cramps, reflex sympathetic dystrophy, thoracic outlet syndrome, carpal tunnel syndrome, or even a combination of several disorders. Frequently, the symptoms are vague. The patient often lacks specific objective physical findings, with only diffuse soft-tissue tenderness being present. Occasionally, however, there may be mild generalized hand swelling and tenderness of the median nerve. Electrical studies may even be abnormal in some patients without any symptoms suggestive of nerve compression. This causes difficulty in arriving at a specific diagnosis (and is misleading if surgery is being contemplated).

Treatment

The usual remedies are tried first: moist heat, splints, rest, and anti-inflammatory medication. The splint should keep the wrist straight, not flexed or cocked, and the patient should avoid extremes of wrist position. If possible, task modification, frequent breaks, and shortening the exposure time improves the situation, although this is not always possible in most job situations. Occasionally, surgery such as carpal tunnel release is indicated if the symptoms are clear-cut, but these procedures sometimes fail to completely resolve the patient's symptoms in this setting in spite of positive nerve conduction studies.

Prognosis

Occasionally, some permanent "injury" does occur as a result of repetitive motion, but it is not common. There is little doubt that discomfort does occur, however. Many patients continue with symptoms in spite of job changes, with pain occurring even with slight domestic tasks. These patients can usually be allowed to work but will frequently experience discomfort with any light job. Unfortunately, very few jobs are available that do not require upper extremity use to at least some degree. Some patients may even have to completely change occupations.

ULNAR NERVE PARALYSIS (CUBITAL TUNNEL SYNDROME)

Paralysis of the ulnar nerve may occur from several causes, but the most common is chronic trauma to the nerve where it passes behind the elbow. The nerve is most superficial at this location and is easily subjected to external pressure. A cubitus valgus deformity at the elbow secondary to a growth plate fracture or infection may also cause paralysis by progressive stretching of the nerve in its groove behind the elbow (Fig 7–15). The nerve may also sublux in and out of its groove, thereby giving rise to symptoms.

Clinical Features

Minimal pressure against the elbow may lead to paresthesias and numbness along the distribution of the ulnar nerve in the forearm and hand (Table 7–1). In contrast to ulnar tunnel syndrome, symptoms are also present on the dorsum of the hand. More severe involvement leads to progressive forearm, hypothenar, and intrinsic motor weakness and atrophy. Nerve conduction studies usually reveal delayed conduction at the elbow.

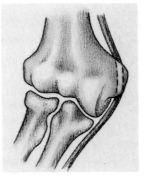

FIG 7–15.
Valgus deformity of the elbow that may stretch the ulnar nerve and lead to paralysis.

TABLE 7–1.

Differential Diagnosis of Common Causes of Forearm and Hand Pain*

Disorder	Findings Present	Findings Absent
Carpal tunnel syndrome	Painful paresthesias along portions of median nerve (i.e., palm side of hand). Index and long often only fingers involved. May have night pain in long-standing cases. Pain may radiate as high as shoulder. Tinel's sign may be positive at wrist	Pain not worsened by resisted motion or stretching. No symptoms on dorsum of hand. Full range of motion
Tenosynovitis	Pain and tenderness usually well localized to site of involvement. Pain may be reproduced by passive stretch or resistance against movement of affected tendon. May be local swelling	No paresthesias. Full range of motion. No night pain
Tennis elbow (most common lateral)	Pain may radiate from elbow to forearm and hand. Localized tenderness at epicondyle. Pain aggravated by resisted dorsiflexion of wrist (if lateral) Pain with gripping activities	Full range of motion, no paresthesias or night pain
Osteoarthritis	Local tenderness, sometimes with swelling of affected joint. Pain with motion. Decreased motion	No paresthesias, Tinel's sign negative
Cubital tunnel syndrome	Painful paresthesias along ulnar nerve distribution in forearm and hand. Tinel's sign may be positive behind medial epicondyle	Full range of motion. Pain not worsened by resisted motion. No night pain

*****NOTES:** Treatment and workup.
  1. NSAID, moist heat, splint, and modification of activities as indicated for 2 to 4 weeks.
  2. Roentgenogram, inject (if appropriate), change NSAID for 2 to 4 weeks.
  3. Nerve conduction studies, referral as indicated

Treatment

Protecting the nerve from pressure may improve the symptoms. Otherwise, the treatment is usually surgical. The ulnar nerve is transferred anterior to the medial epicondyle and any constricting bands are released. The pain is usually relieved immediately, but sensory recovery is often delayed, and motor function may not be completely restored. It is important, therefore, that all compression neuropathies undergo definitive treatment before significant motor weakness becomes manifested.

KIENBÖCK'S DISEASE

Avascular necrosis of the carpal lunate bone is an uncommon disorder that usually follows an injury. The cause is unknown, but the condition is considered to represent a circulatory disturbance to the bone. A similar involvement of the navicular is termed *Preiser's disease*.

Clinical Features

A history is frequently obtained of a single major injury. Multiple minor injuries such as those that occur with certain manual occupations may also lead to symptoms. Chronic pain, tenderness, swelling, and restriction of wrist motion (especially dorsiflexion) are common. The pain may be aggravated by passive dorsiflexion of the long finger in Kienböck's disease or the index finger in Preiser's disease. The initial roentgenogram is usually normal, but eventually the affected bone becomes abnormally dense and white (Fig 7–16). Later, fragmentation and collapse occur. The end result is frequently degenerative arthritis.

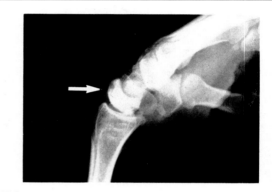

FIG 7–16.
Kienböck's disease. The lunate is dense and sclerotic.

Treatment

In the early stages before collapse has occurred, intermittent plaster immobilization for several months may permit reconstitution of the normal bony architecture. The cast is removed on a daily basis for range-of-motion exercises. In the later stages, surgical excision of the affected bone or arthrodesis of the wrist may be necessary.

SOFT-TISSUE INJURIES

Fingertip Injuries

A variety of fingertip injuries are encountered in daily practice. By definition, these are injuries that occur distal to the distal interphalangeal joint. Bone, skin, and nail may all be involved in varying degrees. Examination and treatment of most of these injuries may be performed with the patient under a metacarpal block using 1% lidocaine anesthesia. The anesthesia is instilled into the web space rather than the digit to prevent pressure on the digital vessels (Fig 7–17). Epinephrine should not be used. A small Penrose drain applied to the base of the finger makes a satisfactory tourniquet. Some general principles in the treatment of these injuries should be followed.

1. Proper healing occurs only in a clean wound. Gentle cleansing and thorough debridement are mandatory.

2. The nail should be retained. It protects the

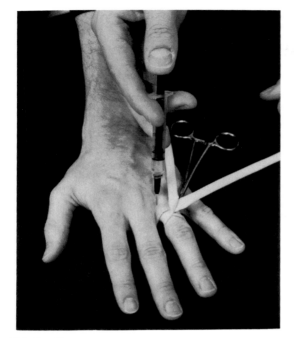

FIG 7–17.
Metacarpal block. The anesthesia should be instilled into the web space. (The tourniquet is added later when the block becomes effective.)

nail bed, acts as a splint for bone and soft tissue, and prevents excessive dorsal scar formation. The partially avulsed nail should be restored to its normal position and held in place with one or two sutures through the nail into the adjacent soft tissue.

3. Repair the nail bed whenever possible. One should use 6-0 chromic or other absorbable suture. Sometimes, this requires elevation or even removal of the nail. Following repair, the nail is replaced and attached. Failure to repair the bed can result in scarring and future nail deformity.

4. Working surfaces should be replaced with as near-normal skin as possible.

5. Preserve length, especially the radial three digits (thumb, index, and long fingers).

The treatment of all fingertip injuries is directed toward coverage of the deeper tissue. This may be accomplished by simple closure, free

grafts, or flaps. *Major* wounds should not be allowed to heal by the "open" treatment method without closure or coverage. Epithelialization of the wound will eventually occur but may take up to 12 weeks, and the resultant skin coverage is often thin and tender and breaks down easily.

Simple Closure

Simple closure is effective when skin loss is minimal and sufficient looseness of the surrounding skin and soft tissue is present to permit suturing of the wound without undue tension. A small portion of the distal phalanx may be removed with a rongeur. The scar line should be kept on the dorsal aspect if possible in order to prevent a tender scar from being present on the volar aspect of the finger. Never trim "dog ears." They will usually disappear with time, and trimming them may compromise healing.

Epithelialization

Many *minor* soft-tissue amputations to the pulp without bone loss that are less than 1 cm^2 in size can be treated by thorough cleansing, debridement, and healing by secondary intention. Dressings are changed regularly, and in 2 to 3 weeks, epithelialization is usually complete.

Free Grafts

Free grafts are usually split thickness or full thickness in nature. The thinner grafts tend to "take" better than do thicker grafts but do not afford the protection of a full-thickness graft. Although they may heal over bone or tendon, secondary revisions are often necessary. Their use should be limited to dorsal wounds or those without exposure of bone or tendon. These thin grafts may be obtained from a number of areas. The donor area often ends up being unsightly after healing, however, and should be chosen carefully. The thigh or lateral aspect of the buttock is a satisfactory donor site.

Full-thickness grafts provide better protection for the volar aspect of the finger but have the same limitations as split-thickness skin grafts when used over bone and tendon. They are less

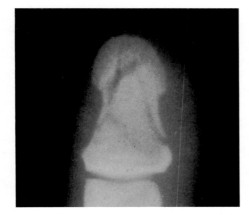

FIG 7–18.
Fracture of the distal phalanx.

sensitive and may be used on volar injuries. The flexor creases of the wrist and elbow are excellent donor sites. The donor wound is easily closed without undue tension in these areas. The graft should include no subcutaneous tissue. As with all grafting procedures, it is wise to plan backward and be certain that the graft will completely cover the area of the wound. If the patient brings in the amputated fingertip, it may be used

as a full-thickness graft if it is in good condition. All fat must be removed prior to application. In children under 5 years of age, defatting the tip is not necessary. As healing progresses, full-thickness grafts may become dark after a few days. This should not be a cause for alarm because the deeper portion is usually viable in spite of the appearance of the more superficial layers.

Flap Grafts

Extensive wounds may require local flaps. A variety of flap grafts are available for use depending on the need. These grafts provide more bulk and protection and are used when subcutaneous tissue is needed, for example, over bone and tendon. They are occasionally used by the experienced surgeon.

Crush Injuries

These injuries are the result of direct violence to the tip of the finger. A painful subungual hematoma or fracture of the distal phalanx may occur (Fig 7–18). The treatment of these injuries is directed at the soft tissues. Isolated painful he-

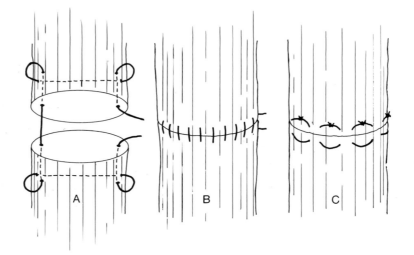

FIG 7–19.
A, the Kessler technique for tendon repair: 4-0 nylon is used. A running suture of 6-0 nylon is added. **B** and **C,** simple horizontal mattress sutures may be used instead of the Kessler technique.

matomas may be drained by gently drilling a hole into the nail with a no. 11 blade. A heated paper clip may also be used. The hematoma should not be drained, however, when a fracture of the phalanx is present.

Fracture fragments are stabilized by the adjacent soft tissue and can usually be ignored. A tube-gauze compression dressing and ice are applied, and the hand is elevated to combat swelling. Warm soaks are started in 48 to 72 hours, and gentle motion is encouraged. Recovery is usually rapid.

Extensor Tendon Injuries

The extensor mechanism of each finger is a complex system, only a part of which is the extrinsic tendon itself. Restoration of normal function requires accurate diagnosis and repair. All skin lacerations over the hand should be thoroughly inspected for tendon injury, but special attention should be paid to lacerations over the metacarpophalangeal joint. Extensor tendon lacerations in this area are particularly difficult to diagnose because the injury frequently occurs with the metacarpophalangeal joint in *flexion,* and the examination is usually carried out with the finger in *extension.* The tendon laceration will then lie at a different level than the skin laceration and often goes undetected. With any extensor tendon injury, there is variable loss of active extension of the finger.

Lacerations in the extensor complex must be repaired accurately, and there should be no hesitation to extend the wound proximally or distally in order to properly visualize the ends of the tendon. Direct end-to-end repair using nonabsorbable suture such as nylon is desirable (Fig 7–19). The finger and wrist are splinted in extension in order to remove tension from the suture line. Immobilization is maintained for approximately 4 weeks.

Partial lacerations consisting of greater than one third of the tendon should also be repaired. Small "nicks" can usually be left alone.

Flexor Tendon Injuries

Flexor tendon injuries are diagnosed by history and examination. Partial or complete loss of finger flexion will be accompanied by a typical posture of the finger (Fig 7–20). There are often associated digital nerve injuries.

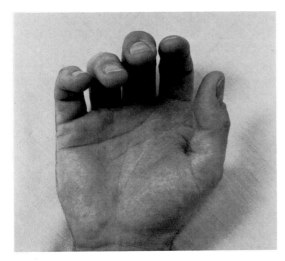

FIG 7–20.
The position of rest. With the hand lying on a flat surface, the fingers will maintain a position of slight flexion. When the flexor tendons are lacerated, the affected finger will rest in extension.

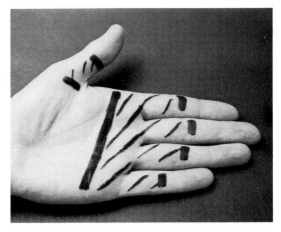

FIG 7–21.
No-man's-land, the critical area of the annular ligaments.

Repair of flexor tendon injuries is a complex problem that should be undertaken only in the operating room by an experienced surgeon. Primary repair of these injuries is indicated when the laceration occurs distal to the sublimis insertion or proximal to the distal palmar crease. Primary tendon repair between these two points, in so-called "no-man's-land," is frequently unrewarding because adhesions are likely to form between the lacerated tendon ends and the flexor sheath and pulleys (Fig 7–21). In selected cases of sharp wounds, primary tendon repair may be undertaken in this area. Otherwise, simple closure of the skin laceration followed by secondary tendon grafting in 6 to 8 weeks is often preferable.

Lacerations of the wrist that involve the palmaris longus tendon should always be carefully evaluated for *median nerve injury* because these two structures are close in this area.

HAND INFECTIONS

Human Bites

These are common injuries that are often mistaken for innocuous lacerations. Serious complications and disability frequently result, however, usually from the inoculation of virulent oral bacteria into the wound.

A variety of organisms may be involved but the most common are mixed anaerobes and aerobes and *Staphylococcus aureus*.

The usual mechanism of injury is a fist fight in which the clenched fist strikes the opponents tooth. Most commonly, the metacarpophalangeal (MCP) joint of the index or long finger is involved. The injury may cause penetration of tendon, MCP joint capsule, and even the metacarpal head. When the finger is extended, the site of injury is often obscured and obliterated. Thus, drainage is hindered, and infection is encouraged. (Laceration of the extensor tendon may also occur but is often overlooked because the finger is examined in the extended position.) The stage is set for spread of the infection into the joint and sometimes throughout the entire hand.

Treatment

Appreciation of the injury is most important so that the initial wound is properly treated. Thorough inspection, cleansing, and debridement are needed. The laceration may need to be enlarged in order to fully visualize the extent of the wound. Cultures are taken, and the wound is left open. No structures are repaired. A wick may be placed in the wound, and a soft bulky dressing is applied.

Antibiotics are administered on an empiric basis. Initially, they are given intravenously followed later by the oral route. They are changed as needed depending on the results of the initial culture and sensitivity.

If a wick is used, it is removed the next day, and daily wound cleansing and dressing changes are begun. The laceration is inspected closely, and if it is not improving, further surgical debridement and intravenous antibiotic therapy may be necessary. If the wound is healing satisfactorily, antibiotic coverage is continued for 2 to 3 weeks. Secondary closure of the wound is usually unnecessary. Complete extensor tendon lacerations may eventually require secondary repair.

Wounds treated within a few hours can usually be managed on an outpatient basis. Older injuries may require hospitalization because cellulitis and abscess formation are often well established.

Felon

A felon is an infection of the closed space of the pulp of the distal phalanx (Fig 7–22). It occurs secondary to a local puncture wound and is characterized by rapidly increasing pressure and pain. Osteomyelitis of the distal phalanx and extension of the infection into the flexor sheath or

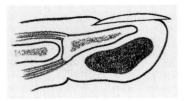

FIG 7–22.
Felon. The pus accumulates in the pulp of the distal phalanx.

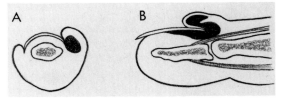

FIG 7–24.
Paronychia. **A,** the abscess is present beneath the eponychium. **B,** the infection has penetrated under the nail and extended proximally.

adjacent joint may result. Early incision and drainage are indicated. A short 24-hour trial of conservative treatment with antibiotics and hot packs may be attempted, but if symptoms do not rapidly diminish, early drainage is advisable. A metacarpal block is adequate anesthesia. A tourniquet is applied to the base of the finger, and a direct incision is made into the point of maximum tenderness and swelling. The incision does not have to be any longer than 5 to 10 mm. If no specific "point" can be detected, a straight lateral incision, which may be extended around the tip of the finger, is made (Fig 7–23). The "fishmouth" incision should not be used. Routine care of the wound after drainage includes dressing changes every 2 to 3 days and maintenance of antibiotic therapy. The wound will usually be healed in 2 weeks.

Paronychia

Paronychia is an infection of the distal phalanx that occurs along the edge of the nail. The organism, usually *Staphylococcus,* is often introduced by biting the nail or by a rough manicure. Local signs of infection such as redness, swelling, and tenderness are invariably present (Fig 7–24).

Acute paronychia will usually require drainage, although antibiotics and local care will occasionally result in a cure. Once the pus has localized, incision and drainage are indicated. This is easily accomplished by passing a scalpel *between* the nail and the adjacent eponychium with the patient under local anesthesia (Fig 7–25). If the infection has penetrated under the nail, a small portion of it may have to be excised. Incision and drainage *through* the eponychium should be avoided.

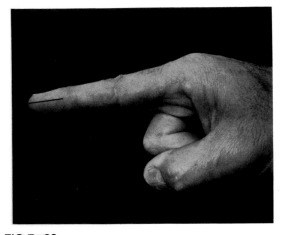

FIG 7–23.
Drainage of a felon. The incision is placed posterior to the neurovascular bundle.

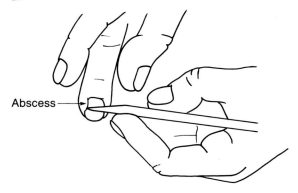

FIG 7–25.
Drainage of acute paronychia. Under digital block, a scalpel blade is passed between the nail fold and the nail. Pus is usually able to be evacuated.

Abscess

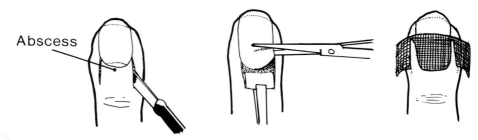

FIG 7-26.
Drainage of paronychia when a subungual abscess is present. Lateral incisions are made through the eponychium, and the base of the nail is removed. Packing is applied, and the eponychium is replaced but not sutured.

Once the infection spreads under the nail, a subungual abscess results. In this case, drainage is only effective if the proximal part of the nail is excised (Fig 7-26). The nail will usually regrow. Chronic paronychia is treated in a similar manner.

Tendon Sheath Infections

Infection may occur inside a flexor tendon sheath from extension of a felon or directly from a puncture wound. The rapid increase in pressure due to the accumulation of pus may obliterate the blood supply to the tendon and result in necrosis and complete loss of function of the tendon. The infection may also spread through the rest of the hand. Early diagnosis and treatment are therefore important.

Clinical Features

The patient with suppurative tenosynovitis is febrile and often in a toxic condition. The disorder can usually be diagnosed by the presence of the four cardinal signs of Kanavel: (1) the finger is uniformly swollen, (2) the finger is held in slight flexion for comfort, (3) intense pain is present on passive extension of the finger, and (4) marked tenderness is present along the course of the inflamed sheath.

Treatment

Early treatment with high doses of antibiotics, elevation, and splinting may result in a cure. In addition, wide incision and drainage are usually necessary to prevent sloughing of the tendon and further spread of the infection.

High-pressure injection wounds of the hand can cause severe infections. These occur when paint, oil, or grease is accidentally injected into the soft tissues of the hand. The puncture wound may be quite small, but extensive debridement and decompression are necessary to control infection and prevent the need for amputation. Paint appears to be the most toxic substance. Prompt recognition of the problem is important.

FRACTURES OF THE FOREARM

Fractures in Adults

Fractures that occur through both bones of the forearm in adults are usually shortened and displaced. Accurate reduction of these injuries by closed methods is difficult, and there is a strong tendency for these unstable fractures to angulate after swelling subsides in spite of a good reduction and cast immobilization. Strong muscular forces acting across the fracture fragments predispose to this loss of correction. Consequently, there is a high rate of nonunion. For these reasons, displaced fractures of both bones of the forearm in the adult are often treated by primary open reduction and internal fixation (Fig 7–27). Closed treatment may be attempted, but if it is unsuccessful the first time, operative intervention is usually indicated. The length of immobilization is shorter with surgery, and there is a more rapid return of function. Undisplaced fractures are treated with a long arm cast for 8 to 12 weeks.

Isolated fractures of either the radius or the ulna are treated in a similar manner. If enough angulation is present to interfere with rotation, closed reduction is attempted. If it is unsuccessful, open reduction and internal fixation are indicated. Undisplaced fractures are treated with a long arm cast for 8 to 12 weeks or until healing is complete.

Fractures in Children

Fractures in children differ from those in adults in that surgery is rarely necessary. Reduction is usually possible by manipulation with the patient under light anesthesia. Angulated fractures are reduced by traction and countertraction, with manual correction of the angulation. It is often necessary to break the opposite cortex of the greenstick fracture in order to prevent reangulation from occurring in the cast (Fig 7–28). Displaced fractures are treated by reduction with traction and countertraction (Fig 7–29). Slight "bayonet" apposition is acceptable in young children if the alignment is satisfactory because subsequent remodeling of growth will correct minor deformities. Children are examined at weekly intervals for 3 weeks in order to determine whether any reangulation of the fracture is occurring after the swelling subsides. If angulation

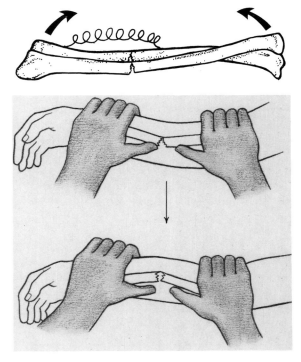

FIG 7–28.
Top, greenstick fracture of the forearm. The tension side of an angulated greenstick fracture of both bones of the forearm will frequently act as a spring and may cause the angulation to recur. *Center,* and *bottom,* these fractures should be manually broken through to prevent recurrence. The periosteum on the concave side will remain intact. Reduction is then accomplished by simple traction.

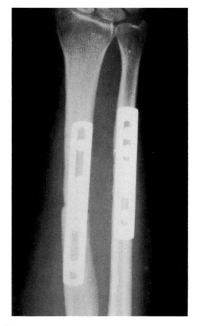

FIG 7–27.
Postoperative roentgenogram of a fracture of both bones of the forearm that was successfully treated by primary open reduction with internal fixation.

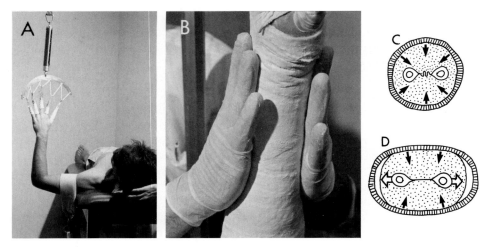

FIG 7−29.
Reduction of a forearm fracture by simple vertical traction and countertraction. **A,** the fingers are incorporated into finger "traps." Countertraction is applied with a weight or water bucket. **B,** a long arm cast is applied with the elbow flexed 90 degrees and molded into an oval shape and straight by placing the hands on the anterior and posterior sides. **C,** an improperly molded circular cast may allow the forearm bones to encroach on the interosseus space, which could limit rotation. A properly molded elliptical cast **(D)** will prevent this from occurring.

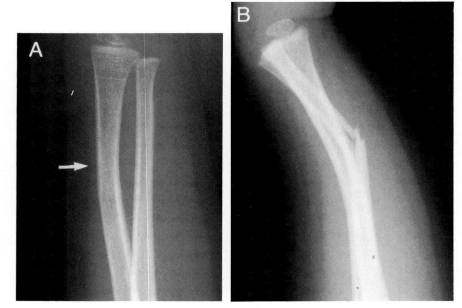

FIG 7−30.
A, Traumatic bowing of the radius *(arrow).* **B,** Fracture of the ulna with bowing of the radius.
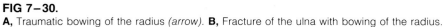

does recur before 2 weeks, it can usually be corrected manually. If more than 2 weeks passes, however, the healing is so rapid in children that the angulation may be permanent. The cast is worn for 7 to 8 weeks.

All forearm fractures in children and adults are immobilized by a long arm cast with the elbow flexed 90 degrees. The forearm portion is always molded to prevent encroachment on the interosseous space.

Traumatic Bowing of the Forearm

This is an unusual clinical entity in which "plastic deformation" of the radius and/or ulna occurs in the absence of typical clinical and roentgenographic findings for fracture (Fig 7–30). The usual cause is a fall on the outstretched hand. There may be a fracture of one bone and bowing of the other or, less commonly, bowing of both bones.

Management of these injuries is controversial. Persistent angulation could limit pronation and supination, although young children (under 5 years old) will undergo bone remodeling and probably do not need reduction. An angulated fracture of one bone is also difficult to reduce until the bowing of the other bone is corrected. In older children, the angulation should be corrected. The reduction may require significant force, and general anesthesia is usually needed.

Galeazzi Fracture-Dislocation

This injury is a fracture of the shaft of the radius with a dislocation of the distal radio-ulnar joint

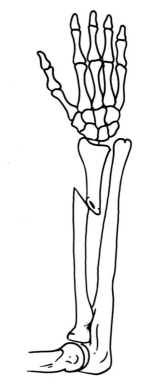

FIG 7–31.
Galeazzi fracture-dislocation. There is a fracture of the distal portion of the radius with shortening. This shortening can only occur if there is injury elsewhere (in this lesion, a radio-ulnar dislocation). On the lateral view, the distal portion of the ulna is usually dislocated dorsally.

(Fig 7–31). It is rare in children. The disorder is sometimes called the reverse Monteggia fracture. Usually the radius is fractured in its distal third, and the radio-ulnar disruption is often missed. Surgery is usually required for repair.

FRACTURES OF THE WRIST

Several common injuries occur in the region of the wrist joint: Colles' fracture, fracture of the distal portion of the radius in children, epiphyseal fractures of the distal aspect of the radius, and fractures of the scaphoid. Treatment of all these injuries is very similar.

Colles' Fracture

Colles' fracture is the most common injury about the wrist. It usually results from a fall on the outstretched hand. The force of the fall fractures the distal portion of the radius and displaces it into the typical "silver-fork" position. In addition to the dorsal angulation, there is shortening and radial deviation of the distal fragment. There is usually an associated injury to the ulnar styloid or ulnar collateral ligament of the wrist (Fig 7–32).

The fracture can usually be reduced with the patient under local anesthesia if reduction is performed within a few hours. If more time passes, a general anesthetic may be necessary because the local anesthetic may not diffuse through the clotted hematoma after several hours have passed. The tip of the ulna should also be injected.

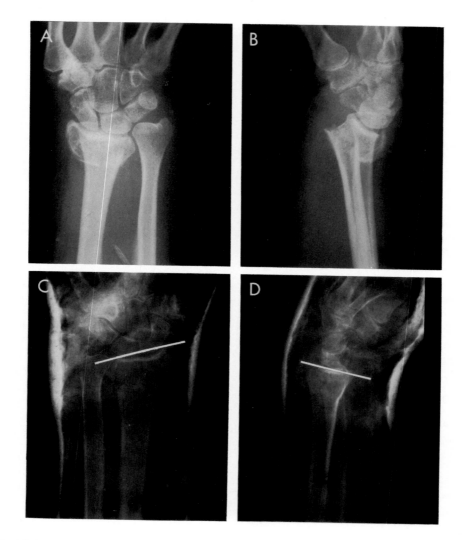

FIG 7–32.
A and **B,** typical Colles' fracture with dorsal and radial displacement. Normally, the tip of the styloid process of the distal portion of the radius extends 1 cm distal to the tip of the ulnar styloid. The articular surface of the lower part of the radius inclines 25 degrees ulnarward and 10 degrees volarward. **C** and **D,** following complete reduction, the length and these angular relationships are restored.

With the assistant grasping the forearm for countertraction, the surgeon grasps the hand of the affected wrist (Fig 7–33). The thumb of the surgeon's other hand is placed over the distal fragment, and the wrist is hyperextended to break up any impaction. Traction and countertraction are then applied, and by using the thumb for pressure on the distal fragment, the

rotation is corrected, and the dorsal cortex of the distal fragment is forced onto the dorsal cortex of the proximal fragment (see Chapter 2). Ulnar and volar pressure over the distal fragment will then correct the radial and dorsal angulation. The radial styloid is palpated to determine whether the length has been restored. With the assistant maintaining volar and ulnar tension on

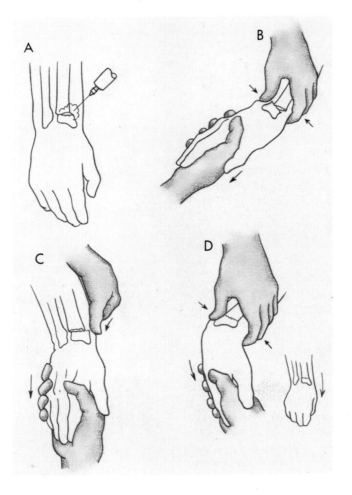

FIG 7–33.
Reduction of Colles' fracture. **A,** the needle is inserted dorsally into the fracture hematoma, and 5 to 10 mL of local anesthesia is injected. **B,** the distal fragment is disimpacted, and longitudinal traction is applied. Thumb pressure is then applied to the distal fragment to correct the dorsal displacement. **C,** the radial displacement is corrected by further digital pressure and ulnar deviation of the wrist. **D,** upward pressure on the proximal fragment and tension on the slightly flexed, ulnarly deviated hand will maintain the reduction. A cast is then applied and properly molded. (Adapted from Compere EL, Banks SW, Compere CL: *Pictorial Handbook of Fracture Treatment,* ed 5. Chicago, Year Book Medical Publishers Inc, 1963.)

the hand, a well-molded cast is applied with the wrist slightly pronated. The cast is well molded over the dorsal and radial aspects of the distal fragments and the volar aspect of the proximal fragment in order to keep the dorsal soft tissue tight. A short arm cast is usually sufficient. Excessive volar flexion of the wrist should be avoided and is unnecessary if the cast is properly applied and molded. Excessive flexion of the wrist may cause median nerve compression. The base of the thumb may be included to the interphalangeal joint to help prevent radial collapse.

An alternative method of treatment is to use the method of traction previously described for forearm fractures. After anesthesia has been obtained, the fracture is disimpacted, and the patient's index finger and thumb are placed in the finger traps. A counterweight is placed on the upper part of the arm, and the fracture is manipulated. A properly molded cast is then applied with the forearm in slight pronation. Roentgenograms are then repeated.

If the reduction is satisfactory, the wrist is elevated, and ice is applied for 48 to 72 hours. Active motion of the fingers is encouraged, and the roentgenogram is repeated in 7 to 10 days. The fracture is immobilized for approximately 6 weeks.

After the cast is removed, some temporary stiffness should be expected for several weeks. This usually subsides gradually as the activity level is increased. A temporary splint that is removed several times a day for exercise is frequently helpful in the transition period between cast removal and full use of the extremity.

Occasionally, some loss of reduction may occur after the swelling subsides. This is particularly true if there is comminution of the dorsal cortex. In the elderly patient, this position should be accepted rather than attempting to remanipulate the fragments in order to improve the roentgenographic appearance. This would only lead to more swelling, stiffness, and loss of function. Accepting the minor cosmetic deformity caused by the slight malunion is preferable in the older pa-

tient. If this occurs in younger patients (especially radial shortening), remanipulation with pinning or an external fixator is indicated.

Smith's Fracture

This fracture has often been called the reverse Colles' fracture (Fig 7–34). One form of this fracture may be considered as such. The type that does not involve the articular surface may be treated by traction, manipulation, and casting in supination. Treatment in supination is important. "Cocking up" the wrist (the reverse of the Colles' treatment) will frequently not hold the reduction.

One type of Smith's fracture has an articular component that results in volar subluxation of the carpal bones. This injury often requires open reduction with internal fixation for satisfactory results.

Barton's Fracture

This is an oblique fracture that is essentially the reverse of the intra-articular Smith's fracture. The injury involves an oblique dorsal rim fracture-dislocation through the articular surface of the distal portion of the radius. Because this fracture

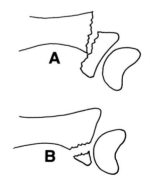

FIG 7–34.
Smith's fracture. Closed reduction is usually successful with the type that does not involve the articular surface **(A),** but surgery is usually necessary for the intra-articular type **(B).**

involves the joint surface, accurate reduction is necessary, and open reduction is often required.

Fracture of the Lower Portion of the Radius in Children

In children and adolescents, a fracture may occur through the distal radial epiphysis. If it is displaced, it is reduced in the same manner as Colles' fracture and immobilized for 5 weeks. If it is undisplaced, the diagnosis may be difficult. It should be kept in mind, however, that sprains of the wrist are very rare in children. This is because the epiphyseal plate is weaker than the surrounding ligamentous structures and trauma will usually produce an epiphyseal fracture rather than a ligamentous sprain. Clinical tenderness over the epiphysis is highly suggestive of a fracture, and a short arm cast should be applied to these injuries for 2 weeks even though the roentgenographic findings may be normal. If a healing callus is present at the end of 2 weeks, the cast is continued for an additional 2 weeks. If no callus is present, the cast is removed, and the "sprain" has had excellent treatment.

Fractures of the distal portion of the radius also occur in children approximately 2.5 cm above the wrist joint. They are treated in the same manner as Colles' fracture. Undisplaced or so-called *torus* fractures also occur in this area (Fig 7–35). No displacement occurs with this injury, but it should be immobilized in a short arm cast for 3 weeks.

A common fracture that is particularly difficult to reduce completely is the displaced, overlapping fracture of the distal part of the radius with either a greenstick fracture of the ulna or an intact ulna (Fig 7–36). Sometimes the radius can be reduced by first maximally supinating the wrist and, by using digital pressure, replacing the distal radial fragment. The wrist is then pronated. Usually, however, the ulnar fracture must be completed before reduction is possible. If the ulna is intact, it should be left alone and the radius realigned as closely as possible. Bayonet ap-

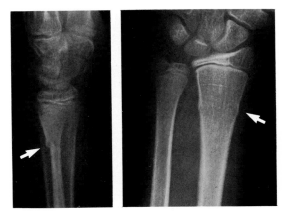

FIG 7–35.
The "buckle" or torus fracture *(arrows)* of the distal portion of the radius.

position of this fracture is acceptable as long as alignment is satisfactory.

Fractures of the Scaphoid

The scaphoid is the carpal bone that is most prone to fracture (Fig 7–37). This injury also occurs as the result of a fall on the out stretched hand.

The blood supply to this bone frequently enters the distal portion. Consequently, fractures that occur through the midportion of the bone may lead to avascular necrosis of the proximal fragment. Nonunion is also more frequent following this injury.

The diagnosis is sometimes difficult. It should be suspected, however, in any patient with a history of a "sprained wrist" who has persistent swelling and pain in the wrist. Clinically, tenderness and swelling in the anatomic snuffbox are characteristic findings.

Initial roentgenographic findings are often normal because there may be little or no displacement of the fracture fragments. The fracture usually becomes visible in 2 to 4 weeks, however, as decalcification around the fracture line occurs.

Whenever this injury is suspected, even if the

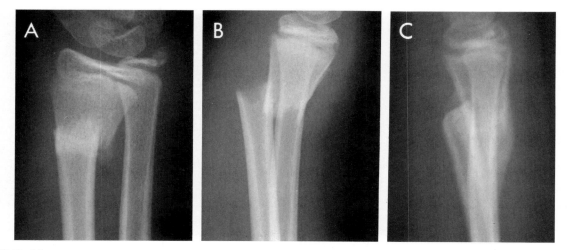

FIG 7–36.
Anteroposterior **(A)** and lateral **(B)** roentgenograms of a displaced fracture of the distal portion of the radius without a fracture of the ulna. End-to-end apposition could not be obtained and bayonet apposition was accepted. **C,** a lateral roentgenogram several months later shows good alignment and early remodeling.

roentgenographic findings are normal, a short arm cast including the thumb should be applied. The roentgenogram is repeated in 2 to 3 weeks. If a fracture is present, the immobilization is continued until the fracture has healed, which in this case may take from 3 to 6 months. A minimum of 6 weeks' immobilization is necessary. If there is any displacement of the fracture fragments, a

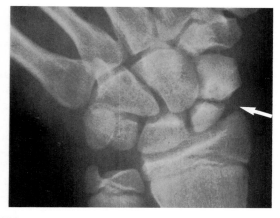

FIG 7–37.
Fractured scaphoid, *(arrow).*

long arm cast should be applied for 6 weeks, followed by a short arm cast for an additional 6 weeks.

Sprained Wrist

Although simple, uncomplicated ligamentous injuries of the wrist do occur, there are a number of conditions that are often misdiagnosed as sprains. Failure to appreciate and properly treat these disorders can lead to permanent disability and chronic pain. Among the more common injuries presenting as "sprains" are (1) fractures of the navicular (usually due to a fall); (2) undisplaced epiphyseal fractures of the distal portion of the radius in children; (3) fracture of the hook of the hamate (often occurring when a baseball bat handle strikes the palm); (4) avulsion fractures of the triquetrum, an injury that may signify serious ligamentous disruption (Fig 7–38); (5) carpal instability, frequently manifested by scapholunate dissociation, a separation of lunate from the scaphoid that may require surgery; and (6) subluxation of the distal portion of the ulna (usually due to complete ligamentous rupture

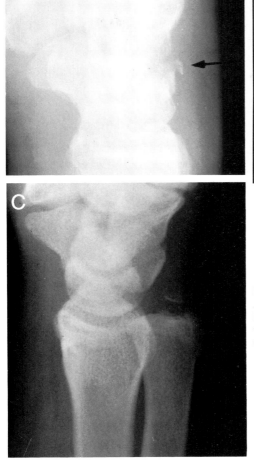

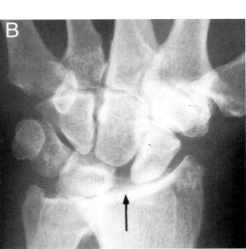

FIG 7–38.
A, avulsion fracture of the triquetrum *(arrow).*
B, scapholunate dislocation *(arrow)* (note the widening between the scaphoid and lunate).
C, dislocation of the distal portion of the ulna.

between the ulna and its attachments to the radius and carpal bones).

Careful clinical examination will usually reveal local tenderness and swelling. Routine wrist roentgenograms are always performed, and special views are added as indicated.

If a serious bony or ligamentous injury is not suspected clinically or roentgenographically, the wrist should be immobilized for 3 to 4 weeks and re-evaluated. Elastic wraps or "light braces" are inadequate. More serious fractures or ligamentous disruptions should be referred.

FRACTURES OF THE HAND

The principles of treatment of finger injuries are similar to other fractures except that the reduction must be more accurate in the hand. With certain exceptions, manipulation and exter-

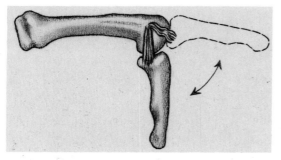

FIG 7–39.
Collateral ligaments of the metacarpophalangeal joint. These ligaments are normally lax in extension and tight in flexion. Prolonged splinting in extension may allow them to shorten slightly, thereby making future flexion difficult.

nal immobilization constitute satisfactory treatment. Principles of treatment include the following:

1. Avoid overimmobilization.
2. Be certain to correct rotational as well as angular malalignment.
3. Early surgery in the form of open reduction and internal fixation is often more "conservative" than are overzealous manipulation and prolonged, improper splinting.
4. Fingers should be immobilized in the position of moderate flexion. Avoid splinting the finger joints in extension, especially the metacarpophalangeal joint (Fig 7–39).
5. Displaced intra-articular fractures involving greater than 25% of the joint surface are unstable and usually require open reduction and internal fixation (Fig 7–40).
6. In the position of grasping, the axes of all flexed fingers point to the navicular bone (Fig 7–41). Failure to appreciate this fact may result in rotational malunion.
7. "Chip" fractures near joints usually have a tendon or ligament attached. These injuries require careful evaluation (Fig 7–42).

Fractures of the Metacarpal

Fractures of the shaft of the finger metacarpal often present with dorsal angulation because of the action of the interosseous muscles (Fig 7–43). Fractures that are in good alignment and apposition will heal satisfactorily in 4 weeks. Slight shortening may be accepted. A short arm plaster cast or splint incorporating an aluminum splint and extending over the finger provides adequate immobilization.

Fractures of the neck of the metacarpal are common in the small finger (Fig 7–44). These commonly occur in fist fights and are sometimes called "boxer's" fractures. Clinically, there is swelling over the fracture site and depression of the "knuckle" of the affected finger. Fractures with minimal angulation are treated with a compression dressing for 1 week followed by gradually increasing active exercises. Fractures with angulation over 40 degrees should be reduced. If closed reduction is successful, the finger is im-

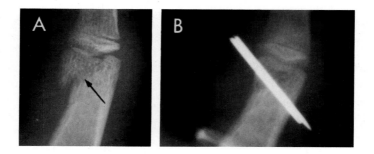

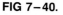

FIG 7–40.
A, a displaced intra-articular IP joint fracture *(arrow).* Open reduction with internal fixation **(B)** was required.

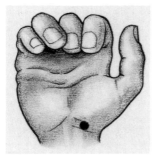

FIG 7–41.
Normally, the axes of the flexed fingers point to the navicular *(dot)*. Malunion with rotation will cause the fingers to overlap when a fist is made. The resultant functional disability may be great.

mobilized in a plaster splint for 4 weeks. Even if fractures of the fourth and fifth metacarpal necks heal with a mild amount of angulation, the functional result is usually good. The same fracture in a child will usually correct itself with further growth. Open reduction is occasionally indicated in severely angulated fractures.

Bennett's fracture is actually a fracture-dislocation that occurs at the carpometacarpal joint of the thumb (Fig 7–45). The metacarpal is usually dislocated proximally because of the pull of the

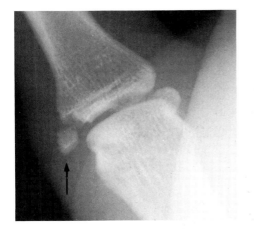

FIG 7–42.
Collateral ligament avulsion fracture, which usually causes instability.

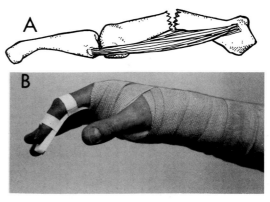

FIG 7–43.
A, fracture of the metacarpal. **B,** reduction is maintained by a metal splint incorporated in a cast or plaster splint.

long abductor muscle that inserts at its base. This injury requires exact reduction in order to avoid disturbing the function of this important joint. Most of these injuries are displaced and require reduction and internal fixation for the best overall results.

A similar fracture-dislocation occurs at the carpometacarpal joint of the small finger (Fig 7–46). While not as potentially serious as the injury to the thumb, reduction and internal fixation are often required, nonetheless. Failure to recognize and properly treat the injury may lead to a weakness in grip because more power is provided by the ulnar side of the hand than the radial side.

The *Rolando fracture* is a comminuted intra-articular fracture of the base of the thumb metacarpal. It is frequently difficult to restore normal anatomic alignment to the fracture, even by open reduction. The prognosis for return of normal use of this joint following a Rolando fracture is often poor.

Fractures of the Phalanges

Fractures of the proximal phalanx usually angulate to the volar aspect of the hand (Fig 7–47). This angulation is produced by the pull of the intrinsic muscles. Oblique fractures of this bone

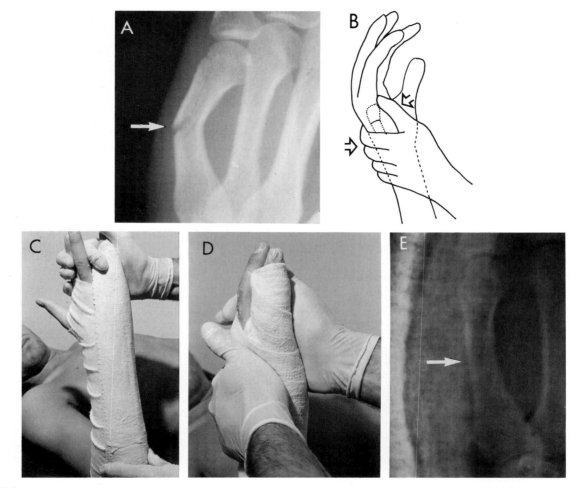

FIG 7–44.
A, fracture of the small finger metacarpal *(arrow).* **B,** reduction is obtained by digital pressure against the distal fragment with counterpressure on the dorsum of the proximal fragment. **C** and **D,** applying and molding the ulnar gutter splint. **E,** the end result.

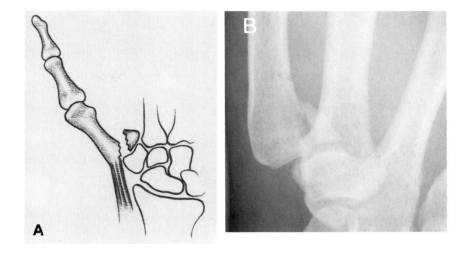

FIG 7–45.
A, Bennett's fracture of the base of the thumb metacarpal. **B,** the roentgenographic appearance.

are the most common cause of rotational deformity of the fingers (Fig 7–48). Reduction of the transverse fracture is usually possible by traction on the flexed finger toward the tubercle of the scaphoid. Immobilization in moderate flexion with a splint for 4 weeks is usually sufficient time for healing to occur. Unstable fractures require open reduction and internal fixation.

The common epiphyseal fracture of the base of the proximal phalanx of the small finger is usually a type II Salter fracture and is usually displaced into abduction (Fig 7–49). It is reduced under local anesthesia by applying traction with

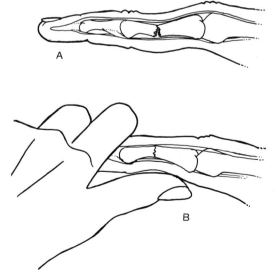

FIG 7–47.
A, fracture of the proximal phalanx. **B,** reduction by flexion of the distal fragment. The position is maintained by a splint.

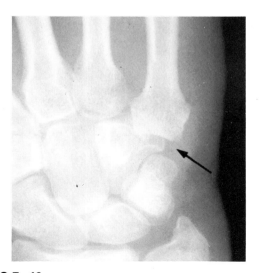

FIG 7–46.
Fracture-dislocation of the small finger CM joint *(arrow).*

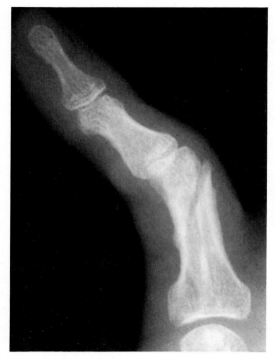

FIG 7–48.
Oblique fracture of the proximal phalanx. Always evaluate for proper rotation.

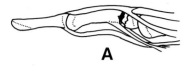

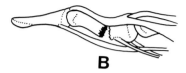

FIG 7–50.
Fracture of the middle phalanx. If the fracture is proximal to the insertion of sublimis tendon, the fracture will tend to angulate into flexion **(A).** This fracture may require treatment in slight extension. Fractures distal to the sublimis insertion **(B)** frequently angulate into extension, and flexion is therefore required for reduction.

the finger in slight flexion and then adducting the finger against a pencil or the physician's finger, which acts as a fulcrum. It is taped to the ring finger and immobilized with a padded splint for 4 weeks.

Fractures of the middle phalanx may angulate volarward or dorsally (Fig 7–50). Traction with manipulation of the fracture will usually effect a reduction. The finger is splinted for 4 weeks.

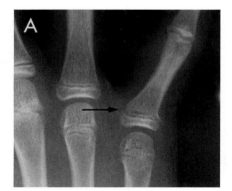

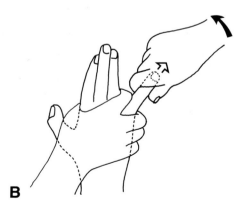

FIG 7–49.
A, epiphyseal fracture of the proximal phalanx of the small finger in the typical position of ulnar deviation. **B,** reduction by traction and pressure against the finger in the web space.

DISLOCATIONS OF THE FINGERS

Metacarpophalangeal (MP) dislocations may be classified as simple or complex. Simple dislocations may be reduced by traction and manipulation (Fig 7–51). The finger is splinted for 3 to 4 weeks. Complex dislocations usually have soft tissue interposed in the joint or the metacarpal neck is buttonholed through a window in the soft tissue (Fig 7–52). It is usually impossible to treat them by closed methods. Some improvement may seem apparent after the manipulation, but the joint does not "snap" back into place and does not feel reduced. Reduction of the complex MP dislocation is prevented by the soft tissue. The more traction and pressure applied to the finger, the tighter the soft tissue becomes. Open reduction is usually necessary.

Interphalangeal (IP) dislocations are also frequent and occur most commonly in the athlete (Fig 7–53). They are usually easily reduced by increasing the angular deformity, applying traction and digital pressure to the distal portion, and manipulating it into flexion. Roentgenograms are always repeated following the reduction to exclude avulsion fractures. If the finger is

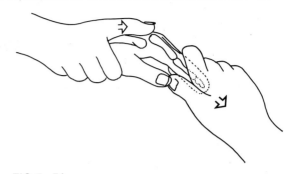

FIG 7–51.
An MP dislocation that may be reduced by simple traction and digital pressure.

stable following reduction, it may be taped to an adjacent finger for 3 to 4 weeks. If the dislocation is unstable, an avulsion fracture may be present, and the injury may represent a fracture-dislocation or ligament rupture rather than a simple dislocation. Examination may reveal some instability in the volar direction or mediolaterally. Special care of this injury is necessary, and surgery is often indicated (see Chapter 15).

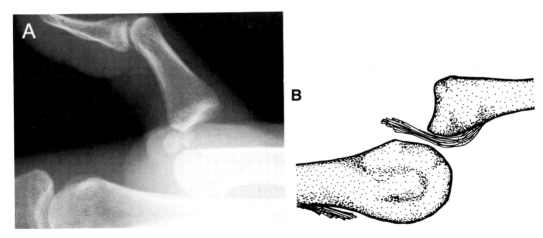

FIG 7–52.
A, Complex MP dislocation. **B,** Soft-tissue interposition that may prevent reduction. (**Remember:** Push rather than pull to reduce most dislocations. Otherwise, a simple one may be converted to a complex one.)

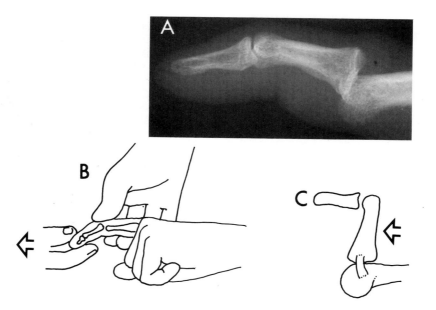

FIG 7–53.

A, PIP dislocation. Traction and digital pressure are usually successful **(B).** Occasionally, the deformity must be increased before reduction is able to be accomplished **(C).**

MISCELLANEOUS DISORDERS

Carpometacarpal Boss

This abnormality is in the same area as the usual ganglion cyst. The deformity is a bony prominence that develops at the base of the index and long finger metacarpals. The etiology is unknown, although repetitive trauma may be a factor. A spur or thickening develops at these CM joints and may become painful. Treatment is usually conservative with splinting and anti-inflammatory medication. Surgical removal is occasionally necessary.

Writer's (Occupational) Cramps

This is a disorder in which the individual develops pain when performing a habitual motor activity. Typically, as the individual begins to write or type, pain develops that increases in severity with more use. Eventually, the activity becomes impossible. The etiology remains unknown, although a variety of neurologic and psychiatric causes have been suggested. The condition may be similar to "spasmodic" torticollis in the neck. Most attempts at treatment fail, including changing pen sizes, desk angles, and even psychological counseling. Sometimes, the only cure is a complete change in jobs.

Mucous Cysts

These are benign lesions that are similar to ganglia. They usually develop on the dorsal aspect of the DIP joints of the index or long fingers and are usually associated with osteoarthritis and osteophytes of the joint. Heberden's nodes are also commonly present. They may produce grooving of the nail of the affected digit. They are characteristically located on one side of the extensor tendon. Treatment ranges from aspiration to excision, and there is a fairly high recurrence rate regardless of treatment.

Raynaud's Disease and Phenomenon

Raynaud's disease is a benign idiopathic paroxysmal vasospasm that occurs mainly in young women and usually affects the fingers and toes. The "attacks" are frequently daily and are often precipitated by cold or emotional stress. They are typically symmetric and bilateral and are relieved by warming. Extreme pallor is followed by cyanosis and then by hyperemia. Serious sequelae are rare, although small areas of gangrene occasionally occur if the disorder is of many years' duration. Treatment is directed at avoiding cold situations that trigger vasoconstriction. Reassurance, dressing sensibly, and avoiding sudden temperature changes are important. Stress management and avoiding tobacco products are also necessary. Medication is usually not required.

Raynaud's phenomenon consists of similar attacks of ischemia of the digits that occur in the course of other diseases, mainly scleroderma. It is often seen before the characteristic skin changes develop. Early on, however, it may be impossible to differentiate benign Raynaud's disease from scleroderma with Raynaud's phenomenon. (β-Blockers like propranolol may cause a similar peripheral vasospasm.)

Hypothenar Hammer Syndrome

Occlusion of the ulnar artery at the wrist may produce symptoms similar to those seen with ulnar tunnel syndrome. This disorder is usually secondary to some repetitive trauma to the ulnar

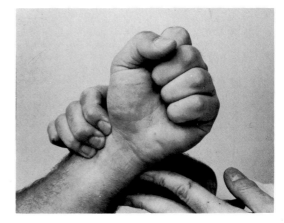

FIG 7–54.
Allen's test. The hand is elevated. The radial and ulnar arteries are occluded, and the patient clenches the fist for 20 seconds. The arteries are released one at a time. Release of either artery will usually allow rapid restoration of the circulation to the hand. If one artery is occluded, however, revascularization of the hand will be delayed or absent.

aspect of the hand such as what occurs when the hand is used as a mallet. This produces a thrombosis of the ulnar artery and results in ischemic manifestations such as pain, pallor, paresthesias, and decreased temperature of the affected digits. Local tenderness may be present, and Allen's test is frequently positive (Fig 7–54).

Treatment is directed at avoiding the offending practice. The symptoms may resolve in many cases without any further treatment. Surgical resection of the thrombosed segment may be necessary if symptoms fail to respond to conservative treatment.

BIBLIOGRAPHY

Allen MJ: Conservative management of fingertip injuries in adults. *Hand* 1980; 12:257.

Barton NJ: Fractures of the hand. *J Bone Joint Surg [Br]* 1984; 66:159.

Bishop AT, Beckenbaugh RD: Fracture of the hamate hook, *J Hand Surg [Am]* 1988; 13:135.

Borden S: Traumatic bowing of the forearm in children. *J Bone Joint Surg [Am]* 1974; 56:611.

Bowers WH, Hurst LC: Gamekeeper's thumb. *J Bone Joint Surg [Am]* 1977; 59:519.

Boyes JH: *Bunnell's Surgery of the Hand,* ed 5. Philadelphia, JB Lippincott Co, 1970.

Conklin JE, White WL: Stenosing tenosynovitis and its possible relation to the carpal tunnel syndrome. *Surg Clin North Am* 1960; 40:531.

DeOliveira JC: Barton's fractures. *J Bone Joint Surg [Am]* 1973; 55:586.

Dias JJ, et al: Suspected scaphoid fractures. *J Bone Joint Surg [Br]* 1990; 72:98.

Dinham JM, Meggitt BF: Trigger thumbs in children. *J Bone Joint Surg [Br]* 1974; 56:153.

Entin MA: Repair of extensor mechanism of the hand. *Surg Clin North Am* 1960; 40:275.

Fisk GR: The wrist. *J Bone Joint Surg [Br]* 1984; 66:396.

Flatt AE: *The Care of Minor Hand Injuries,* ed 3. St Louis, CV Mosby Co, 1972.

Fuhr JE, Farrow A, Nelson HS: Vitamin B$_6$ levels in patients with carpal tunnel syndrome. *Arch Surg* 1989; 124:1329.

Geilberman RH, et al: Current concepts review. Fractures and non-unions of the carpal scaphoid. *J Bone Joint Surg [Am]* 1989; 71:1560.

Hadley NM: Illness in the workplace: The challenge of musculoskeletal symptoms. *J Hand Surg [Am]* 1985; 10:451.

Henderson JJ, Arafa MA: Carpometacarpal dislocation. An easily missed diagnosis. *J Bone Joint Surg [Br]* 1987; 69:212.

Herndon WA, Hershey SL, Lambdin CS: Thrombosis of the ulnar artery in the hand. *J Bone Joint Surg [Am]* 1975; 57:994.

Hill NA: Dupuytren's contracture: Current concepts review. *J Bone Joint Surg [Am]* 1985; 67:1439.

Jones WA: Beware the sprained wrist. The incidence and diagnosis of scapholunate instability. *J Bone Joint Surg [Br]* 1988; 70:293.

Kaplan EB: *Functional and Surgical Anatomy of the Hand,* ed 2. Philadelphia, JB Lippincott, 1965.

Koman LA, Urbaniak JR: Ulnar artery insufficiency: A guide to treatment. *J Hand Surg* 1981; 6:16.

Leddy JP: Infections of the upper extremity. *J Hand Surg* 1986; 11:294.

Louis DS, Huebner JJ, Hankin FM: Rupture and displacement of the ulnar collateral ligament of the metacarpophalangeal joint of the thumb. Preoperative diagnosis. *J Bone Joint Surg [Am]* 1986; 68:1320.

McKerrell J, et al: Boxers fractures: Conservative or operative management. *J Trauma* 1987; 27:486.

Milford L: The hand, in Crenshaw AH (ed): *Campbell's Operative Orthopaedics,* ed 5. St. Louis, CV Mosby Co, 1971.

Muddu BN, Morrias MA, Fahmy NR: The treatment of ganglia. *J Bone Joint Surg [Br]* 1990; 72:147.

Nelson CL, Sawmiller S, Phalen GS: Ganglions of the wrist and hand. *J Bone Joint Surg [Am]* 1972; 54:1459.

Osterman AL: The double crush syndrome. *Orthop Clin North Am* 1988; 19:147.

Putzakis MJ, Wilkins J, Bassett RL: Surgical findings in clenched-fist injuries. *Clin Orthop* 1987; 220:237.

Rang MD: *Children's Fractures,* ed 2. Philadelphia, JB Lippincott, 1983.

Rayan GM, Flournoy DJ: Chronic paronychia due to multiple pyogenic organisms. *J Hand Surg [Am]* 1988; 13:790.

Reckling FW: Unstable fracture-dislocations of the forearm (Monteggia and Galeazzi lesions). *J Bone Joint Surg* 1982; 64:857.

Rockwood CA, Green DP: *Fractures in Adults.* Philadelphia, JB Lippincott, 1984.

Rodrigo JJ, Kiebauer JJ, Doyle JR: Treatment of Dupuytren's contracture. *J Bone Joint Surg [Am]* 1976; 58:380.

Sakellarides HT, DeWeese JW: Instability of the metacarpophalangeal joint of the thumb. *J Bone Joint Surg [Am]* 1976; 58:106.

Scheyer RD, Haas DC: Pyridoxine in carpal tunnel syndrome. *Lancet* 1984; 1:42.

Smith RJ: Post-traumatic instability of the metacarpophalangeal joint of the thumb, *J Bone Joint Surg [Am]* 1977; 59:14.

Spinner RJ, Bachman JW, Amadio PC: The many faces of carpal tunnel syndrome. *Mayo Clin Proc* 1989; 64:829.

Stark HH, et al: Fracture of the hook of the hamate. *J Bone Joint Surg [Am]* 1989; 71:1202.

Upton AR, McComas AJ: The double crush in nerve entrapment syndromes. *Lancet* 1973; 2:359.

Villar RN, et al: Three years after Colles fracture: A prospective review. *J Bone Joint Surg [Br]* 1987; 69:635.

Walsh HP, McLaren CA, Owen R: Galeazzi fractures in children. *J Bone Joint Surg [Br]* 1987; 69:730.

Wehbe MA, Schneider LH: Mallet fractures. *J Bone Joint Surg [Am]* 1984; 66:658.

Zook EG, Guy RJ, Russell RC: A study of nailbed injuries: Causes, treatment and prognosis. *J Hand Surg [Am]* 1984; 9:247.

CHAPTER 8

The Back

Back pain is one of the most frequent conditions requiring medical treatment. It is also the most expensive ailment between the ages of 30 and 60 years and one of the most difficult to treat. Back pain may be due to a variety of disorders, including gynecologic, genitourinary, and gastrointestinal diseases, but the most common causes are lumbar strain and disorders of the lumbar disc.

ANATOMY

The vertebrae, discs, and ligaments of the dorsal and lumbar spine are similar in most respects to their counterparts in the cervical spine. The lumbar vertebrae are larger and thicker, however, due to their weight-bearing function (Fig 8–1). Anterior and posterior longitudinal ligaments are applied to the respective surfaces of the vertebral bodies, and posterior stability is aided by supraspinous and interspinous ligaments and the ligamentum flavum. The discs account for over one third of the total height of the lumbar spine and account for most of the normal lordosis.

Spinal nerves exit the canal by passing through intervertebral foramina, each foramen consisting of the inferior aspect of the pedicle above and the superior aspect of the pedicle below the level of exit. In the lumbar spine, disc disease usually affects the nerve root exiting one level below because that is the nerve that actually passes over the disc (Fig 8–2). Thus, a herniated disc between the fourth and fifth lumbar vertebrae commonly affects the fifth nerve root and not the fourth.

EXAMINATION

Examination of the back is performed with the patient standing, sitting on the examining table, and in the supine position. The patient is first observed in the standing position. Any list or excessive kyphosis or lordosis is noted. Next, the chest is measured in full inspiration and expiration. Normal expansion is greater than 5 cm but may be less than 2.5 cm in ankylosing spondylitis. The iliac crests are then palpated to determine whether they are level. If they are not, footboards

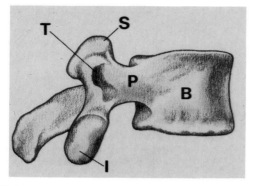

FIG 8–1.
A typical lumbar vertebra: *S* = superior articular facet; *I* = inferior articular facet; *P* = pedicle; *T* = transverse process; *B* = body.

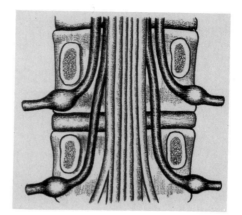

FIG 8–2.
Relationship of nerve roots to discs in the lumbar spine.

of varying thicknesses may be placed under the shorter extremity to assess the amount of shoe lift necessary to level the pelvis. The shoulders are also observed for evenness, although the dominant shoulder is frequently lower in the normal population. The spine and sacroiliac joints are palpated and percussed for spasm and tenderness. Any varicosities in the lower extremities are also noted. The range of motion is then slowly tested. With the patient bending forward as far as possible, flexion is measured as the distance between the fingertips and the floor. This calculation represents a combination of lumbar spine mobility and hamstring flexibility. While the patient is flexed forward, the back is viewed from behind to detect any scoliosis and from the side to detect any persistence of the normal lumbar lordosis that might be present secondary to protective muscle spasm. Extension and right and left bending are then measured. Pain on bending *toward* the affected side frequently signifies disc disease, whereas pain on bending *away* from the affected side frequently denotes muscle strain. The gait pattern is then observed,

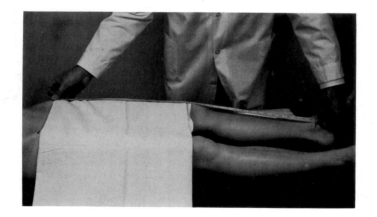

FIG 8–3.
The lower extremities are measured between the anterior superior iliac spines and the medial malleoli with the leg in neutral alignment. Discrepancies under 1 cm are probably not significant.

and the ability to walk on the heels (L5 root) and balls of the feet (S1 root) is tested.

With the patient in the sitting position, a complete neurologic examination of the lower extremities is performed. Reflexes, motor strength, and sensation are tested. The thighs and calves are measured to detect any muscular atrophy. Discrepancies of one-half inch in the thigh and one-fourth inch in the calf are significant. Straight leg raising in the sitting position is also tested and compared with straight leg raising tests that will be performed in the supine position. The peripheral pulses are palpated and any abnor-malities in the vascular status of the extremity noted.

With the patient in the supine position, the hip is placed through a full range of motion and thoroughly tested to rule out primary hip abnormality. The straight-leg-raising tests are then performed, and the leg lengths are measured (Fig 8–3). Next, with the patient on the side, manual pressure is applied to the iliac crest (pelvic compression test). Reproduction of pain in the sacroiliac joints or symphysis pubis with this maneuver may suggest disorders of these areas.

ROENTGENOGRAPHIC ANATOMY

An evaluation of disorders of the lumbar spine should include a standard roentgenographic examination. The roentgenographic features are well visualized by the following: (1) anteroposterior view (Fig 8–4), (2) lateral view (see Fig 8–4), and (3) oblique views in both directions (Fig 8–5). In addition, a spot lateral view of the lumbosacral space may be necessary.

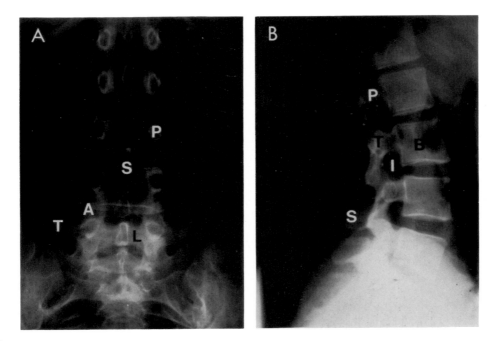

FIG 8–4.
Anteroposterior **(A)** and lateral **(B)** view of the lumbar spine: *S* = spinous process; *P* = pedicle; *T* = transverse process; *L* = lamina; *A* = articular facet joint; *B* = body; *I* = intervertebral foramen.

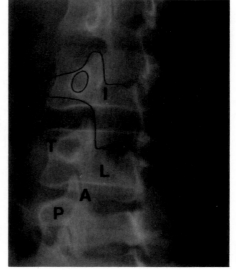

FIG 8–5.
Oblique view: *A* = articular facet joint; *I* = isthmus or pars interarticularis; *T* = transverse process; *L* = lamina; *P* = pedicle. The oblique view visualizes the so-called Scottie dog. Spondylolysis occurs through the isthmus.

LUMBAR DISC SYNDROMES

The intervertebral disc is probably the source of most back pain and the pattern of disc deterioration in the lumbar spine is similar to what occurs in the cervical spine. In the lumbar spine, however, acute soft disc herniation is the most common cause of pain, whereas in the cervical spine, symptoms are usually secondary to spondylosis. Ninety-five percent of disc lesions in the lumbar spine occur at the fourth and fifth spaces, with most of the remainder occurring at the third space. With repetitive trauma, progressive degeneration of the nucleus pulposus occurs, which may lead to protrusion or complete extrusion of a portion of the disc contents into the neural canal. This usually occurs in the area of greatest weakness at the posterolateral aspect of the disc (Fig 8–6). Chronic disc deterioration may also occur and result in spur formation, disc space narrowing, and degenerative changes in the facet joints and between adjacent vertebral bodies.

Disc herniation is most common in the third and fourth decades and is uncommon before the age of 20 years.

A rare but serious complication of lumbar disc disease is the *cauda equina syndrome*. This results from a massive central disc protrusion and may produce variable degrees of permanent paralysis in the lower extremities. Bladder and bowel function may also be severely impaired.

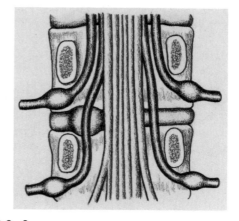

FIG 8–6.
Lumbar disc protrusion. Note that the herniation affects the root that exits one level below.

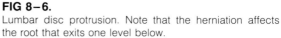

This condition is a true emergency and usually demands immediate surgery.

Clinical Features

The onset of symptoms is variable. One specific traumatic episode may produce symptoms, but because of the progressive nature of the disease process in the disc, the symptoms usually occur gradually. The most common complaint is low back pain, which is often deep and aching in nature. The pain is aggravated by activity and relieved by rest. Coughing, sneezing, or other actions that increase the stress on the disc tend to intensify the pain. The back pain is often localized near the disc and may be referred to the iliac crest or buttock. It is probably the result of stretching of the annulus by the expanding, protruding disc. *Radicular* pain occurs when the disc protrudes far enough to press on the adjacent nerve root. Nerve root pain is usually quite intense. Often, if the disc herniates completely (extrudes), the low back pain may be relieved, but the leg pain intensifies.

Low back pain may occur in combination with radiating pain, or the two pain patterns may occur separately. Radicular pain characteristically spreads over the buttock and passes down the posterior or posterolateral aspect of the thigh and calf and may even spread onto the foot. Both types of pain usually improve with bed rest. If little or no relief of pain occurs with rest, inorganic causes should be considered. Relentless pain that is not relieved or may even be aggravated by recumbency should lead one to suspect a spinal cord tumor.

Paresthesias in the form of numbness and tingling are common and are usually more marked in the distal portion of the extremity. They may follow a specific dermatome pattern (Fig 8–7).

Examination often reveals restriction of low back motion. Bending toward the affected side frequently exacerbates the pain. Variable degrees of local tenderness and muscle guarding are present. In an attempt to relieve tension on the nerve root, the patient may list or bend away from the painful side and stand with the affected

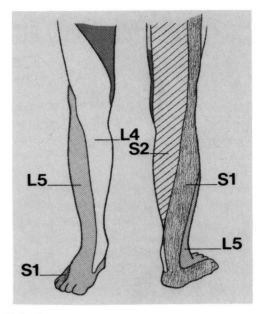

FIG 8–7.
Dermatomes of the lower extremity.

hip and knee slightly flexed. A characteristic clinical picture may be present, depending on the level of nerve root involvement (Table 8–1). The sensory examination may reveal diminished sensation along the affected dermatome. The various tests measuring sciatic nerve root tension are frequently positive (Fig 8–8).

Special Studies

The diagnosis usually becomes apparent on the basis of the history and physical examination. Early disc herniation may be difficult to differentiate from other causes of back pain, however.

1. Plain roentgenograms are indicated within 2 to 4 weeks. They are usually normal.

2. Electromyography, computed tomography (CT), magnetic resonance imaging (MRI), or myelography are used to confirm the diagnosis (Fig 8–9). They are not usually indicated for at least 4 to 6 weeks. The myelogram is not a procedure without some morbidity, and all of these tests are costly. They are indicated under the following

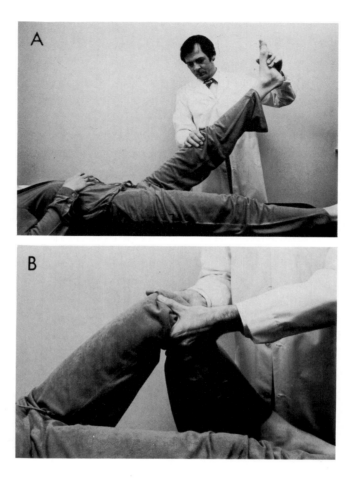

FIG 8–8.
Tests of nerve root tension, the most important examination in herniation of the lumbar intervertebral disc. **A,** the foot is slowly raised, keeping the knee straight, until sciatic pain is produced. A positive test includes the following: (1) pain produced before 70 degrees is reached, (2) aggravation of the pain by dorsiflexion of the ankle, and (3) relief of the pain by flexion of the knee. **B,** the popliteal compression test is then performed by flexing the knee and applying pressure to the popliteal nerve in the fossa. Reproduction of leg pain by this maneuver is further evidence of nerve root irritation. If the patient can extend the leg to 90 degrees while sitting but the same test is impossible in the supine position, malingering should be suspected. If raising the leg on the contralateral side reproduces pain in the affected leg, disc herniation should be strongly suspected.

circumstances: (1) if surgical intervention is being contemplated or (2) if other, more serious spinal pathology is suspected. Myelography is gradually being replaced by the other imaging studies. If it is performed, spinal fluid analysis may show a slight increase in protein content.

3. Discography is considered to be of only limited value.

Note: The number of symptomatic conditions discovered by special studies but not suspected clinically is very small. These tests should only be adjuncts to the clinical assessment.

Treatment

The initial treatment is always conservative. The objective is to "unload" the disc, and this is ac-

TABLE 8–1.

Clinical Features of Common Lumbar Disc Syndromes

Disc	Pain	Sensory Change	Motor Weakness Atrophy	Reflex Change
L3-L4 (L4 root)	Low back, posterolateral aspect of thigh, across patella, anteromedial aspect of leg	Anterior aspect of knee, anteromedial aspect of leg	Quadriceps (knee extension)	Knee jerk
L4-L5 (L5 root)	Lateral, posterolateral aspect of thigh, leg	Lateral aspect of leg, dorsum of foot, first web space, great toe	Great toe extension, ankle dorsiflexion, heel walking difficult (footdrop may occur)	Minor (posterior tibial jerk depressed)
L5-S1 (S1 root)	Posterolateral aspect of thigh, leg, heel	Posterior aspect of calf, heel, lateral aspect of foot (3 toes)	Calf, plantar-flexion of foot, great toe; toe walking weak	Ankle jerk
Cauda equina syndrome (massive midline protrusion)	Low back, thigh, legs; often bilateral	Thighs, legs, feet, perineum; often bilateral	Variable; may be bowel, bladder incontinence	Ankle jerk (may be bilateral)

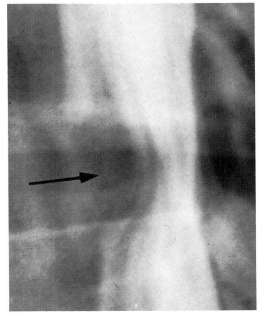

FIG 8–9.
Abnormal lumbar myelogram revealing a large extradural defect *(arrow)* in the dye column that is consistent with disc herniation.

complished only by strict, complete bed rest. Rest for 23 hours a day on a firm mattress is begun and continued for a minimum of 10 to 14 days. While the patient is in bed, the hips and knees are kept moderately flexed. Lying on the abdomen, which increases the lumbar lordosis, is avoided. Hip flexion and pelvic tilt exercises are begun within the limits of pain (Fig 8–10). Salicylates, analgesics, and moist heat are used as necessary. Although of questionable benefit, pelvic traction (10 to 15 kg), diathermy, and massage may be prescribed. If improvement occurs, which it does in the majority of cases, gradual resumption of ambulation is allowed. A lumbosacral corset may be temporarily used, but it is always best to encourage patients to develop their own musculature. The brace is discontinued as soon as possible. Recurrences are prevented by a proper exercise program and the avoidance of stress to the lower part of the back (Fig 8–11).

Caudal or epidural cortisone injections are occasionally used. They are somewhat controversial but may help relieve residual radicular pain. They have no effect on acute leg pain due to disc pressure. The condition of the majority of patients will improve with conservative treatment.

Disc removal is reserved for those patients

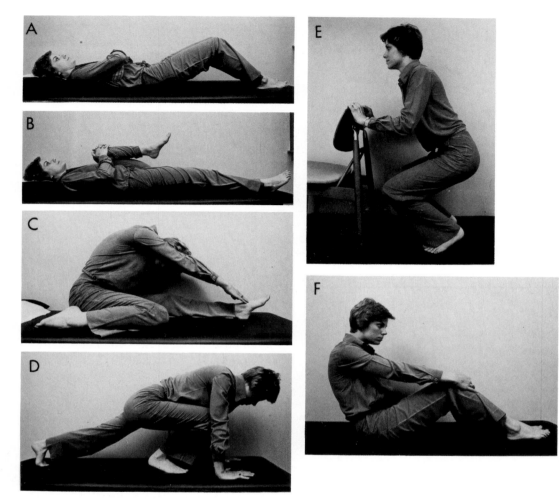

FIG 8–10.
Low back exercises. **A,** pelvic tilt performed to decrease the lumbar lordosis and raise the anterior aspect of the pelvis. The small of the back is pressed to the floor and the abdominal and buttock muscles are tightened. **B,** hip flexion, performed to stretch the tight posterior spinal musculature and unload the posterior disc. Each knee is drawn up and pulled firmly to the chest several times and held for 10 to 20 seconds. The exercise is then repeated with both knees. After the acute pain has subsided, the remainder of the exercises are performed: **C,** hamstring stretching exercises; **D,** hip flexor stretching exercises; **E,** quadriceps strengthening and heel cord stretching exercise; and **F,** abdominal strengthening exercise (sit-ups, which may be partial). All exercises are performed on a carpeted floor and should be repeated in sets of five to ten at least three times daily.

with major or progressing neurologic deficits or those with intractible leg pain who fail to respond to conservative management for at least 6 weeks. There are three general ways of removing disc tissue:

1. *Laminotomy* ("laminectomy"). The disc is removed through a small incision, and the nerve is explored under direct vision. A small portion of the lamina is sometimes removed for better visualization. With a positive history, physical find-

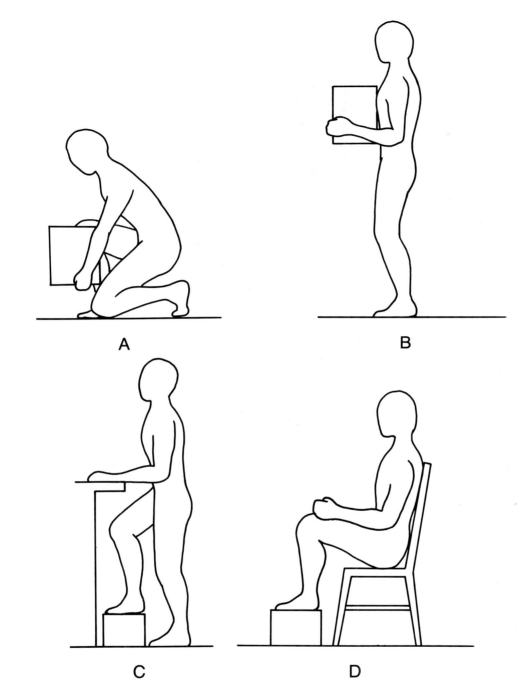

FIG 8–11.
General postural instructions. Patients should be instructed to do the following: **A,** bend the knees and hips and keep the back straight when lifting. **B,** hold objects close to the body when carrying. **C,** place one foot on a stool when standing. **D,** keep the knees higher than the hips when sitting, and keep the back straight when standing by "tucking in" the abdomen and tightening the buttocks to decrease swayback. In addition, they should avoid high-heeled shoes and sleeping on the abdomen, activities that increase lordosis.

ings, myelography (or similar study) and electro-myelography (EMG), there is a 90% to 95% success rate for surgery. In the absence of one or more of these, the cure rate for disc removal by any means declines considerably. Patients must also be cautioned that although their leg pain will usually disappear postoperatively, some mild intermittent low back pain may persist.

Microdiscectomy is the same procedure except that an operating microscope is used and the incision and surgical exposure are minimized. Advocates of this procedure note that there is less postoperative pain and a shorter hospital stay. A disadvantage to the procedure may be the narrower view afforded to the disc, nerve root, and adjacent bony structures.

2. *Automated percutaneous discectomy*. In this procedure, a small suction cutter is used to remove the disc. The instrument is placed through a cannula that has been passed through the flank to the posterolateral aspect of the disc under fluoroscopic control. It is performed through a very small incision, and no dissection or bone removal is needed. The disc is actually removed anterior to the herniation. Its success rate is 70% to 85%. One of the reasons for failure is that portions of the disc extruded or trapped in the spinal canal (or pressing on the nerve root) are never directly removed as they are with posterior surgery (laminectomy, microdiscectomy). An advantage is that the procedure has very few side effects and can often be performed under local anesthesia, which makes recovery very rapid.

3. *Chemonucleolysis*. In 1964, enzymatic dissolution of the nucleus pulposus was introduced for the treatment of a herniated lumbar disc. The procedure involves injecting the affected disc with chymopapain, a derivative of the papaya plant that digests the disc. It was developed partly because of its "noninvasive" nature and partly because of a relatively high rate of poor results in some series following traditional laminectomy and disc excision. Preliminary reports of its use appeared encouraging, but a double-blind study left its efficacy in doubt, and it was removed from general use in the United States. It

continued to be used in other countries and some centers in the United States and has recently been re-released.

Its main advantages are a shorter hospital stay and a short convalescence. The most common complication from the procedure is a relatively severe anaphylactoid reaction in aproximately 1% of the cases. Its main disadvantage is that the pathologic process being treated is never directly visualized and the patient with extruded disc material will certainly not benefit from its use.

Its success rate is about 75%. Enthusiasm for this procedure is waning, partly due to the complication rate and partly to the lower success rate. Like percutaneous discectomy, its "less invasive" nature also carries a greater risk of overuse.

Summary

If there is a large amount of posterior disc extrusion, an open posterior surgical approach is more advisable. This may be as often as 50% of the time. If not, all of the procedures discussed will probably give satisfactory results. The most important point then is not which procedure is chosen but, rather, which patient is selected for the procedure. Regardless of the method of management, the following facts are well known and should be kept in mind:

1. There is no long-term statistical difference in the outcome of most patients treated conservatively (by nature) and those treated surgically. The major benefit to surgery is that the intense pain in the leg is relieved sooner.

2. Disc removal by any means does not cure back pain, only leg pain.

3. Having sciatic nerve root pain does not assume surgery.

4. Before any procedure is contemplated, *radicular* symptoms should have been present for at least 6 weeks and should have failed to improve with at least 2 weeks of complete bed rest. If this rule is strictly followed, the majority of patients will get better on their own without surgery.

5. Cauda equina syndrome (back pain, bilateral sciatica, saddle anesthesia, motor weakness

sometimes with incontinence) is the only absolute indication for disc removal.

Chronic Lumbar Disc Disease

A high percentage of adults over the age of 40 years have degenerative disc disease at one or more levels on roentgenographic examination (Fig 8–12). Significant thinning of the disc accompanied by osteophyte formation is often present. These roentgenographic changes are common in the general population and are present in many asymptomatic individuals. Degenerative changes in the adjacent facet joints and surrounding soft tissues may, however, lead to intermittent low back pain and even nerve root irritation.

Chronic low back pain of this nature will usually respond to conservative management. Salicylates, rest, moist heat, and the use of a lumbosacral corset may be the only treatment necessary. Flexion exercises will correct associated muscular and postural problems. Occasional flare-ups are treated in the same manner. When signs of nerve root irritation with radicular pain are present, compression of the root by a small, acute, soft disc herniation or degenerative spur should be suspected. Surgical intervention is occasionally indicated to relieve nerve pressure under these circumstances. Arthrodesis of the adjacent vertebrae may rarely be indicated to relieve chronic low back pain by stabilizing the degenerated painful disc segment. Conservative treatment is usually successful in most cases, however.

The Facet Syndrome

The small articular facet joints of the spine have occasionally been implicated as a cause of

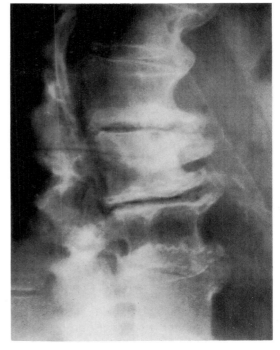

FIG 8–12.
Chronic degenerative disc disease in an adult with only minimal symptoms.

chronic low back pain. They may be affected due to disc thinning and even develop arthritis. The diagnosis is difficult to make, and some doubt its exsistence. The patient is often one who has a long history of chronic spine pain that has not responded to the traditional methods of management. Clinically, there may be local facet tenderness and pain on side bending.

In order to alleviate the symptoms, injection and even denervation of these joints has occasionally been performed. The results of these treatments are only modestly successful.

LUMBAR STRAIN

Muscular or ligamentous injury is a common cause of low back pain. It may follow single or multiple traumatic episodes. Incomplete muscular tears or ligament sprains occur and lead to pain and tenderness over the affected area. These injuries respond well to rest and symptomatic treatment over a 1- to 2-week period. When the injury is superimposed on a chronic pattern of low back pain or lumbar disc disease, the treatment is often more lengthy, however.

A variety of factors predispose to chronic repetitive low back strains. Obesity, poor muscular tone, faulty work habits, the wearing of high-heeled shoes, and the lack of a daily exercise program are among the contributing factors. Most of these cause the center of gravity of the body to be shifted forward, which leads to an increase in the lumbar lordosis. This places an added strain on the discs, ligaments, and muscles in order to maintain an upright posture. The condition is also frequently seen in teenagers who are vigorous weight lifters.

Obesity contributes to chronic low back pain in other ways. First, it is known that intra-abdominal pressure aids the erector spinae muscles in keeping the lumbar spine erect and decreases intradiscal pressure. Obese patients have poor abdominal muscular tone and thus do not benefit from this action. Obese patients also typically have an increase in their lumbar lordosis, which further adds stress to the lower part of the back.

With a daily program of proper postural exercises, weight loss, and a general exercise program, most patients with chronic back pain will be able to rehabilitate the lower part of the back. Full cooperation is necessary.

Note: The term *lumbar strain* is often used as a "wastebasket" diagnosis. An exact diagnosis of low back pain of this nature may be difficult. Muscle strain, ligament sprain, and mild early disc herniation or degeneration may all present with similar clinical findings. Regardless of the cause, the initial treatment is the same. A short (1 to 2 days) period of rest and mild analgesics followed by a gradual return to activities may be all that is needed. Walking or other similar aerobic exercise is started early to prevent generalized cardiovascular and musculoskeletal deterioration. Patients with chronic back pain may benefit from postural back exercises and correction of obesity. Relaxation techniques are sometimes helpful. Active participation by the patient is most important. Proper lifting and bending habits are stressed.

SPONDYLOLISTHESIS

Spondylolisthesis is a term applied to a disorder, usually in the lumbar spine, in which a gradual slipping of one vertebra on another occurs. Several types have been described (congenital, degenerative, pathologic, traumatic, and spondylolytic). Most spondylolisthesis, however, is secondary to spondylolysis, which represents a defect in the pars interarticularis or isthmus of the vertebra (Fig 8–13). This defect has a definite hereditary predisposition and usually becomes manifested as the result of repetitive stresses to the lower part of the back. It is often associated with lumbosacral anomalies such as transitional vertebrae. Spondylolisthesis is classified according to the amount of forward slippage of the affected vertebra (Fig 8–14).

Clinical Features

Spondylolysis may be symptomatic even without spondylolisthesis, and both conditions may be as-

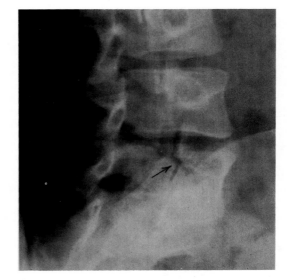

FIG 8–13.
Bony defect *(arrow)* in the isthmus or neck of the "Scottie dog" present in spondylolysis (oblique view).

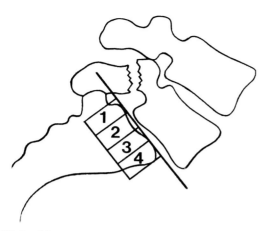

FIG 8—14.
Meyerding's classification of spondylolisthesis. The amount of slippage is graded 1 to 4. Grade 1 represents 25% forward displacement; grade 2, 25% to 50%; grade 3, 50% to 75%; and grade 4, greater than 75%.

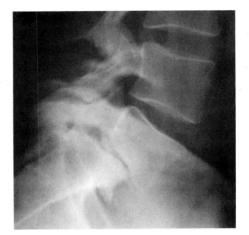

FIG 8—15.
Spondylolisthesis of the lumbosacral junction.

sociated with lumbar disc herniation. The disorder is often asymptomatic, however, and is frequently discovered incidentally on roentgenograms taken for other purposes. The symptoms usually begin gradually in the second or third decade. Low back pain, sometimes radiating into the buttocks, occurs with activity and is relieved by rest. Symptoms of nerve root irritation may also be present, along with radiation of the pain into the extremities. These symptoms often progress in severity, especially in the teenager.

Examination may reveal guarding of the lower part of the back and spasm of the paraspinal muscles. With moderate forward slippage, the lumbar lordosis appears increased, and the buttocks may appear more prominent. A palpable "step-off" in the spinous processes of the lumbar spine may be present. There is usually tenderness in the affected area and hamstring spasm.

Roentgenograms reveal the typical findings of a defect in the pars interarticularis, which may be accompanied by forward slippage (Fig 8—15).

Treatment

Management is usually conservative and consists of rest, weight loss, anti-inflammatory medication, and the use of a lumbosacral corset. Except for abdominal strengthening, back exercises are not advised and may even aggravate the condition. A change in occupation or work habits is sometimes indicated. The spondylolisthesis may increase in degree, but this is usually a gradual process. Progressive symptoms or intractable pain warrant surgical intervention. Decompression with spinal fusion is usually performed to stabilize the affected vertebra by arthrodesing it to the sacrum.

LUMBAR SPINE STENOSIS

Lumbar spinal stenosis is a syndrome in which narrowing of the lumbar spinal canal occurs; this

may lead to vague and unusual symptoms. The disorder occurs secondary to a combination of

disc degeneration, facet joint arthritis, and subluxation and occasionally to a congenitally small
spinal canal.

Clinical Features

The history is highly suggestive. Low back pain,
motor weakness, leg cramping (pseudoclaudica-
tion), and a sensation of "poor circulation" in the
extremities are typical. The patient is usually over
40 or 50 years of age. The symptoms are characteristically aggravated by walking and by extension of the lumbar spine. Improvement usually
occurs with rest or flexion of the back. These
symptoms are often misinterpreted as being vascular in origin. Sphincter disturbances and muscle atrophy may also be present.

Physical findings typical of disc herniation are
usually absent. Neurologic findings are also frequently minimal, and results of a straight-leg-raising test are usually normal. Pain on extension of
the lumbar spine may be severe.

Roentgenographic examination of the lumbar
spine usually reveals degenerative changes
throughout the lower part of the back. Electromyography and myelography may help localize
the disorder, and computerized axial tomography is frequently diagnostic (Fig 8–16). MRI is
also helpful.

Treatment

Treatment is directed at reducing the lumbar lordosis. A light corset is sometimes beneficial, as is
anti-inflammatory medication. Hip flexion and
abdominal strengthening may also be helpful.
Operative treatment consists of wide complete
decompression of the involved area. Spinal fusion may also be necessary.

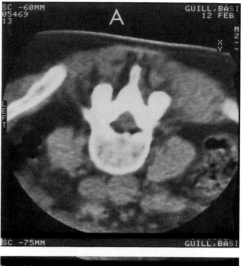

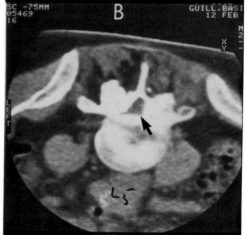

FIG 8–16.
Normal **(A)** and abnormal **(B)** computerized axial tomographic scans of the lumbar spine. Marked narrowing *(arrow)* is present in **B** due to hypertrophic spurring.

BACK PAIN IN THE WORKPLACE

Work-related low back pain is a growing problem in industrial societies, not only from a medical standpoint but also because of its legal and
socioeconomic aspects. Low back pain accounts
for as much as 25% to 30% of workers' compensation payments and the majority of long-term
disability cases.

A variety of terms have been used to describe
this condition, including "chronic benign industrial back pain," "compensation lumbago," and

chronic pain syndrome. This terminology partly reflects the difficulty in assigning a specific diagnosis and cause for the pain. A part of this difficulty, in turn, is due to the fact that low back pain in general and especially back pain in the workplace may be the result of a variety of biomechanical, biochemical, behavorial, socioeconomic, and psychophysiologic disorders.

Evaluation

An accurate history is especially important to determine whether an "injury" actually occurred or if the pain simply developed during or after a job. The pain may be referred to one or both legs, but it is usually not truly *radicular* in nature. Frequently, a description of the location and nature of the pain changes slightly from visit to visit.

Physical findings are often nonspecific. There is usually generalized low back tenderness and diminished range of motion. Often, the physical findings are "nonanatomic" in nature. There is usually no neurologic deficit, and sciatic tension tests are generally normal but often difficult to assess.

Special Studies

All of the anatomic structures of the lower part of the back (discs, ligaments, facet joints, bone, and muscle) can be the source of pain. The intervertebral disc is thought by many to be the source of most low back pain. Unfortunately, as many as 35% of asymptomatic adults will have abnormal findings on myelography, CT, or MRI that are usually related to the disc. This makes evaluation of this problem difficult, and it is felt by many that in the majority of these patients with work-related injuries, the exact underlying pathology probably cannot be determined.

Initially, a routine roentgenographic examination should be performed in 2 to 4 weeks if the patient does not improve, mainly to rule out any serious disorder. Further studies (EMG, CT, MRI, bone scan, myelography) should be performed only as adjuncts to the physical examination history. Subjecting these patients to further extensive testing in a "search" for the exact etiology of their pain is likely to be futile and is certainly costly. The same can be said for the various forms of instrumented back-testing devices. Diagnosing a spinal disorder solely on the basis of any of these tests should be avoided. It is rare that these special tests clearly demonstrate a source for the pain when it is not suspected clinically. In addition, any treatment (surgery, etc.) based solely on a special study will probably fail. In general, myelography and other special studies should be used only under the following circumstances: (1) if surgical disc removal is contemplated for intractable leg pain or a serious neurologic deficit or (2) if other serious spinal abnormality is suspected.

Treatment and Prognosis

Considerable controversy exists regarding the treatment of this problem. Historically, the disorder has always been resistant to traditional medical care. Thus, there has been a proliferation of rehabilitation services, pain centers, work-hardening programs, chiropractic care, and physical therapy services. Patients often prefer this type of "hands-on" treatment, but no scientific proof exists that any of these treatments are any better than nature's own. And while orthopedic and neurologic surgeons are commonly called on to assess and treat this condition, in fewer than 1% of these cases is surgery ever indicated (usually for leg pain associated with severe disc herniation) and not for at least 6 to 8 weeks. Surgery may even become a negative factor for returning the patient to work in that it gives "validity" to the injury.

Fortunately, the natural history of most back problems is that they improve and the end result of conservative management is usually good. Unfortunately, the longer the patient is off of work with benign low back pain, the less likely it is that the patient will ever return to gainful employment, and after 6 months of not working, the chance that the patient will return to *any* work is minimal. Thus, for a number of reasons, the trend for managing this condition has changed.

There has been a de-emphasis on the initial rest period and more encouragement to early exercise and returning to work on a limited basis. This trend has developed largely because of the low success rate with prolonged bed rest and the belief that it causes a deterioration of the musculoskeletal and cardiopulmonary systems. It has also been shown in limited studies that patients who begin exercise programs quickly after minor low back injuries have less pain and are disabled for shorter periods of time. (Only the patient with nerve root impingement due to disc herniation may require more rest). The following approach may be helpful.

1. Reassurance and education. Instructions should be given regarding proper body mechanics and lifting habits.
2. Bed rest for no more than a few days and mild analgesics followed by over-the-counter medication.
3. Temporarily avoid bending and lifting and use a chair with good lumbar support and armrests when sitting.
4. Begin a walking, biking, or swimming program as soon as possible. Back exercises are gradually added as tolerated.
5. Avoid the excessive use of passive treatment (massage, heat, etc.). Encourage active patient involvement, especially with the exercise program. Relaxation techniques may be helpful.
6. Encourage a return to work within the first 2 to 4 weeks (work activities may initially have to be modified).

Patients should be made to understand that the pain may recur if they resume light work, but it is usually not as severe as it is initially and does not mean any damage is occurring. It should not require further time off from work. The patient should continue the exercise program and practice good body mechanics. (A formal education program may be necessary). Active participation by the patient and compliance are extremely important.

If no improvement has occurred in 4 to 6 weeks, referral to a specialist is indicated. Psychosocial factors and work-related conditions may also need investigation. The attitude of the patient to the job and involvement of the employer also play important roles in the length of disability. Workers who like their jobs and employers who promote a good working environment are more likely to have a mutually satisfactory relationship.

THORACIC DISC DISEASE

Symptomatic disc degeneration in the dorsal spine is uncommon. The cause is often traumatic. The most serious sequela of thoracic disc disease is acute or progressive spinal cord compression from central disc herniation. Progressive paralysis is not uncommon. Unilateral nerve root compression from lateral herniation also occurs.

Clinical Features

Dorsal spine pain occurs in most cases. With central herniation, gradually increasing motor weakness in the lower extremities becomes apparent. Sphincter control may be lost, and diffuse numbness is common. Examination usually reveals limited motion in the dorsal spine with spasm. Major neurologic deficits may be present in the lower extremities.

Roentgenographic examination often reveals calcification, narrowing, and spondylosis in the dorsal spine. Myelography may reveal a complete block in central lesions.

Treatment

The treatment is surgical in central lesions. Early cases may respond favorably, but late surgery is of limited value, and residual paralysis is not uncommon.

SCOLIOSIS

By definition, scoliosis is a lateral curvature of the spine in the upright position. The lateral curvature is usually accompanied by some rotational deformity. Scoliosis may be classified as either structural or nonstructural. Structural curves are fixed and nonflexible and fail to correct with side bending. Nonstructural curves, on the other hand, are flexible and readily correct with side bending.

Nonstructural scoliosis is frequently seen as a compensatory mechanism secondary to a leg length discrepancy, local inflammation, or irritation from acute lumbar disc disease. This type of scoliosis tends to disappear when the offending disorder is corrected.

Structural scoliosis may occur from a variety of causes. Congenital abnormalities in the spine with anomalous vertebral formation may lead to asymmetric growth and result in scoliosis. Neurofibromatosis and a variety of neurologic and myopathic conditions may also lead to structural scoliosis. The most common type, however, has no known cause and is usually termed "idiopathic."

Idiopathic scoliosis accounts for approximately 90% of all scoliosis. It appears to represent a hereditary disorder, but the exact mechanism of its production is unknown.

Clinical Features

Genetic or idiopathic scoliosis usually appears clinically between the ages of 10 and 13 years but may be seen at any age. It is more common in females, and serious curvatures are also more frequent in females. In young people, the disease is usually asymptomatic, and subjective complaints are absent. Many cases are diagnosed by nurses in screening clinics or by other family members.

The diagnosis is usually made on routine

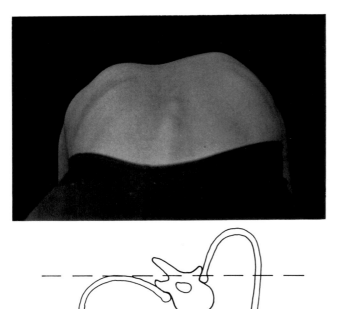

FIG 8–17.
Top, scoliosis with rib prominence due to vertebral rotation best exhibited on forward bending. *Bottom,* cross section of the chest showing rib distortion due to vertebral rotation.

physical examination. Attention should be focused on the problem in all children, but especially in those between the ages of 10 and 14 years, when spinal growth is most rapid. For the examination, the patient should be undressed to the waist or wear a bathing suit, and a routine should be followed. The shoulders and iliac crests are inspected to determine whether they are level. The scapulae, rib cage, and flanks are then observed for symmetry. The spinous processes are palpated to determine their alignment. The patient is then asked to bend symmetrically forward at the waist with the arms hanging free (Fig 8–17). Observation from the back or front will detect the spinal rotation in the form of a rib hump or abnormal paraspinal muscular prominence.

The diagnosis is confirmed by a standing roentgenogram of the spine (Fig 8–18). There is no other method of determining the severity of the curve, and a patient should never leave the office without an accurate roentgenographic measurement of the curvature. The roentgenogram may have to be repeated at intervals in order to determine whether or not the curve is progressive.

Natural History

While it is impossible to accurately predict the outcome of most curves, the following facts are known about scoliosis:

1. Curves under 20 degrees will improve spontaneously over 50% of the time for unknown reasons.
2. There is no accurate method of predicting which curves will get better and which will get worse.
3. Twenty percent of curves under 30 degrees will progress.
4. Progression is more common in young children who are beginning their growth spurt.
5. The larger the curve at detection, the greater the chance of progression.

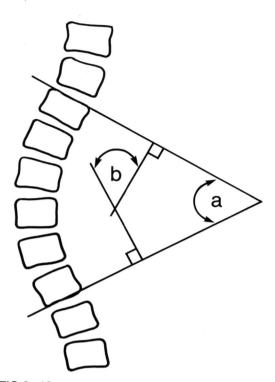

FIG 8–18.
Cobb method of measuring the severity of a curve. The upper and lower end vertebrae are identified. The upper end vertebra is the highest one whose superior border converges toward the concavity of the curve, and the lower end vertebra is the one whose inferior border converges toward the concavity. Lines are drawn along these borders, and the curve is measured directly (a) or geometrically (b).

6. Curves in females and double curves are more likely to progress.

Treatment

The most important aspect in treatment is early detection. A curve that is obviously present when the patient is standing is often already approaching 30 to 40 degrees. Detecting a curve before it reaches 20 degrees is of utmost importance because curves over 20 degrees tend to progress. Prompt referral of all scoliosis patients to a specialist is mandatory. Frequent re-examinations are essential while the child is at an age where progression is common. The failure to diagnose or treat this problem early may result in progressive deformity, pain, cardiopulmonary compromise, and disability. Early discovery and treatment can prevent this progression.

The treatment depends on the age of the patient and the severity of the curve (Table 8–2). In the immature patient, frequent observation is necessary until the curve reaches 20 degrees. Curvatures over 20 degrees require treatment. The curve can be stabilized and, in many cases, improved by spinal bracing. The Milwaukee brace or thoracolumbosacral orthotic (TLSO) are commonly used for this purpose (Fig 8–19). Treatment in the brace is continuous for 23 hours a day, and the brace may have to be worn for 2 years or longer. Exercises are performed in the brace in order to improve the cosmetic appearance and decrease the curvature. Exercises alone will effect no change in the curvature, nor will they prevent any progression without the brace. Excellent results are obtained with proper use of the brace in curvatures between 20 and 40 degrees. It will not fully correct the curve, but it will usually prevent progression to the stage where spinal surgery is necessary.

TABLE 8–2.
Algorithm for Decision Making for Genetic Scoliosis in the Growing Child

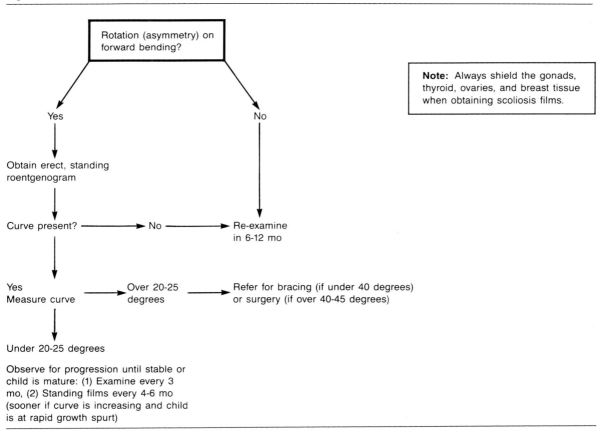

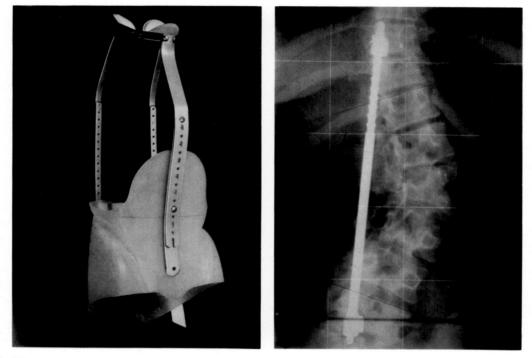

FIG 8–19.
Left, the Milwaukee brace. *Right*, postoperative roentgenogram following instrumentation and spinal fusion for scoliosis.

Surgery is generally reserved for those cases that are over 40 to 45 degrees. Correction of the curvature by intraoperative instrumentation and maintenance of the correction by spinal fusion along the entire length of the curve are usually performed. This may be preceded by corrective casts or traction. Postoperatively, a cast or brace is worn for 6 to 12 months until the fusion mass is solid.

In the adult patient, the spinal deformity may progress and eventually become painful. This is especially true of curves over 40 to 50 degrees. Occasionally, instrumentation and spinal fusion may also be indicated in these cases.

KYPHOSIS

Curvature of the spine in the anteroposterior direction in which the convexity is directed posteriorly is termed *kyphosis.* This curvature exists in the normal spine at the thoracic and sacral regions. Abnormal thoracic angulation can occur from several pathologic states. Diseases of the discs and vertebral bodies are the most common causes. Congenital kyphosis is rare and is usually secondary to a localized malformation of the spine.

Senile Kyphosis

Senile kyphosis results from multiple areas of disc degeneration at the thoracic level. It is relatively common in the elderly patient and may be

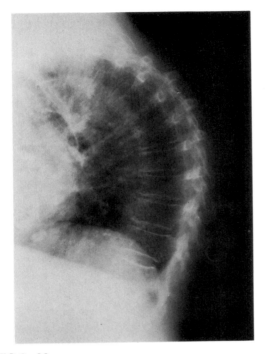

FIG 8–20.
Roentgenogram of an elderly patient with senile kyphosis.

symptomatic. Roentgenograms will often reveal thinning of the discs and osteoporosis with mild wedging deformities (Fig 8–20).

Treatment is directed toward maintaining good posture. Exercises that strengthen the back and abdominal muscles are often helpful. The use of a light spinal brace will frequently relieve the symptoms.

Postural Round Back

Faulty posture is common in adolescents and young children. It probably occurs as a result of minor muscular imbalances and weakness. The typical picture is one in which the patient, often a teenager, shows an increase in the normal dorsal kyphosis, lumbar lordosis, and an increased pelvic inclination. The shoulders are often rounded and drooped, and the abdomen may be protuberant. The scapulae are frequently prominent. The kyphosis is typically supple in contrast to the nonflexible, fixed kyphosis in Scheuermann's disease.

Roentgenograms of the dorsal spine are usu-

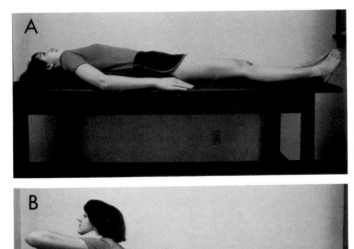

FIG 8–21.
Exercises for postural round back. **A,** the resting position with a pillow under the dorsal spine.
B, scapular adduction and thoracic hyperextension exercise that stretches the pectoral muscles and contracted anterior soft tissues. In addition, the low back exercises previously described are performed to correct excessive lumbar lordosis.

ally unremarkable. No wedging or end-plate irregularities tend to be present.

After ruling out other causes of kyphosis, the patient is started on an exercise program to overcome contractures and decrease the lumbar lordosis (Fig 8–21). The disorder usually responds well to the exercises.

Scheuermann's Disease

Scheuermann's kyphosis is a *fixed* kyphosis that develops near the time of puberty. The cause is unknown, but the deformity is caused by typical wedging abnormalities in the dorsal and dorsolumbar spine that result in a decrease in the anterior height of the vertebrae. Mild forms may clinically resemble postural round back.

Clinical Features

Poor posture is a common complaint, and fatigue and pain usually accompany the deformity. The family history is often positive.

Examination reveals an increase in the normal kyphosis of the dorsal spine that is usually associated with local tenderness. There may be tightness of the hamstring, pectoral, and iliopsoas muscles. In contrast to postural round back, this kyphosis is usually fixed. The abdomen may be protuberant, and there is usually an increase in the lumbar lordosis. The results of neurologic examination are usually normal.

A positive diagnosis is possible only with a roentgenographic examination. Wedging of the vertebrae, irregularity of the end plates and typical Schmorl's nodules are seen on the lateral view, usually between T2 and T12 (Fig 8–22). Synostoses and osteophyte formation are not uncommon in the adult patient.

Treatment

Conservative treatment consisting of a Milwaukee brace and postural exercises will usually result in a cure. The brace is worn for approximately 1

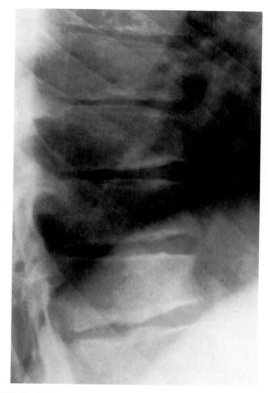

FIG 8–22.
Roentgenogram of Scheuermann's disease. End-plate irregularities and mild wedging deformities are present.

year full time and is used at night for an additional year. Hamstring stretching and pelvic tilt exercises are initiated. Severe deformity with pain or neurologic symptoms are indications for surgery at any age. The surgery is similar to that performed for scoliosis.

Long-term results of conservative treatment are generally favorable when the disease is confined to the dorsal spine. There is an increased incidence of back pain with curves that are low in the dorsal spine or upper lumbar spine. The working capacity for the patient is usually not affected, however.

DISCITIS

Discitis is an infectious or inflammatory disease of unknown cause. An infectious basis is strongly suggested. The process most commonly occurs in the midlumbar spine of children about the age of 6 years. A history of trauma or infection elsewhere may be present.

Clinical Features

The symptoms consist of low back pain that often radiates into the abdomen or lower extremities. The child has difficulty walking and standing and may even refuse to walk or sit at all. A slight limp may be present.

Examination reveals restriction of motion in the lumbar spine in association with hamstring spasm and a flattening of the normal lumbar lordosis. Local tenderness in the midlumbar region is usually present. The child is often irritable and may run a low-grade fever. Nausea and vomiting occasionally occur.

There is a positive blood culture in approximately 50% of patients, and the organism is usually *Staphylococcus*. Needle aspiration of the affected disc will sometimes reveal the same organism. There is usually an increase in the sedimentation rate and white blood cell (WBC) count. The bone scan is usually abnormal, and plain roentgenograms frequently reveal single disc space narrowing with irregularity of the adjacent end plates. Eventually, fusion may even occur between the involved vertebrae.

Treatment

Treatment consists of antibiotics, bed rest, and the application of a body cast. Treatment is continued until the systemic signs of infection, such as the sedimentation rate, temperature, and WBC count, are normal. The prognosis is usually good.

LUMBOSACRAL ANOMALIES

A variety of minor congenital abnormalities may exist in the lumbar spine and at the lumbosacral junction. The majority of these occur at the lumbosacral region, and most are asymptomatic.

Facet joint asymmetry, variations in the number of lumbar vertebrae, spina bifida occulta, and transitional lumbosacral vertebrae are among the more common anomalies seen on routine roent-

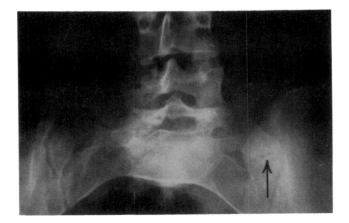

FIG 8–23.
Transitional lumbosacral vertebra. A false joint is present *(arrow)*.

genograms. Only the transitional vertebra appears to be related to low back pain.

The transitional vertebra (lumbarized S1 or sacralized L5) may produce pain at the false joint that forms at the articulation between its elongated transverse process and the sacrum (Fig 8–23). The disc between this vertebra and the sacrum is usually markedly thinned but is rarely the cause of symptoms. The treatment is usually conservative. A lumbosacral corset may be beneficial by restricting motion at this area.

In general, congenital anomalies of the spine in the pediatric age group are seldom causes of back pain. Spina bifida occulta is seldom, if ever a cause of back pain in this age group. Inspection of the back is extremely important to at least identify other congenital anomalies that may have significant neurologic deficits associated with them, such as Faun's beard, which is a doughy, fatty mass in the midline of the back, sometimes covered by excessive hair. This is good evidence for a lipoma that may extend to the spinal cord and produce neurologic symptoms.

MEDICAL CAUSES OF BACK PAIN

Back pain is not only common but may have a number of nonorthopedic causes. It is the purpose of this section to deal with those causes of back pain that are other than musculoskeletal in origin and that may have a relationship to systemic disease.

History

As with all disorders in medicine, an accurate and complete recorded history must be obtained and is of particular importance for those patients presenting with low back pain. A complete history and physical examination may not be possible on the initial visit, but nonmusculoskeletal causes for the back pain must always be kept in mind. The history should proceed in a standard, orderly fashion and include those areas of systemic symptoms that may be related to the patient's chief complaint. There are many history forms available that have been developed to save time, but they should not supplant the one-on-one taking of the history.

Chief Complaint/History of the Present Illness
The history should designate the time of onset of the problem and any associated circumstances as well as previous history of back pain, whether similar or not. The onset of the pain should be coordinated with the type of pain and its relationship to activity or rest. Its response to medication is recorded. The description of the pain, its point of maximum intensity, and areas of radiation should be documented. The change in the patient's ability to take part in work or sports should also be noted. In females, the relationship of the pain to the patient's age, menstrual cycle, and obstetric history is helpful, especially if there was any trauma involved (such as in forceps or breech deliveries or multiple gestations).

Past History/System Review
General systemic symptoms should be sought, especially weight loss, malaise, and fever. Any previous injuries or surgery (especially for cancer) should be recorded. The status of the gastrointestinal and genitourinary systems should be evaluated. Present medications and their doses are recorded. Skin disorders should be assessed, particularly if they suggest psoriasis or collagen vascular disease. Previous hospitalizations and/or procedures such as myelography are noted.

Finally, psychological or socioeconomic factors should be recorded and any positive responses developed as to their relationship to the chief complaint.

Physical Examination

Because the physician is looking for other than musculoskeletal causes for the back pain, the examination must be complete with the patient undressed.

General

Age, height, and weight are recorded, and the patient is observed for general appearance, coordination, and gait. The physician should look for asynchronous arm swing. The skin should be examined not only regarding pallor, clubbing, or cyanosis but also for any diagnostic rashes.

Chest, Heart, and Lungs

Examination of the heart should include auscultation for murmurs, especially that of aortic insufficiency, which may be seen in ankylosing spondylitis. Examination of the lungs should include auscultation for wheezes, especially localized ones, which could suggest tumor obstruction. Diaphragmatic excursion is evaluated for possible air trapping. Diminished excursion may also be due to ankylosing spondylitis, which results in a decrease in chest expansion to less than 2.5 cm. (The average male's expansion is over 5.0 cm.) In addition to measuring chest expansion, the external evaluation should include a breast examination.

Abdomen and Pelvis

Examination should include palpation for aneurysm, hepatomegaly, and/or splenomegaly. Any areas of tenderness are noted, and a rectal examination of the prostate is always included. Evaluation of women should include pelvic and rectal examinations with a Papanicolaou smear, Thayer-Martin culture if indicated and bimanual examination for full evaluation of both tubes and ovaries and rectal shelf area. The external genitalia are always examined, and the rectal examination should include guaiac testing of the stool.

Back and Extremities

The patient is observed getting in and out of a chair and walking across the room. The back is inspected for atrophy, spasm, scoliosis, and masses. The hips and back are examined for range of motion. If the normal lordosis increases with forward flexion, a functional disorder should be suspected. The back, pelvis, and hips are palpated for point tenderness. The peripheral pulses are also evaluated.

A neurologic examination including Babinski tests and tendon reflexes is then performed (Fig 8–24). Since the majority of lumbosacral disc disease takes place at the L5 or S1 level, examination of the Achilles tendon reflex and extensor hallucis longus muscle function is critical in low back examination and in determining the cause of pain in the patient. Examination of the reflexes to show hyperactivity may indicate an intraspinous lesion such as a metastatic lesion in the cord area. Sensory deficits should be tested, but these are sometimes difficult to evaluate because of the patient's subjective assessment of this particular examination. However, the findings of lower extremity numbness, evidence for neurologic deficit in testing the pinprick, and the light touch in the perianal area and the patient's history of incontinence should suggest the possibility of spinal cord compression.

Ankylosing Spondylitis

Ankylosing spondylitis is a chronic inflammatory condition of the joints of the axial skeleton that characteristically manifests itself by morning stiffness in the low back and progressive loss of spinal movement. The disorder is more common in men and is frequently familial. The sacroiliac and spinal apophyseal joints are usually involved first, and the disorder commonly has its onset between the ages of 15 and 30 years. The disorder is also known as Marie-Strümpell disease.

An early diagnosis is often difficult due to the insidious onset of the disease. The pain is usually located low in the buttocks and thigh region but rarely radiates into the hip, calf, or foot. Often the disease is mild, and there may be few systemic symptoms; however, in a severe form, fatigue, weight loss, anorexia, fever, and other systemic complaints may accompany the onset. Even though peripheral joint involvement may be present before the development of pain in the sacroiliac region, the diagnosis can only be presumptive until the sacroiliac joints are involved

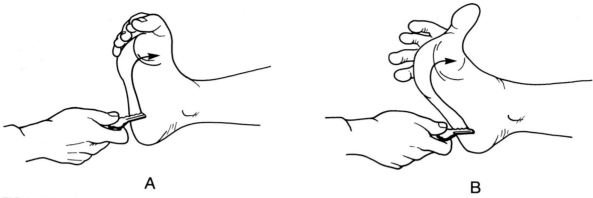

A   B

FIG 8–24.
Babinski test. A sharp instrument is lightly scraped along the plantar aspect of the foot from the calcaneus along the outer border. The leg should be relaxed. If the ankle dorsiflexes or the foot withdraws, reduce the intensity of the stimulus. In a negative response **(A),** the toes bunch together or do not move. An abnormal response **(B)** includes extension of the great toe while the other toes may splay and flex. The Babinski test is normally positive in the newborn but disappears soon after birth. An abnormal response indicates an upper motor neuron lesion. The response may be absent, however, if there is damage to the reflex arc at the nerve or root level.

to such a degree as to be demonstrated roentgenographically. Although this disease is more common in men, women who have ulcerative colitis have an extremely high incidence of developing this disorder.

Clinical Signs
Clinical signs include bilateral sacroiliac tenderness and limited motion of the lumbar spine. An important physical finding is the loss of chest expansion to under 2.5 cm because of rib cage involvement, and this can be easily checked by measuring chest expansion at the nipple line before and after deep inspiration.

Virtually any of the other joints of the skeleton may be involved, but most commonly the hips, shoulders, knees, wrists, metacarpophalangeal, and metatarsophalangeal are the secondary joints usually seen. When there is involvement of the hips and shoulders, permanent damage may develop, but in the other joints the process often resolves without any residual disability or deformity, and this is similar to the arthritis that may be seen with inflammatory bowel disease.

Usually no skin lesions occur with ankylosing spondylitis, but an anterior uveitis occurs in approximately 25% of the patients. There is usually no urethritis that helps distinguish it from Reiter's syndrome.

Roentgenographic Findings
The early roentgenographic features are usually those of bilateral sacroiliitis. Initially, there are erosions of these joints, and they lose their clearcut demarcation because of cystic changes and subchondral sclerosis. The vertebral bodies may also become demineralized, and a typical squaring of the anterior vertebral bodies develops. Apophyseal joint irregularities and paraspinal ligamentous calcifications develop later, and eventually there may be complete fusion of the sacroiliac and hip joints as healing takes place following the inflammation. As the disease progresses, calcifications of the anulus fibrosis and paravertebral ligaments develop, which give rise to the so-called bamboo-spine appearance characteristic of ankylosing spondylitis (Fig 8–25).

Laboratory Findings
The current availability of the HLA-B27 system is important in the diagnosis of ankylosing spondylitis. This antigen occurs in nearly 100%

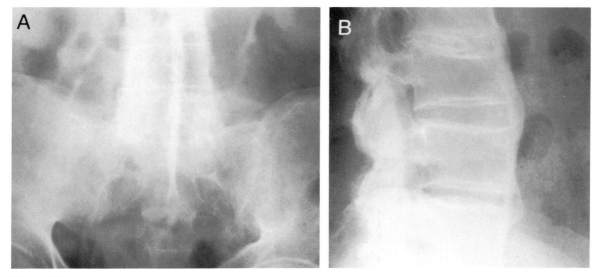

FIG 8–25.
Ankylosing spondylitis. On the anteroposterior view **(A),** the sacro-iliac (SI) joints and the lumbar spine are fused. **B,** a lateral view shows the typical bamboo-spine appearance.

of white patients with ankylosing spondylitis, and the test may provide a useful method to screen those patients with either a familial history of the disease or low back pain suggestive of the disorder.

Other laboratory findings suggestive of the disorder include an elevated sedimentation rate, mild hypochromic anemia, elevation of the level of cerebrospinal fluid (CSF) protein, the presence of IgG antiglobulins, and an elevated creatinine phosphokinase level in the serum.

Extraskeletal Manifestations

The extraskeletal manifestations are those of uveitis, aortic insufficiency, and apical pulmonary fibrosis. Because this is a chronic disease, the development of secondary amyloidosis is not uncommon and should be considered in those patients in whom chronic renal disease develops. Another late but uncommon manifestation of ankylosing spondylitis occurs with the involvement of the cauda equina; the patient may present with incontinence of urine, pain, and sensory loss in the sacral nerve distribution.

Differential Diagnosis

The differential diagnosis of ankylosing spondylitis includes (1) psoriatic arthritis, (2) Reiter's syndrome, (3) arthritis associated with chronic inflammatory bowel disease, and (4) rheumatoid arthritis. *Psoriatic arthropathy,* although similar, usually has late involvement of the sacroiliac joints, involves both the small and the large joints, particularly of the upper extremity, and has very specific skin lesions associated with it. Although aortitis may occur in psoriatic arthropathy, urethritis is absent, as is pulmonary fibrosis.

Reiter's syndrome is similiar to psoriatic arthropathy in that sacroiliac joint involvement usually occurs late. The small and large joints, particularly of the lower extremity, are affected, and skin lesions are usually specific. Uveitis may occur, and urethritis is present at least at some point in the illness. Aortitis may occur, but pulmonary fibrosis has not been reported.

The arthritis associated with *inflammatory bowel disease* usually involves the large joints, particularly hips and shoulders, and sacroiliitis may be present early in the illness. Skin manifestations may be nonspecific or pathognomonic. In the patient with chronic ulcerative colitis, the skin lesion of pyodermic gangrenosum is at least very suggestive of the chronic underlying illness. In chronic inflammatory bowel disease, uveitis may occur but is uncommon. Urethritis is usually not present, and aortitis is rare.

Rheumatoid arthritis usually affects the peripheral joints and is more common in females. The tenosynovium and bursae are also frequently involved with the inflammatory process. It rarely affects the axial skeleton.

Treatment

1. Medication. In general, the drugs utilized in the treatment are all anti-inflammatory agents. The salicylates should be tried first since these are the least expensive and may offer dramatic relief.

2. Exercise. Next to drug therapy, exercise is the most important aspect of care. Swimming, general sports activities, and maintenance of ideal body weight are all important.

3. Postural training is especially important. Patients must be instructed to avoid stooping and to sit in an erect position. Otherwise, a flexion contracture of the spine may develop and cause the patient to be unable to look straight forward. The chair should have a hard, straight back and seat. Sleeping should be in the supine position on a firm mattress, and pillows should not be placed under the head or knees.

4. Surgery. Despite optimal management, the disease may progress to irreversible deformities of the spine and hips. Surgical techniques are available to correct the flexion deformity of the spine, and hip replacement is used for relief of the chronic hip pain. Re-ankylosis may occur following hip surgery, and the decision to undergo hip arthroplasty must be made with this possibility in mind.

Prognosis

Early diagnosis, good long-term management, frequent follow-up examinations (including help-ing the patient understand the disease), exercise, and the appropriate medications will usually provide the patient with a normal life span. Death may occur as a result of the development of aortic insufficiency or secondary amyloidosis with chronic renal disease. If valvular disease develops, the patient should be educated as to the use of prophylactic antibiotics to prevent subacute bacterial endocarditis. The usual course of the disease is not life-threatening, however, and a relatively normal life-style and work load are generally possible.

Multiple Myeloma

This disorder, sometimes called plasma cell myeloma, is a neoplastic proliferation of the plasma cell of the bone marrow. It may present as a systemic process or, less commonly, as a "solitary" lesion. Multiple myeloma is found in increasing incidence in patients over 40 years of age, and men are affected twice as often as women. It is usually associated with a rise in serum globulin content, often due to abnormal globulins. It is the most common primary tumor of bone.

Clinical Features

The early manifestations of the disorder are weakness, anorexia, weight loss, and bone pain. The majority of patients present initially with back pain. Commonly, this leads to the detection of a destructive skeletal lesion. As the disease progresses, other organ systems become involved and result in more bone pain, anemia, renal insufficiency, and/or bacterial infections. The infections, often recurrent bouts of pneumonia or urinary tract infection, are usually due to the dysproteinemia. They are often pneumococcal in origin and are apparently related to the patient's inability to synthesize normal amounts of specific antibody in response to the bacterial challenge.

Secondary amyloidosis is also sometimes associated with the disorder. Amyloid deposition may be manifested in several patterns. Involvement of the heart or kidney may lead to cardiac failure or nephrotic syndrome.

Roentgenographic Features

The classic finding is the "punched-out" lesion with sharply demarcated edges (Fig 8–26). Usually, multiple lesions are found, but in 10%, only a single skeletal defect may be present. Diffuse osteoporosis due to generalized demineralization is the only finding in about 25% of cases. The typical lesions may occur in any part of the skeleton but are most common in the spine, skull, ribs, and pelvis. Pathologic fractures are common. Intervertebral body collapse may result in nerve root or cord compression. Diffuse bony involvement may even result in hypercalcemia.

Using the bone scan to assess the disorder is helpful, but a negative scan can be misleading. This tumor is often "cold" on a bone scan due to its rapid destruction. Plain films are often better for evaluation.

Laboratory Findings

In approximately half of the cases, the urine contains the Bence Jones protein, which has the

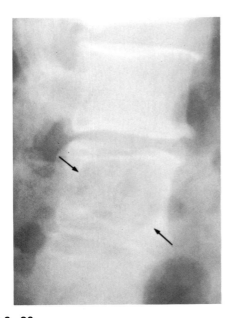

FIG 8–26.
Multiple myeloma *(arrows)*. (This patient had a normal bone scan.)

unique property of precipitating in an acid pH when the temperature is between 4.4 and 15.6°C and redissolving when the temperature is 32.2° C. Anemia is often present, and the sedimentation rate is usually elevated. Serum protein electrophoresis usually displays the characteristic dysproteinemia. The serum calcium concentration is occasionally elevated, but the alkaline phosphatase level is usually normal.

Treatment and Prognosis

Since patients with multiple myeloma may have hypercalcemia, hypercalciuria, and hyperuricemia, the importance of ambulation and adequate hydration in their treatment cannot be overstressed. Every effort should be made not to immobilize the patient and allow him to become bedridden with pain. Since plasma cell tumors are characteristically radiosensitive, x-ray therapy has been shown to be of extreme help in the control of localized symptomatic lesions. Of the therapeutic drugs presently available, melphalan (Alkeran), cyclophosphamide (Cytoxan), and prednisone are the most useful for long-term treatment. An oncologist should be consulted since the treatment of these patients is long term and requires the expertise of more than one physician. Recently it has been shown that in a few patients who become refractory to continuous melphalan or cyclophosphamide therapy, some remissions have been achieved with a combination of cyclophosphamide and doxorubicin (Adriamycin). The physician can measure response to chemotherapy by objective signs of improvement, including decrease in concentration of abnormal M-type serum globulins, decreased Bence Jones proteinuria, hematologic improvement of the anemia, and cessation of further skeletal destruction.

The prognosis remains poor, even with newer therapies such as α-interferon. Complete remissions are uncommon. Most patients succumb after a median of 3 years, although a small percentage will survive 10 years. At present, no treatment is curative.

Osteoporosis

Osteoporosis is the most commonly seen metabolic disease in the United States. It is almost universally found in the elderly and, like atherosclerosis, develops slowly over a period of many years.

By definition, osteoporosis is a disorder of the skeleton in which the total skeletal mass is decreased. The shape, composition, and structure of the bone are normal. It is one of the conditions commonly classified as "osteopenias," the others being osteomalacia, endocrine disorders (such as hyperparathyroidism, cortisone overuse), and marrow-packing conditions (such as multiple myeloma and leukemia).

Etiology

There are many relatively uncommon types of osteopenia. Lack of activity and immobilization may result in osteoporosis. In elderly patients, intestinal lactase deficiency may also be associated with osteoporosis. Osteoporosis may also occur with developmental disturbances such as osteogenesis imperfecta or nutritional disturbances such as a lack of protein or vitamin C. Endocrine disorders such as hypopituitarism, acromegaly, thyrotoxicosis, Cushing's disease, and long-standing diabetes may also be causes of osteoporosis.

The most common types of osteoporosis are postmenopausal and "senile." There is often some overlap between these two disorders. The postmenopausal type is also the most common symptomatic form of osteoporosis. This disorder becomes increasingly more frequent with age, and recent estimates are that approximately 18 million women in the United States will have a significant degree of vertebral atrophy and that approximately 2 million will have asymptomatic fractures of the dorsal and lumbar vertebra. Based on these findings, it is estimated that approximately 1 million fractures will be experienced by women over the age of 45 years on a yearly basis and, of these, 75% will have osteoporosis as the underlying problem. The disorder is relatively uncommon among black men of any age, and black women seem to be less vulnerable than white women. The actual causes for postmenopausal and senile osteoporosis are unknown. Bone destruction seems to increase due to the loss of estrogen restraint on bone breakdown. It is known that pregnancy, the use of contraceptives, and the use of postmenopausal estrogens lead to less osteoporosis. It is also known that normal women have a decreasing bone mass after the age of 20 years that may be due to a poor dietary intake of calcium.

Clinical Features

The disease is often insidious in its onset. Spontaneous fractures, vertebral collapse, and osteoporosis are often discovered as incidental findings on roentgenograms (Fig 8–27).

Symptomatic vertebral fractures may cause nonradicular midline pain. Loss of overall body height is common. A characteristic dorsal kyphotic vertebral deformity, called dowager's hump, is often present. Local tenderness will

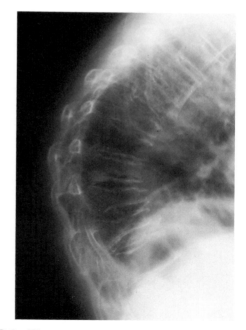

FIG 8–27.
Osteoporosis. Multiple compression fractures are present.

usually accompany an acute compression fracture.

The results of laboratory analysis are usually normal. Urinary calcium levels may be slightly increased early in the disorder due to increased breakdown of bone.

There have been many investigative techniques proposed to diagnose this generalized demineralization of bone, including attempts at direct measurement of vertebral demineralization and calcium balance studies. Often, the definite diagnosis of osteoporosis is still made by finding advanced disease or inferred by the presence of fractures of the vertebral bodies with a history of minimal trauma.

A particularly interesting form of regional osteoporosis is so-called *Sudeck's atrophy,* a form of reflex sympathetic dystrophy that is commonly found in the hands and feet. This particular type of localized osteoporosis is characterized by atrophic, glossy, tight skin with swelling, tenderness, and sweating over the affected area. Usually this disease is self-limited, but at times, stellate ganglion sympathetic blocks or the use of corticosteroids are often necessary.

Roentgenographic Findings

The previously mentioned dorsal kyphotic vertebral deformity may often be present. Roentgenograms may also show areas of demineralization in the spine and pelvis. This is usually less marked in the skull and long bones. Typically, there is a loss of the horizontal trabeculae of the vertebral bodies and prominence of the end plates. The discs may bulge into the adjacent vertebrae. There are usually no osteophytes or cortical erosions. In particular, pathologic changes in osteoporosis lead to a wedge-type deformity, and importantly, the apex of the wedge fracture is anterior (posterior wedging should suggest a different disease such as Paget's disease, trauma, or metastatic malignancy).

Treatment

Just as the cause of osteoporosis remains unknown, there is also uncertainty regarding its prevention and treatment. Among the currently available therapeutic measures are the following:

1. Exercise. Although there is no clear evidence regarding the role of exercise in the prevention or treatment of osteoporosis, it is reasonable to include a regular *weight-bearing* program. General conditioning regimens, especially those designed to develop better body mechanics, may be useful in that they may improve balance and thus decrease the chance of falling.

2. General nutrition. If the patient's dietary intake is inadequate, calcium (1 to 1.5 g/day) and vitamin D (400 to 800 IU/day) should be added. This is as important in the premenopausal female as it is in the older individual, and an accurate dietary history is therefore important. The diet should also contain adequate protein.

3. Estrogen. Hormone therapy has been proved to be the most effective means of preserving bone mass and decreasing fracture rates. It is usually started at menopause but may still be effective if begun as late as 10 to 15 years after menopause. The duration of therapy is unknown, but 10 years seems appropriate.

Estrogen therapy has a number of risks as well as other benefits. Endometrial carcinoma is one of the potential adverse effects of long-term estrogen therapy. The addition of progesterone in the last days of the cycle appears to negate this risk. The question of whether or not to use progesterone in patients who have had hysterectomies remains unanswered.

Another risk of estrogen therapy may be the possible increased risk of breast cancer, and women with a personal or strong family history of breast cancer should not receive estrogen replacement. All patients receiving hormone therapy should have regular examinations.

4. Calcitonin. This is a polypeptide hormone secreted by the thyroid gland in mammals. It appears to act mainly on bone and can cause an inhibition of the normal ongoing resorptive process. It is most effective on bone disorders with an accelerated rate of resorption, such as Paget's disease, but also appears helpful in preventing the bone loss associated with osteoporosis. The

clinical trials are unfortunately of short duration. It is available as the synthetic salmon or synthetic human product.

At this time, it is only available by injection, although intranasal preparations are used in other countries. It is very expensive, and side effects of nausea, vomiting, flushing, and injection site pain occur in 10% to 20% of cases. Its most appropriate use may be in patients who cannot take estrogens. It is effective in preserving bone mass for short durations (under 2 years). Its long-term benefits are unknown.

5. Fluoride. By an unknown mechanism, fluoride appears capable of increasing bone mass. Unfortunately, the bone produced is abnormal bone. It appears to have different effects on different types of bone. While increasing trabecular bone in vertebrae, it may actually decrease mineral content in cortical bone, such as the upper part of the femur. As a result, the rate of vertebral compression fractures appears to decrease significantly, but the hip fracture rate increases. Further studies are needed to determine whether it has any role in the management of osteoporosis.

6. Others. Among the products being investigated are diphosphonates, thiazide diuretics, and anabolic steroids. Like fluorides, they are being used mainly in research centers, and their effectiveness is unknown.

Summary

Once a fracture has occurred, overimmobilization should be avoided. Analgesics should always be used in large enough doses for good pain relief in order to maintain a high level of activity. Light braces may be needed temporarily for compression fractures. Other factors affecting general health should be addressed (nutrition, smoking, alcoholism, exercise, etc.)

Specific measures that may be effective include (1) adequate calcium and vitamin D intake, (2) estrogen replacement therapy, (3) weight-bearing exercise, and (4) calcitonin. The risks of the treatment are weighed against the risks of osteoporosis on a case-by-case basis.

Tumors of the Spine

Primary

Excluding multiple myeloma, primary tumors, benign or malignant, of the spinal column are relatively rare. Of the benign tumors, osteoid osteoma, eosinophilic granuloma, aneurysmal bone cyst, and osteoblastoma occur occasionally. Osteoid osteoma is an interesting benign vascular lesion characterized by night pain that is often relieved by aspirin.

Malignant tumors are quite rare, with sarcomas of several origins being the most common.

In young patients, spinal neoplasms frequently cause local discomfort and scoliosis, and therefore, any young patient with a painful spinal curvature should be carefully assessed for tumor.

Metastatic Bone Disease

Bone is the third most common site for distant spread of neoplastic disease behind only the liver and lung. The major sources are myeloma and breast, lung, kidney, prostate, and thyroid carcinomas. The tumor usually disseminates by the hematogenous route, frequently through Batson's plexus, a vertebral venous system.

Pain is the most common complaint and is usually due to the expanding nature of the lesion and/or a pathologic fracture. There may be a referred or radicular element to the discomfort that gives the problem the appearance of a herniated disc. *Night pain,* aggravated or not relieved by rest, occurs frequently. With progression of the disease, neurologic dysfunction may progress to complete paralysis.

Roentgenographs will often reveal the lesion, but 30% to 50% of the bone must be destroyed before the lesion is visualized. The bone scan is positive in 90% of cases. False negatives commonly occur in myelomas and many carcinomas. This is because these produce such rapid and extensive bone destruction that new bone formation and the reparative process does not occur. CT and magnetic scans will usually reveal the lesion.

Laboratory studies commonly reveal an elevated alkaline phosphatase level. Acid phosphatase levels are usually increased in prostate metastases. Serum calcium levels may also be elevated. Bone marrow aspiration or biopsy is usually necessary to establish the diagnosis.

Treatment of the skeletal metastasis depends on biopsy confirmation of the type of tumor that is present and the appropriate use of radiation therapy, chemotherapy, or hormonal therapy as indicated.

Back Pain of Abdominal or Pelvic Origin

Visceral pain is often referred to the more posterior parts of the spine that innervate the diseased organ. In general, disease of the upper portion of the abdomen may refer pain to the shoulder and dorsolumbar spine, lower abdominal disorders refer pain to the lower lumbar spine, and pelvic disease refers pain to the sacrum. Usually, there are no findings related to the back such as loss of motion.

Abdominal Disorders

Peptic ulcer disease or tumor of the stomach or duodenum may induce pain in the lower thoracic and upper lumbar spine if the posterior wall is involved. If intense, it may radiate around to the front of the abdomen. The ulcer pain tends to retain its original character of response to antacids and food.

Thoracolumbar and left shoulder pain referral is not uncommon from pancreatitis. The pain may be quite intense. Previous episodes may have occurred, and a recent history of alcohol or dietary excess may be present. Tumor and peptic ulceration with extension to the pancreas commonly cause back and flank pain. The patient may seek relief by bending forward. The pain is more likely to be to the left of the spine if the tail of the pancreas is involved and to the right if the head is involved. Nausea, vomiting, prostation,

and diaphoresis may be present, and the abdomen is usually distended and tender. There is commonly a leukocytosis and elevation of serum and urinary amylase levels.

An aneurysm of the aorta may also cause not only acute abdominal pain and collapse with abdominal rigidity but also back pain. Generally, the pain is thoracic but may be higher or lower depending on location. There may be an absence or reduction of pulses in one of the lower extremities, and a pulsatile mass is often present.

In addition to aneurysms, disorders of other retroperitoneal structures may evoke back pain. The pain commonly radiates to the lower portion of the abdomen, groin, labia or testicles and anterior aspect of the thighs. Iliopsoas tumors or abscess, lymphomas, or acute bleeding due to anticoagulation may all produce symptoms sometimes confused with hip, back, or abdominal disorders. Frequently, there is pain with hip motion in extension but not in flexion.

Colon disorders (tumor, colitis, diverticulitis) may cause pain felt in the lower portion of the abdomen, lumbar spine, and groin. Transverse colon lesions may refer to L2 or L3 and sigmoid lesions to the sacrum.

Genitourinary Disorders

Renal diseases are among the most common nonorthopedic disturbances to simulate back disease. The pain of renal colic, caused by the passage of a small stone, clot, pus, or crystals, is usually ipsilateral and felt in the flank and lumbar area. It often radiates into the corresponding groin and testicle or vulva. Vomiting and restlessness are common, and there may be frequency and pain on urination. It is sometimes accompanied by hematuria. A positive Murphy's punch is diagnostic. Renal stones are rare in children, and when they occur, the patient should be evaluated for underlying metabolic disorders such as cystinuria.

Acute pyelonephritis frequently causes low back pain, but systemic and urinary symptoms usually clarify the diagnosis. Chills, fever, urinary frequency and urgency, and pain and tenderness in the costovertebral angle are usually present.

Renal vein thrombosis may also present as back and flank pain. Compression or invasion by local or metastatic tumor, proximal extension of a distal thrombus, and severe dehydration are among the common causes. The presence of unexplained edema (especially if unilateral) and the development of collateral abdominal veins may suggest the diagnosis. Recurrent pulmonary emboli may also occur. Palpable enlargement of the kidney, hematuria, and proteinuria are usually present. The proteinuria sometimes leads to nephrotic syndrome.

Back pain occasionally accompanies prostate disorders. Prostatitis may evoke sacral pain, sometimes radiating into one leg. It is usually accompanied by frequency, and there may be prostatic discharge. Prostate carcinoma with metastases to the lower portion of the back is another cause of lumbar or sacral pain. Most prostatic disorders are diagnosed by rectal examination, which should always be performed, especially for those patients whose back pain is unexplained.

Low back pain is also a common complaint in gynecologic practice. Simple menstrual pain may cause low lumbar and sacral pain. It is frequently crampy and radiates down the legs. Uterine colic or dysmenorrhea may cause similar symptoms. Vomiting sometimes occurs. Pain from endometriosis may also cause cyclical discomfort. The menstrual history is often suggestive of these disorders.

Retrodisplacement of the uterus, especially if associated with retroflexion, may cause a nagging sacral pain, particularly after the patient has been upright for several hours. Tension on the uterosacral ligaments is the usual etiology of back pain due to enlargement, tumors, or malposition of the uterus. Large posterior pelvic tumors may be painful by virtue of pressure or involvement of the sacral plexus. Backache of this type in conjunction with pelvic malignancies (especially carcinoma of the cervix) usually indicates that the disease has advanced to involve the iliac nodes. This pain often becomes more severe and worse at night.

Pregnancy, ectopic or otherwise, should always be ruled out in women of childbearing years, especially if invasive or roentgenographic studies are being planned. A well-performed pelvic examination will help separate the majority of these disorders (Tables 8–2 and 8–3).

TABLE 8–3.

Algorithm for Low Back and/or Leg Pain

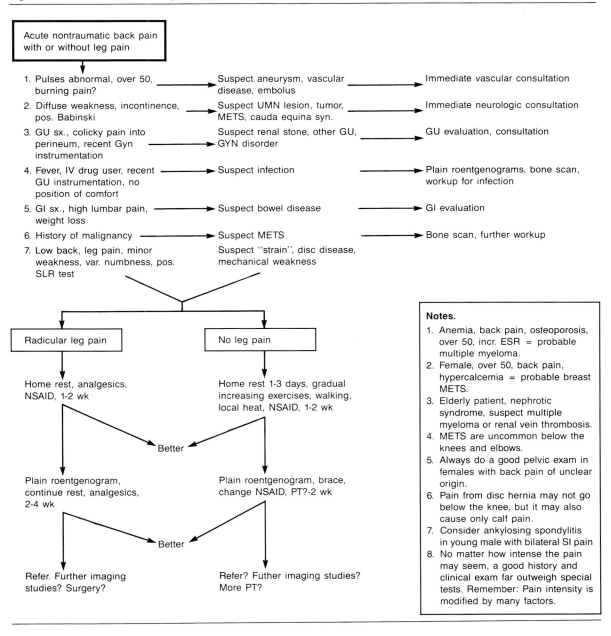

Acute nontraumatic back pain with or without leg pain

1. Pulses abnormal, over 50, burning pain? → Suspect aneurysm, vascular disease, embolus → Immediate vascular consultation

2. Diffuse weakness, incontinence, pos. Babinski → Suspect UMN lesion, tumor, METS, cauda equina syn. → Immediate neurologic consultation

3. GU sx., colicky pain into perineum, recent Gyn instrumentation → Suspect renal stone, other GU, GYN disorder → GU evaluation, consultation

4. Fever, IV drug user, recent GU instrumentation, no position of comfort → Suspect infection → Plain roentgenograms, bone scan, workup for infection

5. GI sx., high lumbar pain, weight loss → Suspect bowel disease → GI evaluation

6. History of malignancy → Suspect METS → Bone scan, further workup

7. Low back, leg pain, minor weakness, var. numbness, pos. SLR test → Suspect "strain", disc disease, mechanical weakness

Radicular leg pain

Home rest, analgesics, NSAID, 1-2 wk

Better

Plain roentgenogram, continue rest, analgesics, 2-4 wk

Better

Refer. Further imaging studies? Surgery?

No leg pain

Home rest 1-3 days, gradual increasing exercises, walking, local heat, NSAID, 1-2 wk

Plain roentgenogram, brace, change NSAID, PT?-2 wk

Refer? Futher imaging studies? More PT?

Notes.

1. Anemia, back pain, osteoporosis, over 50, incr. ESR = probable multiple myeloma.
2. Female, over 50, back pain, hypercalcemia = probable breast METS.
3. Elderly patient, nephrotic syndrome, suspect multiple myeloma or renal vein thrombosis.
4. METS are uncommon below the knees and elbows.
5. Always do a good pelvic exam in females with back pain of unclear origin.
6. Pain from disc hernia may not go below the knee, but it may also cause only calf pain.
7. Consider ankylosing spondylitis in young male with bilateral SI pain
8. No matter how intense the pain may seem, a good history and clinical exam far outweigh special tests. Remember: Pain intensity is modified by many factors.

BIBLIOGRAPHY

Aho K, et al: HLA antigen 27 and reactive arthritis. *Lancet* 1973; 2:157.

Ansell BM: Rheumatic disorders in childhood. *Clin Rheum Dis* 1976; 2:303.

Appelrouth D, Gottlieb NL: Pulmonary manifestations of ankylosing spondylitis. *J Rheumatol* 1975; 2:446.

Arnett FC: The implications of HL-A W27. *Ann Intern Med* 1976; 84:94.

Avioli LV: Osteoporosis, pathogenesis and therapy, in Avioli LV, Vrane SM (eds): *Metabolic Bone Disease.* New York, Academic Press, 1977.

Avioli LV: Senile and post-menopausal osteoporosis. *Adv Intern Med* 1976; 21:391.

Bargolie B, et al: Plasma cell myeloma—new biological insights and advances in therapy. *Blood* 1989; 73:865.

Benson MKD, Byrnes DP: The clinical syndromes and surgical treatment of thoracic intervertebral disc prolapse. *J Bone Joint Surg [Br]* 1975; 57:471.

Bernat JL: A dangerous backache. *Hosp Pract* 1977; 12:36.

Berstein DS, et al: Prevalence of osteoporosis in high and low fluoride areas of North Dakota. *JAMA* 1966; 198:499.

Bingham WF: The role of HLA B27 in the diagnosis and management of low back pain and sciatica. *J Neurosurg* 1977; 47:561.

Blount WP, Moe JH: *The Milwaukee Brace.* Baltimore, Williams & Wilkins, 1973.

Blumberg B, Ragan C: The natural history of rheumatoid spondylitis. *Medicine (Baltimore)* 1956; 35:1.

Boden SD, et al: Abnormal magnetic resonance scans of the lumbar spine in asymptomatic subjects. *J Bone Joint Surg [Am]* 1990; 72:403.

Bolender NF, Schonstrom NSR, Spengler DM: Role of computed tomography and myelography in the diagnosis of central spinal stenosis. *J Bone Joint Surg [Am]* 1985; 67:240.

Bondilla KK: Back pain: Osteoarthritis, *J Am Geriatr Soc* 1977; 25:62.

Bough B, et al: Degeneration of lumbar facet joints. *J Bone Joint Surg [Br]* 1990; 72:275.

Bradford DS, et al: Scheuermann's kyphosis and roundback deformity: Results of Milwaukee brace treatment. *J Bone Joint Surg [Am]* 1974; 56:740.

Bradford DS, et al: Scheuermann's kyphosis: Results of surgical treatment by posterior spine arthrodesis in 22 patients. *J Bone Joint Surg [Am]* 1975; 57:439.

Brewerton DA, et al: Reiter's disease and HLA-27. *Lancet* 1973; 2:996.

Brown MD: Diagnosis of pain syndromes of the spine. *Orthop Clin North Am* 1975; 6:233.

Brown MD: *Intradiscal Therapy With Chymopapain or Collagenase.* Chicago, Year Book Medical Publishers Inc, 1983.

Buchanan JR, et al: Assessment of the risk of vertebral fracture in menopausal women. *J Bone Joint Surg [Am]* 1987; 69:212.

Bulkey BH, Roberts WC: Ankylosing spondylitis and aortic regurgitation, *Circulation* 1973; 48:1014.

Calabro JJ, Amante CM: Indomethacin in ankylosing spondylitis. *Arthritis Rheum* 1968; 11:56.

Caldwell AB, Chase C: Diagnosis and treatment of personality factors in chronic low back pain. *Clin Orthop* 1977; 129:141.

Calin A: Raised serum creatine phosphokinase activity in ankylosing spondylitis. *Ann Rheum Dis* 1975; 34:244.

Carman DL, et al: Measurement of scoliosis and kyphosis radiographs. Intraobserver and interobserver variation. *J Bone Joint Surg [Am]* 1990; 72:328.

Curtis P: Low back pain in the primary care setting. *J Fam Pract* 1977; 4:381.

Dickson RA: Conservative treatment for idiopathic scoliosis. *J Bone Joint Surg [Br]* 1985; 67:176.

Dyck P, et al: Intermittent cauda equina compression syndrome. *Spine* 1977; 2:75.

Eisenstein SM, Perry CR: The lumbar facet arthrosis syndrome: Clinical presentation and articular surface changes. *J Bone Joint Surg [Br]* 1987; 69:3.

Eismont FJ, Currier B: Current concepts review: Surgical management of lumbar intervertebral disc lesions. *J Bone Joint Surg [Am]* 1989; 71:1266.

Engleman EG, Engleman EP: Ankylosing spondylitis: Recent advances in diagnosis and treatment. *Med Clin North Am* 1977; 61:347.

Ferris B, Edgar M, Leyshon A: Screening for scoliosis. *Acta Orthop Scand* 1988; 59:417.

Fost A: Low back disorders: Conservative management. *Arch Phys Med Rehabil* 1988; 69:880.

Godfrey RB, et al: A double-blind crossover trial of aspirin, indomethacin and phenylbutazone in ankylosing spondylitis. *Arthritis Rheum* 1972; 15:110.

Guck TP, et al: Prediction of long term outcome of multidisciplinary pain treatment. *Arch Phys Med Rehabil* 1986; 87:293.

Haddad JG, et al: Effects of prolonged thyrocalcitonin administration in Paget's disease of bone. *N Engl J Med* 1970; 283:549.

Hart FD: The ankylosing spondylopathies. *Clin Orthop* 1971; 74:7.

Harvey MA, James B: *Differential Diagnosis.* Philadelphia, WB Saunders Co, 1972.

Heaney RP: A unified concept of osteoporosis. *Am J Med* 1965; 39:877.

Henley EN, Shapiro DE: The development of low back pain after excision of a lumbar disc. *J Bone Joint Surg [Am]* 1989; 71:719.

Hensinger RN: Current concepts review. Spondylolysis and spondylolisthesis in children and adolescents. *J Bone Joint Surg [Am]* 1989; 71:1098.

Hurme M, Waranta H: Factors predicting the result of surgery for lumbar intervertebral disc herniation. *Spine* 1987; 12:933.

Jackson RP, et al: Facet joint injection in low back pain: A prospective statistical study. *Spine* 1988; 13:966.

Jausey J, et al: Some results of the effects of fluoride on bone tissue in osteoporosis. *J Clin Endocrinol* 1969; 28:869.

Jayson MIV, Bouchier LAD: Ulcerative colitis with ankylosing spondylitis. *Ann Rheum Dis* 1968; 27:219.

Kertez A, Karmos R: Low back pain in the workmen in Canada. *Can Med Assoc J* 1976; 115:901.

Kiel DP, et al: Hip fractures and the use of estrogen in postmenopausal women: The Framingham study. *N Engl J Med* 1987; 317:1169.

Kostiuk JP, et al: Cauda equina syndrome and lumbar disc herniation. *J Bone Joint Surg [Am]* 1986; 68:386.

Krupp MA, Chatton MJ: *Current Diagnosis and Treatment.* Los Altos, Calif, Lange Medical Publications, 1972.

Lane JM, Vigorita VJ: Osteoporosis: Current concepts review. *J Bone Joint Surg [Am]* 1983; 65:274.

Leutwek L, Whedon GD: Osteoporosis. *DM,* April 1963.

Macnab I: *Backache.* Baltimore, Williams & Wilkins, 1977.

Malpas JS: Problems in the management of myeloma. *Postgrad Med J* 1989; 65:468.

Manniche C, et al: Clinical trial of intensive muscle training for chronic low back pain. *Lancet* 1988; 24:1473.

McBryde AM, McCollum DE: Ankylosing spondylitis in women. *N C Med J* 1973; 34:34.

McCullock JA: Chemonucleolysis. *J Bone Joint Surg [Br]* 1977; 59:45.

McEwen C, et al: Ankylosing spondylitis and spondylitis accompanying ulcerative colitis, regional enteritis, psoriasis, and Reiter's disease. *Arthritis Rheum* 1971; 14:391.

McGoey BV, et al: Effect of weight loss on musculoskeletal pain in the morbidly obese. *J Bone Joint Surg [Br]* 1990; 72:322.

Meyerding HW: Spondylolisthesis. *Surg Gynecol Obstet* 1932; 54:371.

Miller GM, Forbes GS, Onofrio BM: Magnetic resonance imaging of the spine. *Mayo Clin Proc* 1989; 64:986.

Moe JH, Kettleson DN: Idiopathic scoliosis. *J Bone Joint Surg [Am]* 1970; 52:1509.

Montgomery SP, Erwin WE: Scheuermann's kyphosis: Long-term results of Milwaukee brace treatment. *Spine* 1981; 6:5.

Mooney V: Percutaneous discectomy. *Spine* 1989; 3:103.

Mooney V, et al: Chronic low back pain: Evaluation and therapy. *Orthop Clin North Am* 1978; 9:543.

Morrisey RT, et al: Measurement of Cobb angle on radiographs of patients who have scoliosis. Evaluation of intrinsic error. *J Bone Joint Surg [Am]* 1990; 72:320.

Nachenson AL: The lumbar spine, and orthopedic challenge. *Spine* 1976; 1:59.

Nash CL: Scoliosis bracing. *J Bone Joint Surg [Am]* 1980; 62:848.

Nelson MA: Lumbar spinal stenosis. *J Bone Joint Surg [Br]* 1973; 55:506.

Novak RE, Jones SG, Jones MW: *Novak's Textbook of Gynecology,* ed 8. Baltimore, Williams & Wilkins, 1970.

Ogryzlo MA: Ankylosing spondylitis, in Hollander JL, McCarty DJ Jr (eds): *Arthritis and Allied Conditions,* ed 8. Philadelphia, Lea & Febiger, 1972.

Ogryzlo MA, Rosen PS: Ankylosing (Marie-Strümpell) spondylitis. *Postgrad Med* 1969; 45:182.

Radin EL: Reasons for failure of L5–S1 intervertebral disc excisions. *Int Orthop* 1987; 11:255.

Ramirez LF, Thisted R: Complications and demographic characteristics of patients undergoing lumbar discectomy in community hospitals. *Neurosurgery* 1989; 25:226.

Recker RR, et al: Effect of estrogen and calcium carbonate on bone loss in post-menopausal women. *Ann Intern Med* 1977; 87:649.

Resnick NM, Greenspan SL: "Senile" osteoporosis reconsidered. *JAMA* 1989; 261:1025.

Riggs R, et al: Short- and long-term effects of estrogen and synthetic anabolic hormone in post-menopausal osteoporosis. *J Clin Invest* 1972; 51:1659.

Riggs BL, Melton LJ III: Involutional osteoporosis. *N Engl J Med* 1986; 314:1676.

Riggs BL, Melton LJ III: *Osteoporosis. Etiology, Diagnosis and Management.* New York, Raven Press, 1988.

Rosenberg E, et al: Effect of long-term calcitonin therapy on the clinical course of osteogenesis imperfecta. *J Clin Endocrinol Metab* 1977; 44:346.

Ruge D, Wiltse LL: *Spinal Disorders: Diagnosis and Treatment.* Philadelphia, Lea & Febiger, 1977.

Scheuman DJ Nagel DA: Low back and leg pain. *Primary Care* 1974; 1:549.

Schlosstein L, et al: High association of an HL-A antigen, W27, with ankylosing spondylitis. *N Engl J Med* 1973; 288:704.

Sewell KL: Modern therapeutic approaches to osteoporosis. *Rheum Dis Clin North Am* 1989; 15:583.

Simons GW, Sty JR, Storshak RJ: Retroperitoneal and retrofascial abscesses. *J Bone Joint Surg [Am]* 1983; 65:1041.

Singer FR: *Paget's Disease of Bone.* New York, Plenum Publishing Corp, 1977.

Smith L: Enzyme dissolution of the nucleus pulposus in humans. *JAMA* 1964; 187:137.

Spiegel PS, et al: Intervertebral disc-space inflammation in children. *J Bone Joint Surg [Am]* 1972; 54:284.

Steinbach HL, Dodds WJ: Clinical radiology of Paget's disease. *Clin Orthop* 1968; 57:277.

Steinbach ML: The roentgen appearance of osteoporosis. *Radiol Clin North Am* 1964; 2:191.

Turner PG, Green JH, Galasko CS: Back pain in childhood. *Spine* 1989; 14:812.

Turner RH, Bianco AJ: Spondylolysis and spondylolisthesis in children and teen-agers. *J Bone Joint Surg [Am]* 1971; 53:1298.

Waldenstrom J: *Diagnosis and Treatment of Multiple Myeloma.* New York, Grune & Stratton Inc, 1970.

Walson AH, Rohwedder JJ: Upper lobe fibrosis in ankylosing spondylitis. *AJR* 1975; 124:466.

Wedgewood RJ, Schaller JG: The pediatric arthritides. *Hosp Pract* 1977; 12:83.

Weinerman SA, Bockman RS: Medical therapy of osteoporosis. *Orthop Clin North Am* 1990; 21:109.

Weinstein SL: Adolescent idiopathic scoliosis: Prevalence and natural history. *Am Acad Orthop Surg Lect* 1989; 38:115.

Wenger DR, Bobechko WP, Gilday DL: The spectrum of intervertebral disc-space infection in children. *J Bone Joint Surg [Am]* 1978; 60:100.

Wheeler M: Osteoporosis. *Med Clin North Am* 1976; 60:1213.

Williams PC: The conservative management of lesions of the lumbosacral spine. *Am Acad Orthop Surg Lect* 1953; 10:90.

Wiltse LL, Widell EH, Jackson DW: Fatigue fracture: The basic lesion in isthmic spondylolisthesis. *J Bone Joint Surg [Am]* 1975; 57:1722.

CHAPTER 9

The Pelvis and Sacrum

Painful disorders of the pelvis, except for anky-losing spondylitis, are uncommon. Most are secondary to trauma and usually respond to conservative treatment.

ANATOMY

The bony pelvis is formed by the innominate bones, the sacrum, and the coccyx. Each hip (innominate) bone is composed of three elements: the ischium, the ilium, and the pubis. These three components meet at the acetabulum and are united by the triradiate cartilage until the age of 16 years, when fusion takes place. The sacrum is composed of five vertebrae, and the coccyx usually consists of four. The coccyx and sacrum are situated more posteriorly in women than in men and thus are more exposed to trauma.

Very little motion occurs at the sacroiliac and interpubic joints because of strong ligamentous structures at these areas. Some motion occurs at the sacrococcygeal joint, but little is present between coccygeal segments.

ROENTGENOGRAPHIC ANATOMY

The pelvis is well visualized by a routine antero-posterior roentgenogram (Fig 9–1). In addition, the sacrum and coccyx may be studied by lateral views and anteroposterior views angled 15 degrees cephalad and caudad.

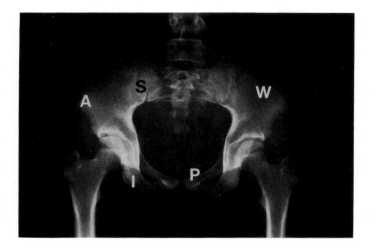

FIG 9–1.
Roentgenogram of the normal pelvis: *S* = sacroiliac joint; *A* = anterior superior iliac spine; *P* = pubic symphysis; *I* = ischium; *W* = wing of the ilium.

OSTEITIS PUBIS

Osteitis pubis is a painful inflammation of the pubic symphysis that is usually self-limited. The cause is unknown, but the condition frequently develops after urologic procedures or infections, after childbirth, or following repetitive stresses associated with certain athletic activities.

Clinical Features

The onset is gradual, with symptoms developing a few days after the traumatic event. Pain and tenderness over the symphysis pubis are usually present. Coughing may aggravate the pain, which radiates along the adductor and rectus abdominis muscles. Stretching these muscles is painful.

Examination reveals local tenderness over the symphysis pubis and adjacent soft tissue. Passive abduction of the hips and active adduction of the hips against resistance are painful.

Roentgenograms of the pelvis taken early in the disease may be normal. Later, variable amounts of spotty demineralization, widening of the symphysis pubis, and sclerosis are noted (Fig 9–2). Reossification eventually occurs over several months.

Treatment

Treatment consists of anti-inflammatory drugs and rest. This may be supplemented by diathermy or ice packs. A local injection of a steroid/lidocaine mixture may also be helpful. The disease has a tendency toward spontaneous recovery, but this may take several weeks. The activity level of the patient is allowed to increase as tolerated.

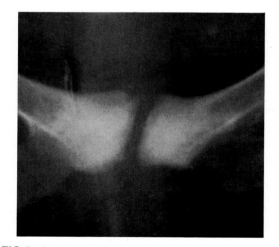

FIG 9–2.
Osteitis pubis.

OSTEITIS CONDENSANS ILII

This is a lesion in which sclerosis of a fairly large area of ilium adjacent to the sacroiliac joint occurs (Fig 9–3). It is most common in multiparous women. Its importance lies in distinguishing it from ankylosing spondylitis (Marie-Strümpell disease). Ankylosing spondylitis is usually associated with an increase in the sedimentation rate and roentgenographic involvement on both sides of the sacroiliac joint. It occurs primarily in men and is associated with pain. There is disagreement, however, as to whether osteitis condensans ilii is ever a painful condition.

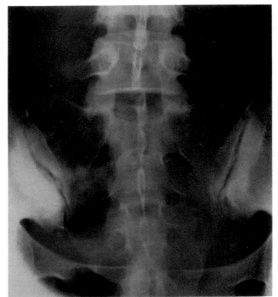

FIG 9–3.
Osteitis condensans ilii. The iliac portions of the sacroiliac joints are sclerotic and white. The joints themselves are not involved.

COCCYGODYNIA

The coccyx consists of from three to five segments and usually angulates forward to a variable degree. In the normal, erect sitting position with weight on the thighs, the coccyx does not have pressure against it. With flattening of the lumbar lordosis and sitting in the slumping position, however, the coccyx can reach the seat, and pain may develop over its tip.

During childbirth, injury to the coccyx frequently occurs and leads to fibrosis and stiffness. Manipulation or fracture of this stiffened segment may be required in future deliveries.

Chronic strains and osteoarthritis may also result from repetitive trauma. Joint motion is usually restricted, and activities that move the coccyx are painful. Complete bony ankylosis may even result, with the coccyx fusing in a deformed position. Fractures of the tip of the sacrum or coccyx also occur but usually do not produce long-term symptoms unless a painful pseudarthrosis or traumatic arthritis ensues. "Tailbone" (sacrum or coccyx) fractures are actually quite uncommon.

The roentgenogram is often misinterpreted due to the normal sacrococcygeal and intercoccygeal spaces.

The sacrum and coccyx may also be the site of pain referral from visceral structures or lumbar disc degeneration.

Clinical Features

Pain on sitting is the most common complaint. This pain is aggravated by slumping, sitting on a hard seat, or activity. Many symptoms begin with an injury and may be aggravated by constipation or rectal disease. The symptoms are more common in women.

Local pain and tenderness at the sacrococcygeal joint and adjacent soft tissues are common physical findings. A rectal examination should always be performed and often reveals pain on sacrococcygeal motion. This pain often radiates into the buttocks.

Depending on the history, the roentgenogram may reveal recent injury or degenerative arthritis.

Fractures, when they occur, usually involve the lower part of the sacrum or first sacrococcygeal segment (Fig 9–4). Osteoarthritis may be noted at the sacrococcygeal joint. The alignment or configuration of the sacrum or coccygeal segments visualized roentgenographically seems to have little importance in coccygodynia.

Treatment

Recent fracture or dislocation should be reduced by manipulation with the patient under local anesthesia. Redisplacement is common, however. All forms of painful coccyx are treated with warm sitz baths and a soft doughnut-shaped pillow. Constipation should be avoided. Analgesics and anti-inflammatory drugs are prescribed as necessary. A local injection of steroid is often beneficial for chronic strain or osteoarthritis. Massage may also be beneficial in the treatment of chronic sprain.

The coccyx is frequently the site of functional pain in psychoneurotic individuals. Surgery is rarely indicated in these patients. The occasional patient with painful osteoarthritis or a rigid deviated coccyx who does not respond to conservative measures will benefit greatly from coccygectomy. Acute injuries are all treated conservative-

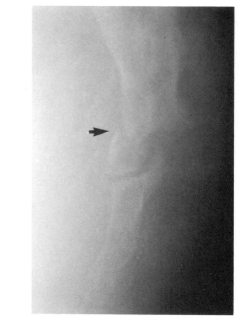

FIG 9–4.
Fracture of the lower portion of the sacrum *(arrow)* just above the sacrococcygeal joint.

ly for at least 6 months, however, even when significant anterior angulation of the coccyx is present.

FRACTURES OF THE PELVIS

The pelvic ring is essentially a rigid circle with very little motion at the interpubic or sacroiliac areas. Fractures involving the ring are generally classified as stable or unstable (see Chapter 16). Stable fractures are those in which the ring is completely broken only at one point (e.g., superior and inferior pubic ramus fractures on the same side). With unstable fractures, the ring is broken in two or more areas (e.g., both pubic rami on the same side plus a sacroiliac (SI) dislocation).

Stable fractures commonly result from minor falls, especially in elderly, osteoporotic females. These fractures may be treated symptomatically with a short period (1 to 2 days) of rest followed by ambulation and weightbearing as tolerated, usually with a walker.

Unstable fractures (Fig 9–5) are often serious and potentially life-threatening. They may be accompanied by genitourinary or other visceral injuries. Posterior fractures in particular may damage the adjacent venous and arterial system and produce massive retroperitoneal bleeding. The initial care is therefore directed at general stabilization of the patient. The fracture usually requires prolonged immobilization and occasionally surgical repair.

Fractures of the acetabulum occasionally in-

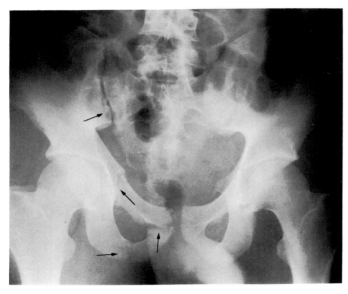

FIG 9–5.
An unstable fracture of the pelvis. In addition to the fractures of the pubic bones, a sacroiliac separation is present on the ipsilateral side. Whenever displacement is present in a fracture at the pubic ramus, injury to another point in the pelvic ring is likely.

volve the main weight-bearing surface of the hip joint (Fig 9–6). Reduction, either surgically or by traction on the femur, may be needed to restore a smooth surface and prevent the development of traumatic arthritis.

Pelvic Insufficiency Fractures

This injury is a type of stress fracture that almost always occurs in elderly females. Stress fractures can be of two types: fatigue and insufficiency. Fatigue fractures develop when unusually high stress is applied to a normal bone. Insufficiency fractures occur in abnormal bone undergoing normal stress.

Osteoporosis is the usual predisposing cause,

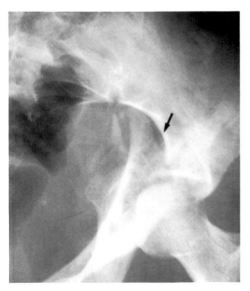

FIG 9–6.
Fracture of the acetabulum *(arrow)*. Reduction of the weight-bearing portion was able to be obtained by skeletal traction.

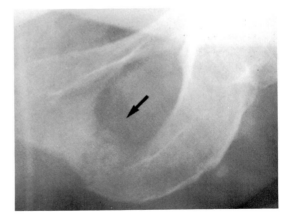

FIG 9–7.
Insufficiency fracture of the pubic bone *(arrow)* in a middle-aged, inactive, obese, osteoporotic female receiving steroids for asthma.

but inactivity, long-term steroid use, and other types of metabolic bone disease may also play a role. The usual sites of fracture are the pubic bones, ilium, and sacrum (Fig 9–7). Because there is usually no history of trauma, the injury is often overlooked or misinterpreted as metastatic disease. Multiple areas may even be involved. (Compression fractures of the vertebrae and femoral neck fractures may act in a similar fashion but are generally easier to recognize.)

Roentgenographic Findings

When the fracture involves the sacrum, it is usually vertical and may be bilateral. The findings of early resorption or late sclerosis may be easily missed due to superimposed bowel gas as well as the subtle appearance of the fracture. Iliac involvement is usually above the acetabulum.

Bone scanning is extremely sensitive for this injury as well as other similar conditions. Fractures may be detected as early as three days after the onset. (Scans may also remain slightly positive for 1 to 2 years.) Computed tomographic evaluation will usually allow differentiation from metastatic disease.

BIBLIOGRAPHY

Dittrich RJ: Coccygodynia as referred pain. *J Bone Joint Surg [Am]* 1951; 33:715.

Hauge MD, Cooper KL, Litin SC: Insufficiency fractures of the pelvis that simulate metastatic disease. *Mayo Clin Proc* 1988; 63:807.

Howorth B: The painful coccyx. *Clin Orthop* 1959; 14:145.

Macnab I: *Backache*. Baltimore, Williams & Wilkins, 1977.

Postacchino F, Massobrio M: Idiopathic coccygodynia: Analysis of 51 operative cases and a radiographic study of the normal coccyx. *J Bone Joint Surg [Am]* 1983; 65:1116.

Resnik CS, Resnik D: Radiology of disorders of the sacroiliac joints. *JAMA* 1985; 253:2863.

Schnute WJ: Osteitis pubis. *Clin Orthop* 1961; 20:187.

Shipp FL, Haggart GE: Further experience in the management of osteitis condensans ilii. *J Bone Joint Surg [Am]* 1950; 32:841.

Traycoff RB, Crayton H, Dodson R: Sacrococcygeal pain syndromes: Diagnosis and treatment. *Orthopedics* 1989; 12:1373.

CHAPTER 10

The Hip

The hip is a ball-and-socket joint in which the femoral head articulates deeply into the acetabulum. This deep fit, combined with thick ligamentous and muscular supporting structures, makes the hip extremely stable but relatively inaccessible. Therefore, the diagnosis of disorders of the hip is sometimes difficult.

ANATOMY

The proximal portion of the femur consists of a head, neck, and greater and lesser trochanters. The axes of the neck and femoral shaft form an angle in the anteroposterior plane: the neck-shaft angle, or "angle of inclination." This normally measures 125 degrees to 130 degrees. An increase in this angle is termed coxa valga, and a decrease is termed coxa vara. The neck and shaft also form an angle in the transcondylar plane that is referred to as the angle of femoral torsion (Fig 10–1). Normal femoral torsion is 40 degrees in the child, and this decreases to 15 to 20 degrees in the adult. Excessive femoral torsion is termed anteversion or antetorsion and is sometimes responsible for in-toeing. A decrease in the normal femoral torsion is termed retroversion or retrotorsion and may cause an out-toeing gait.

The vascular anatomy of the femoral head is of critical importance in many disorders of the hip.

The main sources of blood supply are the retinacular and intramedullary vessels, both of which course from the intertrochanteric region proximally to nourish the femoral head (Fig 10–2). Diseases or injuries that compromise the

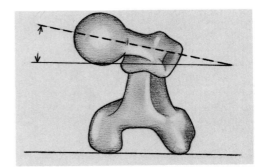

FIG 10–1.
The angle of femoral torsion.

circulation may damage the viability of the femoral head and lead to avascular necrosis.

Among the nerves that supply the hip joint is the obturator nerve. This nerve also supplies a sensory branch to the medial side of the thigh and motor supply to some of the hip adductors. Irritation of this nerve from hip joint disease may result in referred pain along the inner aspect of the knee and thigh that may cause confusion with disorders of the knee joint. Therefore, complaints of pain in this area in the absence of physical findings in the knee should always draw attention to the hip joint.

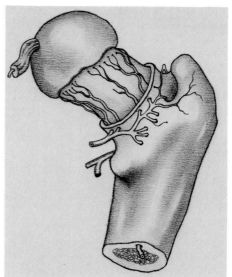

FIG 10–2.
Blood supply to the head of the femur.

EXAMINATION

Several bony landmarks are available for orientation on physical examination. The anterior and posterior superior iliac spines and iliac crest are easily palpable because they are not crossed by any muscles (Fig 10–3). The proximal portion of the iliac crest lies at the level of the fourth lumbar vertebra. The greater trochanter is palpable laterally, and the pubic symphysis is palpable anteriorly.

The femoral head itself lies approximately 2.5 cm distal and lateral to the point where the femoral artery passes beneath the inguinal ligament. This relationship should be recalled when performing venipuncture from the femoral vein. A needle passed through the vein may enter the hip joint and introduce infection into the hip. All femoral venipuncture sites should therefore be meticulously scrubbed and prepared prior to needle insertion.

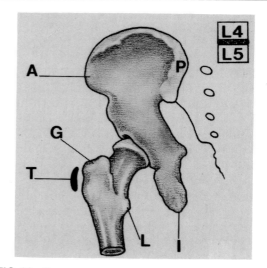

FIG 10–3.
Bony landmarks of the hip: *A* = anterior superior iliac spine; *G* = greater trochanter; *T* = trochanteric bursa; *P* = posterior superior iliac spine; *L* = lesser trochanter; *I* = ischial tuberosity. The upper level of the iliac crest lies at the level of the fourth lumbar vertebra. Adjacent to the posterior superior iliac spine is the sacroiliac joint.

ROENTGENOGRAPHIC ANATOMY

The roentgenographic study of the hip joint should include views in the anteroposterior and lateral planes (Fig 10–4). The lateral view may be either a "true" lateral or a "frog-leg" exposure that is taken with the hips in maximum external rotation.

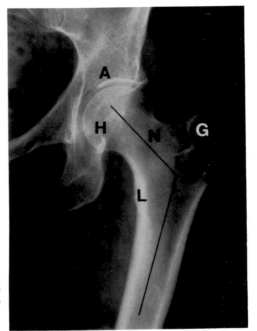

FIG 10–4.
Anteroposterior roentgenogram of the normal hip: A = rim of the acetabulum; H = head of the femur; N = neck of the femur; L = lesser trochanter; G = greater trochanter; I = intertrochanteric region. The angle of inclination is marked.

CONGENITAL DYSPLASIA OF THE HIP

Congenital dysplasia of the hip is a common disorder in which displacement of the femoral head out of the acetabulum occurs. The condition is frequently bilateral, and although the cause is unknown, heredity appears to play a role. Females are affected nine times more often than males, and firstborn children or children born by breech deliveries also have a higher incidence of the disorder. It is occasionally present in association with clubfoot and congenital muscular torticollis deformities.

Pathologically, abnormalities are seen in both the acetabulum and femoral head. The acetabulum may be more shallow in contour and more vertically inclined than normal and result in insufficient coverage and inadequate containment of the femoral head. The femur is often excessively anteverted, and the hip joint capsule may also be lax.

Clinical Features

The clinical picture ranges from mild dysplasia with minimal clinical findings, to subluxation, and even to frank dislocation. Complete dislocation is rarely present at birth, however, but may develop with weight bearing. The physical findings vary according to the amount of instability and the age of the patient.

In the newborn child, dysplasia is much more common than dislocation. The most important physical finding in this age group is limitation of abduction of the flexed hip (Fig 10–5). Any limitation of abduction to less than 50 to 60 degrees is considered abnormal. The newborn child nor-

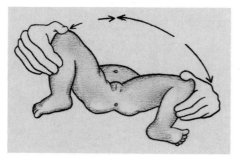

FIG 10–5.
Restricted abduction of the right hip.

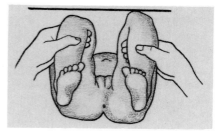

FIG 10–7.
Galeazzi's or Allis' sign. The child is placed on a firm surface with the hips and knees flexed. The knee will appear lower on the dislocated side.

mally has a slight flexion contracture of the hip and knee, but the hips should be able to be fully abducted to lie flat on the examining table. If this is not possible, congenital hip dysplasia should be suspected. Asymmetry of the gluteal skin folds may also be noted. The various tests denoting hip instability are frequently positive (Fig 10–6). When positive, these tests suggest that the dysplasia may progress to dislocation if the condition is not treated.

When complete dislocation is present, there is frequently loss of the normal flexion contracture of the hip, and the affected extremity appears shorter (Fig 10–7). If weight bearing has begun, a painless limp is often the initial symptom. Hip motion, especially abduction, is limited, and abnormal piston mobility or "telescoping" may be present. The Trendelenburg test is usually posi-

tive. This test takes advantage of the fact that normally, when standing on one leg, contraction of the abductor muscles on the side bearing weight will cause the opposite side of the pelvis to be elevated. If the hip is dislocated, these muscles no longer work effectively, and when the child stands on the affected leg, the opposite side of the pelvis drops downward instead.

The roentgenographic examination is usually not very helpful when the patient is under 3 months of age unless a complete dislocation is present. After this age, a delay in the ossification of the femoral head is frequently noted (Fig 10–8). The acetabulum may be more inclined vertically, and the acetabular index is often increased. If subluxation or dislocation has occurred, upward and outward displacement of the femoral head will be seen.

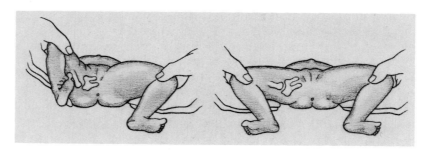

FIG 10–6.
Ortolani's test for congenital dislocation of the hip. A "click" is palpable or audible as the hip is reduced by abduction. If the test is negative, the examination should always be repeated in 2 to 4 months.

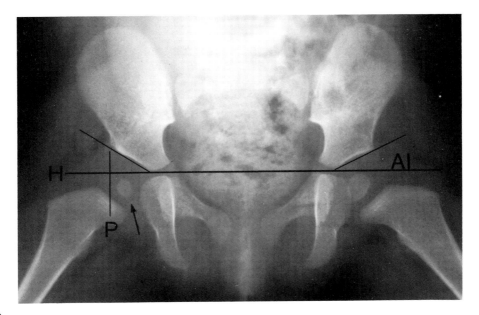

FIG 10–8.
Roentgenogram of the pelvis: *P* = Perkin's vertical line; *H* = Hilgenreiner's horizontal line, *AI* = acetabular index. The ossification center of the capital femoral epiphysis should lie in the inferior medial quadrant formed by Perkin's and Hilgenreiner's lines. The *AI* normally measures less than 30 degrees. Here, ossification of the capital epiphysis on the dysplastic hip *(arrow)* has been delayed as compared with the left.

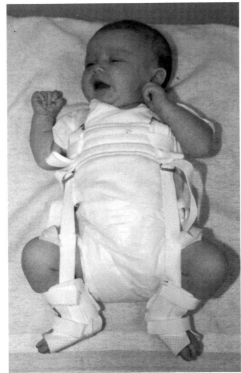

FIG 10–9.
The Pavlik harness.

Ultrasonography is becoming increasingly useful and reliable in congenital hip dysplasia, especially in high-risk infants (breech delivery, positive family history, etc.) or those with uncertain clinical findings. Among its benefits is the elimination of exposure to radiation. Magnetic resonance imaging (MRI) may eventually be helpful, but the diagnosis can usually be established by other means.

Treatment

Any suggestion of instability or stiffness in the hip of the newborn warrants treatment. The treatment is initiated as soon as possible and varies with the age of the patient and the degree of dysplasia. Early detection is of utmost importance because conservative treatment is more likely to succeed in the infant. The older the child is over the weight-bearing age, the more likely surgery will be necessary, and the less likely a normal functional result will ensue. Whenever any doubt exists, treatment and follow-up are indicated.

The objective of treatment is to reduce the femoral head into the acetabulum and maintain that reduction. By maintaining the hip in the reduced position, normal development of the hip joint structures and acetabulum is encouraged. A variety of external devices are available for the treatment of the hip with moderate instability and stiffness. The most functional is the Pavlik harness, which maintains the hip in a more natural "human" position, allows active motion, and prevents full extension in the adducted position (Fig 10–9). The harness is usually worn for 6 weeks plus 1 week for each week in which the diagnosis has been delayed. This device does not force the hip into the excessive abduction that can occur when using triple diapers or many of the other abduction splints. This position of extreme abduction may actually be harmful to the hip by exerting too much pressure on the femoral head, which may lead to avascular necrosis.

Failure to obtain or maintain a stable reduction necessitates surgical intervention. The objective is to reduce the hip by either closed or open methods and maintain the reduction by casting or osteotomy.

LEGG-CALVÉ-PERTHES DISEASE

Perthes' disease, or coxa plana, is a self-limited disorder of the hip in which a portion of the ossific nucleus of the femoral head undergoes avascular necrosis. Eventually, the infarcted, necrotic bone is absorbed and replaced by normal bone. The cause of this condition is unknown, but some cases follow transient synovitis of the hip. The disorder usually occurs between the ages of 4 and 10 years, and males are more commonly affected. Fifteen percent of cases are bilateral, and the condition is rare in blacks.

The disease is frequently divided into three stages. The early stage of the disease is characterized by inflammation and synovitis of the hip joint and early ischemic changes in the ossific nucleus of the femoral head. Roentgenograms taken at this stage reveal joint swelling that may result in lateral displacement of the femoral head. An increase in the opacity of the ossific nucleus is usually present (Fig 10–10).

In the second, regenerative or fragmentation stage, the necrotic area begins to be replaced by viable bone. This phase lasts from 1 to 2 years. The roentgenographic appearance during this stage is one of fragmentation and compression of the femoral head with secondary widening of the femoral neck.

Reossification and healing occur in the third stage, which varies in duration beyond 1 year. The roentgenogram in this stage shows a disappearance of the rarefaction while normal bone continues to re-form. The final roentgenographic appearance depends on several factors, including the age of the patient, the degree of involvement,

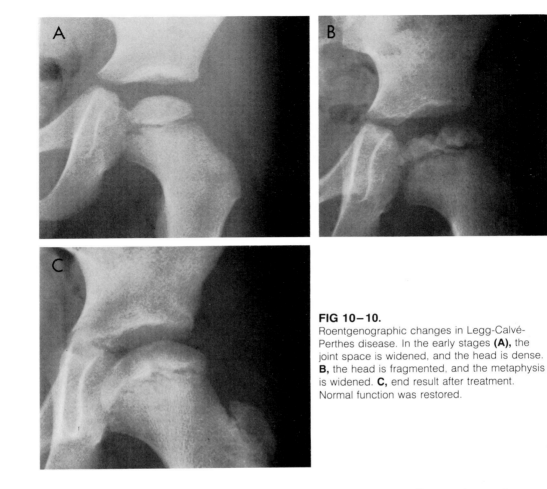

FIG 10-10.
Roentgenographic changes in Legg-Calvé-Perthes disease. In the early stages **(A),** the joint space is widened, and the head is dense. **B,** the head is fragmented, and the metaphysis is widened. **C,** end result after treatment. Normal function was restored.

and the adequacy of treatment. The femoral head may be normal in shape or irregular and flat (coxa plana).

Clinical Features

The onset is gradual, and the initial complaint is usually a mildly painful limp. The pain is often referred down the inner aspect of the thigh to the knee. The discomfort is frequently relieved by rest and aggravated by weight bearing.

Examination reveals moderate restriction of motion secondary to the synovitis. Abduction and internal rotation are especially limited. Pain is present at the extremes of motion, and tenderness is usually noted over the anterior hip joint.

Treatment and Prognosis

The ultimate goal of treatment is to prevent deformity of the femoral head from occurring while healing is progressing. If deformity can be prevented, the chances of degenerative joint disease developing at a later date are lessened. The immediate goals of treatment are the relief of pain, maintenance of joint motion, and containment of the femoral head in the acetabulum. If the head is contained in the acetabulum while it is re-forming, the acetabulum will "mold" the

head and prevent significant deformity from occurring. These goals of treatment are usually accomplished by the use of a brace that allows motion but contains the head in the acetabulum (Fig
10–11). The brace must be worn continuously
for two to three years.

Surgery may be necessary in certain selected
cases, but it is usually reserved for those patients
who fail to respond to conservative treatment. An
osteotomy of the femur or innominate bone is
performed in an attempt to provide "coverage"
of the femoral head.

The prognosis is dependent on the age of the
patient, the degree of involvement, and the adequacy of treatment. Young patients with minimal
involvement who are treated early do very well
with few sequelae. Older patients, over the age
of 8 years, frequently have some permanent restriction of motion, a slight limp, and a more irregular or flattened femoral head. A few patients
will later develop degenerative arthritis.

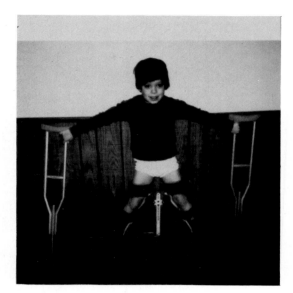

FIG 10–11.
Abduction brace.

SLIPPED CAPITAL FEMORAL EPIPHYSIS

Slipped capital femoral epiphysis is a disorder of
unknown cause in which weakening of the epiphyseal plate of the upper portion of the femur
occurs and results in upward and anterior displacement of the femoral neck. The actual
amount of displacement will vary. In most cases,
the slippage is gradual, and some elements of
healing are usually present.

The condition is seen most commonly in boys
between the ages of 11 and 16 years during their
rapid growth spurt. The disorder is bilateral in
25% of cases and frequently occurs in two distinct body types. The first is the slender, tall, rapidly growing boy, and the second is the large,
obese boy with underdeveloped sexual characteristics. The presence of the disorder in these
two body types suggests a hormonal cause, but
none has ever been proved.

Clinical Features
The onset is generally gradual, and symptoms
usually occur even when little displacement is

present. Discomfort in the hip and knee and a
painful limp with activity are the most common
initial complaints.

Examination reveals tenderness over the hip
joint capsule. An external rotation deformity of
the lower extremity may be present, and internal
rotation, abduction, and flexion are usually restricted. Pain is present at the extremes of motion, and the hip tends to rotate externally and
abduct as it is flexed (Whitman's sign).

In the early "preslipping" stage, the roentgenogram characteristically reveals irregular widening of the epiphyseal plate and joint swelling (Fig
10–12). As displacement occurs, a line drawn
along the superior or anterior neck of the femur
will transect less of the femoral head than normal. This may be more readily seen on the lateral view. More severe degrees of slippage are
usually easily diagnosed.

A condition similar to slipped capital femoral
epiphysis is termed *acute traumatic separation*
of the upper femoral epiphysis (Fig 10–13). This

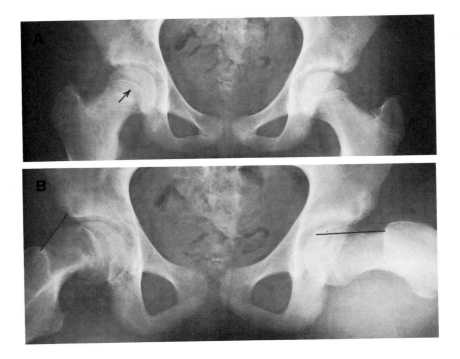

FIG 10–12.
Slipped capital femoral epiphysis. Widening of the epiphyseal plate *(arrow)* and displacement of the femoral head are present.

is actually an epiphyseal fracture and has a much poorer prognosis than the gradual slippage that occurs in slipped capital femoral epiphysis.

Treatment

As soon as the diagnosis is made, surgery is indicated. The patient is immediately placed on crutches, and weight bearing is prohibited. Traction in the hospital may be necessary to reduce the acute component of the slippage. In order to prevent further slippage from occurring, the femoral head is fixed to the neck, generally by using small pins (Fig 10–14). Weight bearing is prohibited for several months until the epiphyseal plate closes. Severe deformities may also require osteotomy of the femur.

The prognosis is usually good, except in those cases with acute traumatic separation. Slight shortening of less than 1.25 cm may result, along with a mild external rotation deformity. The internal fixation devices are usually removed after

the epiphyseal plate closes in 1 to 2 years. In cases with acute traumatic separation, avascular necrosis of the femoral head is a common complication, and this usually results in severe traumatic arthritis of the hip (Fig 10–15).

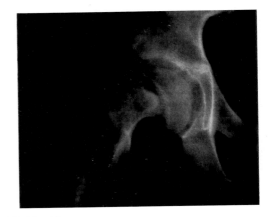

FIG 10–13.
Acute traumatic separation of the upper femoral epiphysis.

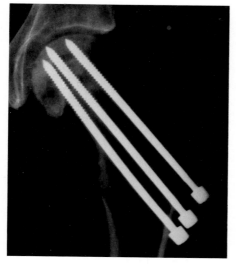

FIG 10–14.
Postoperative roentgenogram following pinning for slipped capital femoral epiphysis.

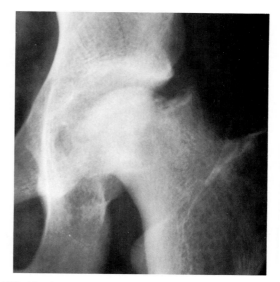

FIG 10–15.
Avascular necrosis and osteoarthritis following acute traumatic slipped capital femoral epiphysis. Reconstructive surgery was eventually required.

Acute Cartilage Necrosis

An occasional complication of slipped capital femoral epiphysis is acute necrosis or lysis of the articular cartilage of the hip joint. The articular surfaces of both the acetabulum and femoral head may be involved up to 1 year after the slippage. This condition appears to be directly re-lated to the severity of the slippage. The cause of this process is unknown, but destruction and degeneration of the hyaline cartilage occur. A painful fibrous ankylosis of the hip joint is frequently the end result.

TRANSIENT SYNOVITIS

Transient or "toxic" synovitis is a self-limited, nonspecific inflammation of the synovium of the hip joint that occurs in children. It is a common cause of pain in the hip in children under 10 years of age. The cause is unknown, but a viral infection is suspected. Its importance lies in its similarity to other hip joint disorders, especially septic arthritis.

Clinical Features

The onset is frequently acute and may follow a traumatic event or a recent upper respiratory infection. A painful limp is characteristic, and the pain is frequently referred to the inner aspect of the thigh and knee joint. A few patients will have night pain.

The hip is typically held in a position of slight flexion, abduction, and external rotation so that the hip joint capsule is under the least amount of tension. Pressure and discomfort are thereby reduced. Passive motions, especially internal rotation and abduction, are restricted. Temperatures of 37.3° C to 38.3° C may be present.

The roentgenogram may reveal swelling of the capsule and adjacent soft tissue. Slight widening of the joint space may also be present, but there are no changes in bone texture.

Laboratory findings are usually minimal, although there may be a slight increase in the white blood cell count. Aspiration and culture of the hip joint fluid are negative.

Treatment

Bed rest, gentle skin traction, and the elimination of weight bearing are indicated. The relief of pain and discomfort is usually rapid, and motion is restored in 2 to 4 days. Crutches are used for 2 to 4 weeks, and the patient is observed closely for up to 2 years because Perthes' disease will develop in a significant percentage (5% to 10%). Antibiotics are used only when the disorder is associated with an infection elsewhere.

SEPTIC ARTHRITIS IN CHILDHOOD

Pyogenic infection of the hip may result from an osteomyelitis of the femoral neck or a bacteremia. It may even develop from contamination by a faulty femoral venipuncture. If improperly

TABLE 10–1.

The Limping Child—Differential Diagnosis of Common Causes*

Disorder	Symptoms/History	Findings
Congenital dislocated hip	Painless. Usually noticed when child first begins to walk (12–18 mo). May be bilateral	Trendelenburg sign positive. Leg shortened if unilateral. "Telescoping" of leg at hip. Abnormal roentgenogram
Perthes disease (or other AVN)	Minimal pain (groin, anteromedial thigh) Age 4–8 yr. Family history positive if due to rare sickle cell or other hereditary anemia. No fever	Decreased hip ROM, especially abduction, and IR. Roentgenogram may show early joint widening. Later (2–4 wk) bony changes. Lab normal (except if due to blood disorder)
Toxic synovitis	Irritable. Slight fever, groin and anteromedial thigh pain. Age 4–8	Diminished hip movement. Slightly painful with motion. Roentgenogram may show slight joint space widening, fluid. Slight increase in ESR, WBC. Hip aspirate shows increased WBC, no bacteria
Septic hip	Painful! Septic, febrile, unable to ambulate. Groin pain (may be difficult to localize findings in young child)	Pain on slightest hip movement. Roentgenogram shows hip joint swelling. Hip aspirate positive for bacteria. Lab reflects infection
Slipped upper femoral epiphysis	Age 10–14 yr. Mild ache in groin, thigh. Leg often externally rotated	Limited IR. Roentgenogram shows slippage
"Low-grade" osteomyelitis, lower limb	Fever, irritable. Moderate pain with weight bearing (may be difficult to localize findings in young child)	Local bony tenderness and soft tissue swelling. Protected motion. Early plain roentgenogram normal. Bone scan abnormal
Inflammatory joint disease	Single or multiple joints. May be mildly febrile	Joint swelling, heat. Some limitation of motion. Serum studies sometimes abnormal. Often diagnosis of exclusion
Neurologic disorders (CP, etc.)	Often bilateral. No pain. Gait is wide based. Delay in motor development. History of perinatal problems	Abnormal neurologic findings

*Notes: Always consider (1) battered child (especially if history of prior injuries, burns), (2) tumor, and (3) occult fractures.
IR = internal rotation; ROM = range of motion.

treated, complete destruction of the hip joint may occur.

Clinical Features

The onset is usually rapid and develops over 24 hours. The child appears acutely ill and refuses to bear weight. The hip is held flexed and externally rotated, and movement is painful.

Fever, leukocytosis, and an elevated sedimentation rate are common. Plain roentgenograms may show only widening of the joint space due to swelling, and bone scanning is usually not helpful in the initial stages.

Treatment

Hip sepsis in the child is an *emergency*. Aspiration of the hip before the administration of antibiotics is the most diagnostic procedure. This is usually performed under fluoroscopic guidance and general anesthesia. *Staphylococcus aureus,* *Streptococcus, Pneumococcus,* and *Haemophilus influenzae* are the most common offending organisms. If infection is confirmed, intravenous antibiotics are started, and the hip is usually drained surgically.

Differential Diagnosis

Differentiation of mild cases from toxic or rheumatoid synovitis may be difficult. A child with toxic or rheumatoid synovitis generally appears well except for the hip, the fever is usually mild, and the hip is more "irritable" than painful. The white blood count and sedimentation are only slightly elevated. The hip aspirate may show an increase in white blood cells, especially polymorphonucleocytes, but the Gram stain and culture will be negative. Complete bed rest and symptomatic care usually cause considerable improvement in 24 hours, in contrast to a septic hip, which usually gets worse (Table 10–1).

COXA VARA

Coxa vara is an abnormality of the upper portion of the femur that consists of a decrease in the normal angle of inclination below 110 to 125 degrees (Fig 10–16). This may result from a wide variety of acquired and congenital conditions and usually results in a shortened extremity.

Acquired Forms

These are the most common types of coxa vara. Included in this category are Perthes' disease, slipped capital femoral epiphysis, rickets, osteomalacia, and various injuries to the upper part of the femur. Each disease has its own clinical and roentgenographic features.

Congenital Forms

Congenital local disturbances in the growth of the proximal aspect of the femur may also lead to shortening and a significant coxa vara deformity. These disorders usually fall into three distinct classifications.

Congenital Coxa Vara (Infantile, Cervical, Developmental)

This disorder is the result of faulty development of the femoral neck, which leads to the varus deformity. The cause is unknown. The disorder is frequently bilateral and becomes manifested after weight bearing has begun.

The child usually presents with a painless limp. If the disorder is bilateral, a "duck-waddle" gait may be present. In this gait pattern, the body sways from side to side. Abduction and internal rotation of the affected extremity are usually restricted, and the leg may be from 2.5 to 5 cm shorter than normal. The lumbar lordosis is usually exaggerated, and with continued weight bearing the varus deformity may progress.

Roentgenographic examination usually reveals a decrease in the neck-shaft angle. In addition, a

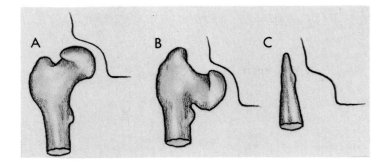

FIG 10–16.
A, the normal neck-shaft angle. **B,** coxa vara. **C,** proximal focal femoral deficiency.

triangular defect in the inferior aspect of the femoral neck may be present.

The treatment of mild deformities in which the neck-shaft angle is greater than 100 degrees consists of a shoe lift, exercises to release contractures, and periodic re-examination. A brace that prohibits weight bearing may be necessary. More severe deformities require an osteotomy of the upper portion of the femur to correct the angulation.

Congenital Bowed Femur With Coxa Vara

This type of coxa vara is characterized by lateral bowing of the femur. The coxa vara is usually not as severe as that found with congenital coxa vara,

but the shortening of the extremity may reach 10 to 15 cm. Treatment consists of equalizing the extremities by shoe lifts.

Congenital Short Femur With Coxa Vara

This uncommon disorder is also known as proximal focal femoral deficiency. Portions of the proximal aspect of the femur are either completely absent or severely underdeveloped, and shortening of the limb may reach 25 to 37.5 cm by adulthood. Bracing is necessary in the young child, and amputation of the lower part of the leg, followed by prosthetic fitting to equalize the leg lengths, is usually the definitive treatment.

DEGENERATIVE ARTHRITIS

Degenerative arthritis confined to the hip joint is a common affliction in the middle and later years of adult life. The cause is not completely understood, but obesity, trauma, congenital hip dysplasia, avascular necrosis of the femoral head, and slipped capital femoral epiphysis are all factors in its onset.

Pathologically, the articular cartilage becomes progressively thinned and worn away. New bone proliferation around the femoral head and acetabulum occurs, and the synovium becomes chronically thickened and congested.

Clinical Features

The clinical course is gradual, and both hips may be affected. The onset of symptoms may be precipitated by a relatively minor injury. Pain after activity and stiffness after rest are characteristic. The stiffness frequently subsides with activity, and the pain frequently subsides with rest. The pain is often referred to the knee joint region. With the passage of time, the pain increases, sometimes even occurring at rest. Crepitus and grating in the hip may develop, and a painful limp is common.

Examination reveals tenderness over the anterior and posterior hip joint and restriction of motion, especially internal rotation and abduction. Pain is usually present at the extremes of motion. A flexion contracture frequently develops. This can be measured by the Thomas test. In this test, the patient is placed in a supine position and the opposite thigh is flexed up to the chest to eliminate motion at the pelvis and lumbar spine. The angle formed between the affected thigh and the examining table is the amount of flexion contracture of the hip.

The roentgenographic findings are characteristic (Fig 10–17). Irregular sclerosis, joint space narrowing, and osteophyte formation are prominent features.

Treatment

Conservative treatment will frequently eliminate symptoms and improve motion. The regimen requires a cooperative patient. Salicylates are prescribed in sufficient doses to relieve pain and reduce the inflammatory response. Ten to 12 tablets are usually required daily. Obesity must be corrected, and the joint placed at rest. Intermittent bed rest and the use of a cane when ambulatory are frequently sufficient. The cane is usually used in the hand opposite the affected extremity (although it may be used in the ipsilateral hand), and pressure is applied to the cane at the same time that weight is being borne on the painful hip. Buck's traction and moist heat are also helpful. Gentle range-of-motion exercise

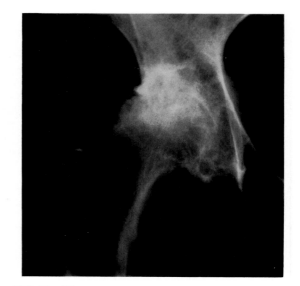

FIG 10–17.
Degenerative arthritis of the hip.

such as swimming will often overcome contractures and restore motion. The treatment plan may have to be repeated at intervals.

A variety of surgical procedures are available for those patients who fail to respond to conservative treatment. The most common procedures are arthrodesis, especially in the young patient, and total hip arthroplasty. The goal of each of these procedures is the elimination of pain. In addition, joint replacement will often improve hip joint motion. The indications for each procedure will vary according to the age and occupation of the patient.

AVASCULAR NECROSIS

Avascular or aseptic necrosis of the femoral head is an uncommon condition that occurs in the third to fifth decade. It is characterized by the development of an area of bone necrosis in the anterosuperior weight-bearing portion of the femoral head. The cause is unknown, but the condition is frequently bilateral and is more common in men. It is often seen in association with gouty arthritis, chronic alcoholism, and chronic renal disease; in divers and workers who use compressed air; and in those patients who have undergone long-term steroid therapy. It probably occurs secondary to a circulatory disturbance to the femoral head. Following the initial infarction,

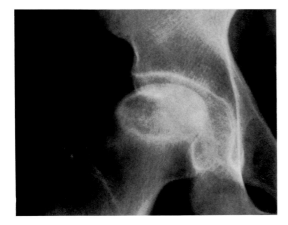

FIG 10–18.
Avascular necrosis of the femoral head.

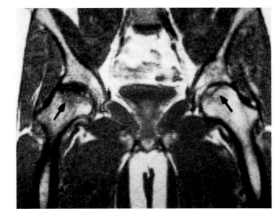

FIG 10–19.
MRI showing bilateral avascular necrosis.

collapse and fragmentation may occur, which lead to deformity of the femoral head and degenerative arthritis.

Clinical Features

The onset is gradual, with pain and a slight limp being common. A history of trauma is usually absent. Joint motion becomes progressively restricted.

The roentgenogram reveals an increase in the density of the superior portion of the femur (Fig 10–18). A radiolucent zone is frequently present between the avascular segment and the surrounding bone. The joint space is usually well preserved until late in the disease, when degenerative arthritis intervenes. Avascular necrosis is one of the main indications for MRI, which usually reveals the lesion quite clearly (Fig 10–19).

Treatment

The goal of treatment is to prevent collapse of the femoral head and encourage repair of the necrotic area. With minimal involvement, prolonged abstinence from weight bearing by the use of crutches may allow replacement of the avascular segment, but bone grafting to hasten this reconstitution is frequently necessary. Later in the disease, when collapse has occurred, prosthetic replacement is indicated.

BURSITIS

Several bursae are present about the hip joint. The one most subjected to irritation and pain is the trochanteric bursa. This sac lies between the greater trochanter and the overlying tendinous portion of the gluteus maximus muscle. Inflammation of the sac is common in the elderly patient and is characterized by local pain over the trochanter that frequently radiates down the lateral aspect of the thigh to the knee. This pain pattern may cause confusion with lumbar disc disease. Local tenderness is usually present, and hip motion, especially internal rotation and abduction, may be painful. It is difficult for the patient to lie on the affected side.

Treatment consists of moist heat, rest, and anti-inflammatory agents. Ultrasound to the affected area may be beneficial, and a local injection of a steroid/lidocaine mixture into the area of maximum tenderness is frequently curative.

MERALGIA PARESTHETICA

Meralgia paresthetica is an uncommon disorder characterized by pain and paresthesias occurring along the course of the lateral femoral cutaneous nerve of the thigh. This nerve enters the leg beneath the inguinal ligament and supplies sensation to the anterolateral aspect of the thigh (Fig 10–20). Painful involvement of the nerve may be confused with hip and low back disorders. The cause of this condition is unknown, but direct pressure or constriction of the nerve at its point of exit into the thigh is thought to play a role.

Clinical Features

The disorder is sometimes seen in obese patients or those who wear tight corsets or undergarments. Hypersensitivity, burning, tingling, and pain that occurs with activity or direct pressure over the nerve are characteristic. The symptoms are often relieved by rest.

The pain may be aggravated by passive extension of the hip. A slight decrease in sensation over the anterolateral aspect of the thigh is sometimes noted, and pain may be reproduced with pressure on the nerve medial to the anterior superior iliac spine.

Treatment

Symptoms often subside spontaneously over a variable length of time. Weight loss and the

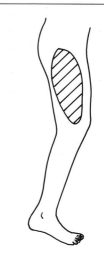

FIG 10–20.
Sensory area of the anterolateral thigh affected in meralgia paresthetica.

avoidance of constricting garments are advised. Injection of the nerve distal to the inguinal ligament 1.25 cm medial and 2.5 cm below the anterosuperior iliac spine with a local anesthetic may relieve symptoms. Surgical release or even removal of the nerve may occasionally be necessary for intractable cases, but the surgical results are only fair.

PROTRUSIO ACETABULI (OTTO PELVIS)

Abnormal intrapelvic protrusion of the acetabulum is a relatively uncommon disorder of unknown cause. It may be present on a congenital basis or develop secondary to trauma or arthritis. It is frequently bilateral and is characterized by abnormal deepening of the acetabulum, which allows the femoral head to be displaced further into the pelvis.

Clinical Features

The onset is usually gradual, with progressive restriction of hip motion occurring over several years. Eventually, with the onset of degenerative arthritis, pain becomes a prominent symptom. Complete ankylosis of the joint frequently occurs.

The roentgenogram reveals abnormal protrusion of the medial wall of the acetabulum with thinning and degenerative changes (Fig 10–21).

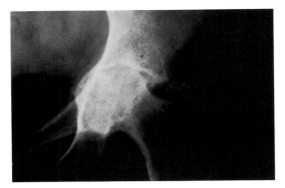

FIG 10–21.
Protrusio acetabuli. The medial acetabular wall protrudes and the femoral head has migrated medially.

DISLOCATIONS OF THE HIP

Dislocations of the hip are the result of severe trauma and are usually posterior in direction (Fig 10–22). They commonly result from the knee being struck while the hip and the knee are in a flexed position. This force drives the femoral head out of the joint posteriorly. These injuries are frequently associated with fractures of the posterior acetabular wall. Anterior dislocations are less common and usually result from a force on the knee with the thigh abducted. The neck of the femur impinges on the posterior rim of the acetabulum, and the head is levered out the front.

Treatment
Traction and the avoidance of weight bearing are indicated in early cases. Arthrodesis in the unilateral case or total hip replacement may be necessary for disabling pain.

Clinical Features
With posterior dislocation, the hip is characteristically held in a position of flexion and internal

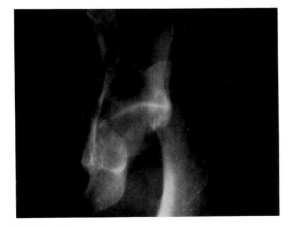

FIG 10–22.
Posterior dislocation of the hip.

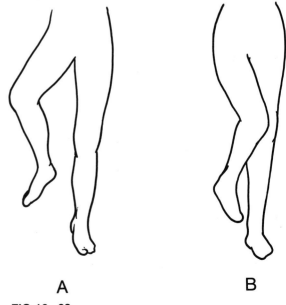

FIG 10–23.
Appearance of hip dislocations. **A,** anterior. **B,** posterior.

rotation (Fig 10–23). All motions are painful. There may be an associated injury of the ipsilateral knee. In anterior dislocations the leg usually rests in external rotation.

Treatment

In the dislocated position, great tension is placed on the blood supply to the femoral head. Avascular necrosis may even result if the dislocation is not promptly reduced. In order to prevent this complication, early reduction within 6 to 12 hours is indicated. The reduction of the posterior location can usually be accomplished by traction on the flexed hip with countertraction on the pelvis. A general anesthetic is usually necessary. If closed reduction fails or an acetabular fragment is present that is of sufficient size to produce instability, open reduction is indicated.

The reduction is frequently maintained by skeletal traction until sufficient soft-tissue and bony healing have occurred to prevent redislocation. Weight bearing is prohibited for an additional 2 to 3 months.

FRACTURES OF THE HIP

The femoral head receives its blood supply from vessels that course proximally up the femoral neck. Fractures that occur distal to these vessels (intertrochanteric) do not disturb the blood supply to the femoral head, but fractures that occur proximally (intracapsular) may destroy the blood supply. With disruption of the blood supply, nonunion of the fracture and avascular necrosis of the femoral head are much more common.

Intracapsular and intertrochanteric fractures are both common in the elderly patient and usually result from a fall on the hip. Both fractures are characterized by shortening and external rotation of the affected leg with pain in the region of the hip joint (Fig 10–24). Osteoporosis clearly plays a significant role. Occasionally, the patient may actually fracture the hip before falling, the fracture representing the completion of an insufficiency injury. Femoral neck fractures may also be occult and show up only with repeated examinations or bone scan.

Treatment

If external immobilization or prolonged bed rest were required in the treatment of these fractures in this age group, the mortality would be high. For this reason, early surgery within 24 to 48 hours is indicated in order to allow the patient to be out of bed at the earliest possible time. Displaced intracapsular fractures in the elderly are best treated by early prosthetic replacement (Fig 10–25). This allows early weight bearing and eliminates the possibility of nonunion and avascular necrosis that could necessitate secondary surgical procedures. Undisplaced or impacted fractures are often treated nonoperatively or by

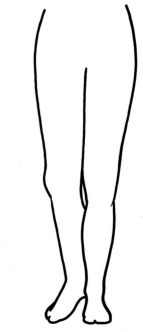

FIG 10–24.
External rotation deformity typical of hip fractures.

simple internal fixation to add stability. These fractures have a much better prognosis regarding healing and avascular necrosis. Young, healthy patients are treated by reduction of the fracture and internal fixation. It is best to try to preserve the femoral head in this age group if it is possible because the long-term results are better than with prosthetic replacement.

Intertrochanteric fractures are treated by open reduction and internal fixation (Fig 10–26). This allows early activity by eliminating the pain at the fracture site. Nonunion in this fracture is much less common than with the intracapsular fracture. Weight bearing is usually restricted for 3 months until union of the fracture has occurred, however.

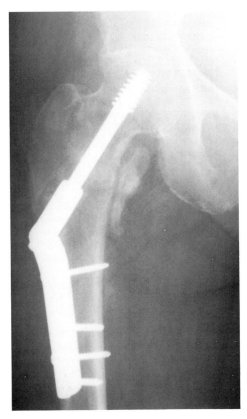

FIG 10–26.
Roentgenogram following reduction and nailing of an intertrochanteric fracture.

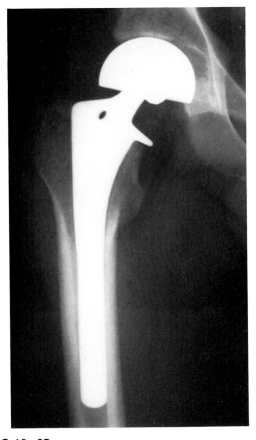

FIG 10–25.
Roentgenogram of the hip following replacement of the femoral head with a prosthesis.

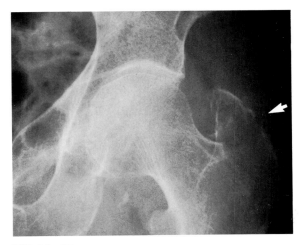

FIG 10–27.
Avulsion fracture *(arrow)* of the greater trochanter.

Occasionally, an isolated fracture of either trochanter may occur following a minor injury (Fig 10–27). Treatment is symptomatic, with crutches and weight-bearing activity as tolerated.

DIFFERENTIAL DIAGNOSIS OF BACK AND LEG PAIN (see TABLE 10–2)

TABLE 10–2.

Differential Diagnosis of Common Causes of Back, Hip, and Leg Pain

Disorder	Common Pain Location or Radiation	Findings Present	Findings Absent
Disc disease	Low back, high buttock. May radiate to posterior thigh (posterior or lateral calf if nerve root impingement). May have paresthesias in foot (Fig 10–28)	Limited low back movement. Often no history of injury. May have positive SLR. Neurologic deficit if nerve root under pressure	Normal hip movement. No local tenderness other than low back.
Hip disease (osteoarthritis, AVN, etc.)	Groin, low buttock. Anteromedial thigh to knee	Groin pain with hip movement. Decreased hip movement	No back pain, no pain below knee. No neurologic symptoms or findings
Hamstring strain	Posterior thigh	Painful SLR but local tenderness, swelling, and hemorrhage in hamstring. History of acute strain to muscle	Back motion normal. No low back pain. No paresthesias or pain below knee
Trochanteric bursitis	Lateral hip, lateral thigh to knee	Tender greater trochanter. May have pain on adduction with IR	Full range of hip and back motion. No paresthesias. No low back pain
Spinal stenosis	Variable. Both buttocks, legs. Older patient. "Pseudoclaudication" pain—worse with walking, better with rest. Long history of back pain. Pain often relieved by flexion of spine	Back extension may reproduce pain. May have minimal variable neurologic abnormalities. Usually advanced degenerative disc disease on roentgenogram	Straight leg raising usually negative. Hips move normally

AVN = avascular necrosis; SLR = straight leg raising; IR = internal rotation.

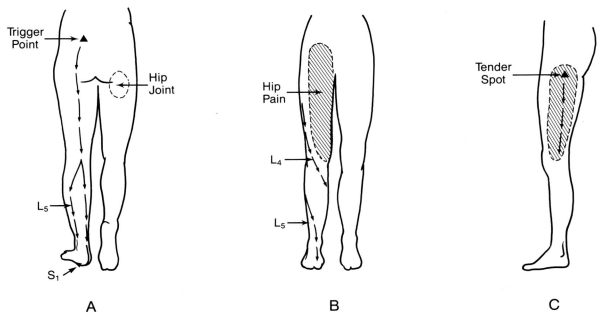

FIG 10–28.
A, typical lumbar disc pain when herniation is far enough to cause radicular (L5 or S1) pain. If herniation is minor, only unilateral low back pain may occur. **B,** anterior distribution of hip joint pain. (Hip disease may also cause low buttock pain.) Also shown are nerve roots L4 and L5. **C,** pain distribution of trochanteric bursitis. **Note:** Calf or general leg symptoms may be the first and only sign of lumbar disc herniation with radiation.

BIBLIOGRAPHY

Aadalen RJ, et al: Acute slipped capital femoral epiphysis. *J Bone Joint Surg [Am]* 1974; 56:1473.

Aegerter E, Kirkpatrick JA: *Orthopedic Diseases,* ed. 3. Philadelphia, WB Saunders Co, 1968.

Allwright SJ, Cooper RA, Nash P: Trochanteric bursitis: Bone scan appearance. *Clin Nucl Med* 1988; 13:561.

Amstutz HC, Wilson PD Jr: Dysgenesis of the proximal femur (coxa vara) and its surgical management. *J Bone Joint Surg [Am]* 1962; 44:1.

Bos CF, Bloem JL: Treatment of dislocation of the hip, detected in early childhood based on magnetic resonance imaging. *J Bone Joint Surg [Am]* 1989; 71:1523.

Bowen JR, Foster BK, Hartzell CR: Legg-Calvé-Perthes disease. *Clin Orthop* 1984; 185:97.

Cattaral A: The natural history of Perthes' disease. *J Bone Joint Surg [Br]* 1971; 53:37.

Clarke NM, et al: Real-time ultrasound in the diagnosis of congenital dislocation and dysplasia of the hip. *J Bone Joint Surg [Br]* 1985; 67:406.

Coleman BG, et al: Radiographically negative avascular necrosis: Detection with MR imaging. *Radiology* 1988; 168:528.

Coleman SS: Treatment of congenital dislocation of the hip. *J Bone Joint Surg [Am]* 1965; 47:590.

Curtis BH, et al: Treatment for Legg-Perthes' disease with the Newington ambulation-abduction brace. *J Bone Joint Surg [Am]* 1974; 56:1135.

Davies SJM, Walker G: Problems in the early recognition of hip dysplasia. *J Bone Joint Surg [Br]* 1984; 66:479.

Engesaeter LB, et al: Ultrasound and congenital dislocation of the hip. *J Bone Joint Surg [Br]* 1990; 72:202.

Epstein HC: Posterior fracture-dislocations of the hip. *J Bone Joint Surg [Am]* 1974; 56:1103.

Ficat RP: Idiopathic bone necrosis of the femoral head. *J Bone Joint Surg [Br]* 1985; 67:3.

Friedenberg ZB: Protrusio acetabuli. *Am J Surg* 1953; 85:764.

Gage JR, Winter RB: Avascular necrosis of the capital femoral epiphysis as a complication of closed reduction of congenital dislocation of the hip. *J Bone Joint Surg [Am]* 1972; 54:373.

Genez BM, et al: Early osteonecrosis of the femoral head. Detection in high risk patients with MR imaging. *Radiology* 1988; 168:521.

Gore DR: Iatrogenic avascular necrosis of the hip in young children. *J Bone Joint Surg [Am]* 1974; 56:493.

Grant JCB: *A Method of Anatomy,* ed 6. Baltimore, Williams & Wilkins, 1958.

Hauzeur JP, et al: The diagnostic value of magnetic resonance imaging in non-traumatic osteonecrosis of the femoral head. *J Bone Joint Surg [Am]* 1989; 71:641.

Hermel MB, Albert SM: Transient synovitis of the hip. *Clin Orthop* 1962; 22:21.

Ilfeld FW, Makin M: Damage to the capital femoral epiphysis due to Frejka pillow treatment. *J Bone Joint Surg [Am]* 1977; 59:654.

Iwasaki K: Treatment of congenital dislocation of hip by the Pavlik harness. *J Bone Joint Surg [Am]* 1983; 65:760.

Kennie DC, et al: Effectiveness of geriatric rehabilitative care after fractures of the proximal femur in elderly women: A randomized clinical trial. *Br Med J* 1988; 297:1083.

Landin LA, Danielson LG, Wattsgard C: Transient synovitis of the hip: Its incidence, epidemiology and relation to Perthes disease. *J Bone Joint Surg [Br]* 1987; 69:238.

Marcus ND, Enneking WF, Massan RA: The silent hip in idiopathic aseptic necrosis (treatment by bone-grafting). *J Bone Joint Surg [Am]* 1973; 55:1351.

Meyers MH: *Fractures of the Hip.* Chicago, Year Book Medical Publishers Inc, 1985.

Mitchell GP: Problems in the early diagnosis and management of congenital dislocation of the hip. *J Bone Joint Surg [Br]* 1972; 54:4.

Petrie JG, Bitenc I: The abduction weight-bearing treatment in Legg-Perthes' disease. *J Bone Joint Surg [Br]* 1971; 53:56.

Ramsey PL, Lasser S, MacEwen GD: Congenital dislocation of the hip: Use of the Pavlik harness in the child during the first six months of life. *J Bone Joint Surg [Am]* 1976; 58: 1000.

Smith K, Bonfiglio M, Dolan K: Roentgenographic search for avascular necrosis of the head of the femur in alcoholics and normal adults. *J Bone Joint Surg [Am]* 1977; 59:391.

Solomon L: Drug-induced arthropathy and necrosis of the femoral head. *J Bone Joint Surg [Br]* 1973; 55:246.

Somerville EW: Perthes' disease of the hip. *J Bone Joint Surg [Br]* 1971; 53:639.

Stewart MJ, Milford LW: Fracture-dislocation of the hip. *J Bone Joint Surg [Am]* 1954; 36:315.

Sunberg SB, Savage JP, Foster BK: Technetium phosphate bone scan in the diagnosis of septic arthritis in childhood. *J Pediatr Orthop* 1989; 9:379.

Tachdjian MO: *Pediatric Orthopedics.* Philadelphia, WB Saunders Co, 1972.

Terjesen T, Bredland T, Berg V: Ultrasound for hip assessment in the newborn. *J Bone Joint Surg [Br]* 1989; 71:767.

Tinetti ME, Speechly M, Ginter SF: Risk factors for falls among elderly persons living in the community. *N Engl J Med* 1988; 319:1701.

Viere RG, et al: Use of the Pavlik harness in congenital dislocation of the hip. An analysis of failures of treatment. *J Bone Joint Surg [Am]* 1990; 72:238.

Williamson DM, Glover SD, Benson MK: Congenital dislocation of the hip presenting after the age of three years. *J Bone Joint Surg [Br]* 1989; 71:745.

Wilson NI, DiPaola M: Acute septic arthritis in infancy and childhood. *J Bone Joint Surg [Br]* 1986; 68:584.

Wopper JM, et al: Long-term followup of infantile hip sepsis. *J Pediatr Orthop* 1988; 8:322.

CHAPTER 11

The Knee

The knee is the largest joint in the body. The lower portion of the femur and upper aspect of the tibia articulate at only two points where the rounded femoral condyles bear weight on the flat tibial plateaus. The knee joint is subject to a wide variety of traumatic, mechanical and inflammatory disorders. Traumatic and mechanical disorders are often loosely termed "internal derangements."

ANATOMY

The knee joint consists of medial and lateral, femoral and tibial condyles and the patella. The knee has no intrinsic bony stability and depends completely on its ligaments, muscles, menisci,

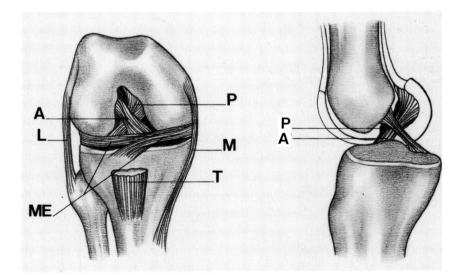

FIG 11–1.
Ligaments of the knee: *A* = anterior cruciate ligament; *P* = posterior cruciate ligament; *L* = lateral collateral ligament; *M* = medial collateral ligament; *T* = patellar tendon; *ME* = medial and lateral menisci.

and capsule for support. The most important ligaments of the knee are the medial and lateral collateral ligaments and the anterior and posterior cruciate ligaments (Fig 11–1). The medial collateral ligament originates below the adductor tubercle and attaches to the upper medial tibia. It limits abduction and assists in controlling rotation. The lateral collateral ligament attaches to the lateral epicondyle of the femur and head of the fibula and controls adduction. The cruciate ligaments attach to the intra-articular portions of the femur and tibia. The anterior cruciate ligament prevents anterior displacement of the tibia and helps control rotation of the tibia on the femur. The posterior cruciate prevents backward displacement of the tibia on the femur and is the major stabilizer of the knee joint.

The muscles about the knee also play important roles in its function. The quadriceps group is the most important. These muscles control extension and prevent dislocation of the patella. The medial and lateral hamstrings provide posterior support to the knee and control flexion. Additional support is provided by the popliteus muscle and the iliotibial band.

Normal knee motion consists of a combination of rotation and either extension or flexion.

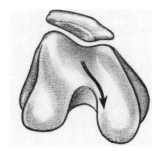

FIG 11–2.
Excursion of a patella with knee flexion.

Normally, as the knee flexes, the tibia internally rotates. Extension of the knee is accompanied by lateral or external rotation of the tibia. These rotational motions are controlled by the ligaments and menisci of the knee. This rotation is reflected in the course that the patella takes with flexion and extension movements (Fig 11–2). Thus, damage to the knee such as a torn meniscus, which prevents normal tibial rotation, can cause patellar symptoms due to abnormal patellar excursion. These patellar symptoms are typically aggravated by walking up and down stairs, an activity that puts the greatest strain on the patella and knee extensors.

ROENTGENOGRAPHIC ANATOMY

Anteroposterior and lateral views are essential in the diagnosis of knee disorders (Fig 11–3). A tunnel view will visualize the intercondylar notch, and tangential views are helpful in diagnosing patellar disorders.

LESIONS OF THE MENISCUS

Injuries of the Meniscus

The menisci, or semilunar cartilages, are two "C"-shaped structures composed of fibrocartilage that act as cushions between the femur and tibia. They also assist in the control of normal knee motion. If the normal rotation of the tibia is forcibly prevented as the knee is flexed or extended, a tear in the meniscus can occur, that is, if flexion occurs with external rotation or extension occurs with internal rotation.

Meniscus tears are the most common of all

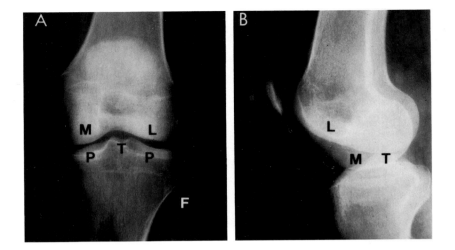

FIG 11–3.
Roentgenograms of a normal knee: *M* = medial femoral condyle; *L* = lateral femoral condyle; *T* = tubercles of the inter-condylar eminence; *P* = medial and lateral tibial plateaus; *F* = head of the fibula. Note that the medial femoral condyle projects more distally on both views.

knee injuries, and the pathologic characteristics of the tear are variable (Fig 11–4). When an injury occurs that produces free fragments or tears, healing to the main body of the meniscus does not take place. The fragment often remains permanently detached but viable because nourishment for the meniscus is provided by the joint fluid. This joint fluid circulates around the tear and prevents healing from taking place. Persistent symptoms are the result. The medial meniscus is injured ten times more frequently because it is more firmly attached and less mobile than the lateral meniscus. In long-standing disease, ar-

ticular cartilage erosion and degenerative changes at the tibiofemoral and patellofemoral joints may even result.

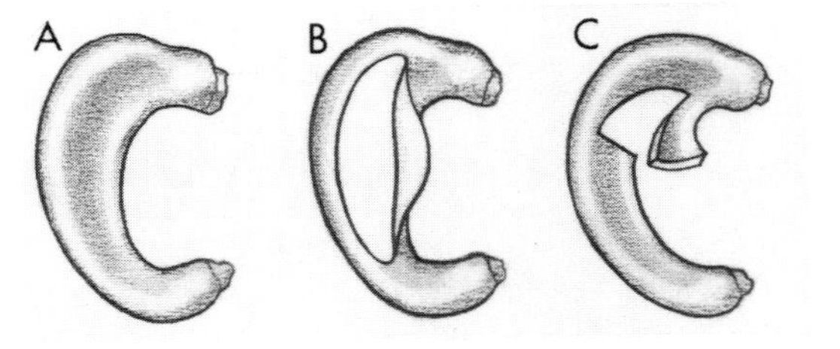

Clinical Features

The history is usually one of a twisting injury to the knee with the foot in the weight-bearing position. Occasionally, the injury is slight. A "popping" or "tearing" sensation is often felt, followed by severe pain. The pain is frequently well localized medially or laterally, depending on which meniscus is injured. Locking, from mechanical blockage of motion by the meniscus, may occasionally occur, but restricted motion after meniscus injury is usually due to other causes, such as hamstring spasm or swelling, that produce a pseudolocking effect. Swelling from joint effusion gradually occurs over several hours. This is in contrast to ligamentous injury, where the swelling is immediate due to hemorrhage. The swelling from meniscus injury is frequently maximum on the day following the injury.

The acute symptoms may subside within a few days only to be replaced by intermittent episodes of locking, buckling, giving out, swelling, and

FIG 11–4.
A, normal meniscus. **B,** longitudinal or "bucket-handle" tear. **C,** tear of the posterior horn.

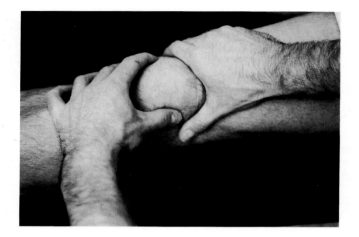

FIG 11–5.
Checking for joint effusion. Milking the suprapatellar pouch with downward pressure will frequently reveal fluid that might not otherwise be apparent. Pressure against the patella may produce a "click" as the patella strikes the femur.

mild pain. Walking up and down stairs is frequently difficult, and squatting may be painful.

The examination usually reveals a joint effusion (Fig 11–5). Its presence indicates acute or chronic synovial irritation. Its absence by history or examination should cause another diagnosis to be considered. This fluid may cause the patella to be ballotable. A click may also be present when the patella is pressed against the femur.

Pain and tenderness at the joint line either medially or laterally may be present. The range of motion is frequently limited. This may be due to swelling, spasm, or, occasionally, the interposition of the torn meniscus. In long-standing disease, atrophy of the quadriceps muscle, especially the vastus medialis, occurs rapidly (Fig 11–6).

The McMurray test is frequently helpful in detecting a meniscus tear, although it is difficult to perform on a painful, swollen knee (Fig 11–7).

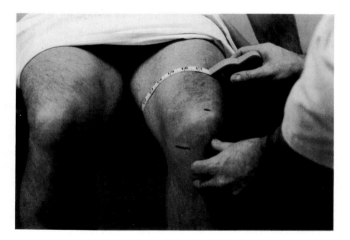

FIG 11–6.
The circumference of the thigh is measured 10 cm above the proximal pole of the patella (the medial joint line is marked).

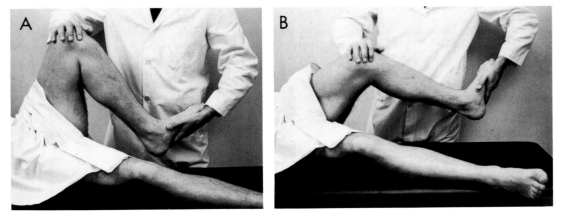

FIG 11–7.
McMurray test. To test for medial meniscus injury, the hip and knee are flexed maximally, and a valgus (abduction) force is applied to the knee **(A).** The foot is externally rotated, and the knee is passively extended **(B).** An audible or palpable snap during extension suggests a tear of the medial meniscus. To test for lateral meniscus injury, the procedure is performed with a varus, internal rotation stress applied.

Special Studies

1. Plain roentgenograms are usually normal but should always be performed to rule out other disorders.
2. Arthrographic examination of the knee remains a valuable tool in assessing the status of the meniscus. (It is less helpful in evaluating ligamentous injuries.) Its disadvantage is its invasive nature. It is usually not indicated until conservative treatment has failed for 3 to 4 weeks.
3. Magnetic resonance imaging (MRI) will probably replace most of the special studies used to evaluate knee pathology. Ligament and meniscal injuries as well as osteonecrosis are accurately visualized. It should not be used as a "screening test," however, and meniscus injuries should first have an adequate clinical trial of conservative management for several weeks.

Treatment

The initial treatment is conservative, except for those cases in which the knee is truly locked. Many meniscus tears, especially peripheral ones, can heal spontaneously in a few weeks. A bulky compression dressing and ice are applied, and the knee is elevated. The patient is placed on crutches and started on quadriceps-strengthening exercises (Fig 11–8). These exercises will compress out the joint effusion, and they should always be performed with the knee in the extended position in order to prevent patellofemoral pain from developing. Gentle range-of-motion exercises are started in 2 to 3 days. Swimming is an excellent exercise for increasing motion and decreasing muscle spasm and discomfort. As pain subsides and motion returns, weight-bearing activities are gradually resumed, but quadriceps exercises are continued for 2 to 4 weeks.

There are few indications for aspiration of the knee and even fewer indications for the injection of steroids in the treatment of an acute injury. The protective responses of the patient should be maintained, and it is better to reduce swelling by quadriceps contractions and to rehabilitate the knee through exercises.

Surgery is reserved for those cases of true irreducible locking or cases with recurrent or persistent signs and symptoms of meniscus injury. The meniscus is removed or repaired, often arthroscopically, in order to prevent irreversible articular damage from occurring and to relieve

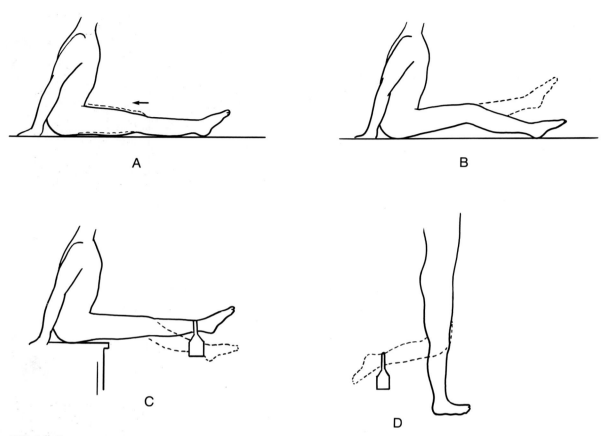

FIG 11–8.
Knee exercises. **A,** isometric quadsetting. The muscle is tightened and the knee stiffened and relaxed several times. **B** and **C,** isotonic short-arc knee extension. The knee is straightened through the last 30 degrees (to prevent peripatellar pain). Weights are gradually added beginning with 2 kg and progressing to 10 kg. **D,** isotonic knee curls for hamstring strengthening. Weight is increased as with quad strengthening. All exercises are performed as five sets of ten lifts each, three times a day. Exercises should not cause pain or swelling.

symptoms. The results are usually excellent, and most patients are able to resume normal activities 3 to 6 weeks after surgery.

Discoid Meniscus

Because of a failure in normal development, a meniscus, usually the lateral, may be elliptical rather than semilunar. The most common clinical finding in this disorder is an audible click that occurs with motion of the knee joint. The click may be present in infancy, but the disorder is usually not otherwise symptomatic at this age. The meniscus frequently wears away, so the clicking disappears.

Occasionally, however, symptoms persist into adulthood, with clicking and aching pain at the lateral joint margin being common complaints. A palpable degenerative *cyst* may even form in the meniscus. Local tenderness at the lateral joint space is usually present.

Meniscectomy may be necessary in an adult

with persistent symptoms. Infants usually require no treatment.

Calcification of the Menisci

The meniscus can become calcified from a variety of causes (Fig 11–9), the most common being degeneration and trauma. However, calcification can also occur in several other conditions, including degenerative arthritis, ochronosis, and pseudogout. The calcification itself is usually not painful. The symptoms are those that result from the primary disorder, and treatment is directed at that disorder.

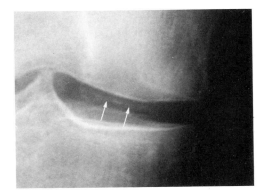

FIG 11–9.
Calcification of the meniscus.

CYSTS

Only two types of cystic lesions, the popliteal cyst and the cyst of the semilunar cartilage, occur with any frequency around the knee joint. The *popliteal* or *Baker's cyst* is an enlargement of the semimembranous bursa that is normally present in the medial aspect of the popliteal space. It may occur in any age group. In children, the cyst appears to be a primary lesion, in contrast to adults in whom most of these cysts are secondary to an intra-articular abnormality of the knee. This intra-articular abnormality, frequently a posterior tear of the medial meniscus or rheumatoid arthritis, causes an increase in joint fluid. This chronic effusion opens the normal anatomic communication between the joint and cyst and allows fluid to escape into the semimembranous bursa.

Clinical Features

In children, the symptoms are usually related to the effects of direct pressure of the cyst on the adjacent soft tissues. Local discomfort is common. In adults, the symptoms are related not only to the effects of the pressure of the cyst but also to the primary intra-articular abnormality. (Many cysts are asymptomatic, however.) The cyst commonly changes in size, depending on

the activity of the patient and the amount of swelling in the knee.

Examination will reveal a cystic mass of variable size lateral to the medial hamstrings in the popliteal fossa. Local tenderness may be present.

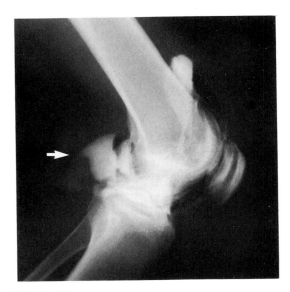

FIG 11–10.
Arthrogram revealing a large popliteal cyst.

Other findings of primary joint disease may be present, especially in adults.

The roentgenogram is usually normal. Arthrographic and ultrasound studies, however, will usually reveal the cyst (Fig 11–10).

Treatment

In children with primary cysts, treatment should be conservative. There is a high rate of spontaneous disappearance of the cyst in this age group and an equally high rate of recurrence following surgical excision. Aspiration and injection of the cyst may be attempted, but it is usually not necessary because the cyst frequently disappears in 1 to 2 years.

In symptomatic adults, every attempt should be made to detect any underlying joint abnormality. Cyst excision without correction of the intra-articular abnormality is followed by a high rate of recurrence of the cyst. Correction of the intra-articular disease will also frequently make cyst excision unnecessary because the cyst becomes asymptomatic following elimination of the cause of the chronic effusion. Older patients are often treated successfully by aspiration alone.

Cysts may also develop in a *meniscus,* usually the lateral, as a result of degeneration or trauma. The patient is generally a young adult who has a history of pain and a gradually enlarging mass over the lateral joint line. A knee effusion may be present. Treatment consists of meniscectomy and cyst excision if the patient is symptomatic.

LESIONS OF THE LIGAMENTS

Ligamentous injuries to the knee are among the most serious of all knee disorders. Because of the importance of the ligaments in stabilizing the joint, early diagnosis of the injury is mandatory. Any delay in diagnosis and treatment may lead to a chronically unstable knee, which predisposes it to early traumatic arthritis.

The mechanism is usually one of forceful stress against the knee when the extremity bears weight. A valgus stress against the knee may sprain or tear the medial collateral ligament, and a varus stress will injure the lateral collateral ligament. Tears of the cruciate ligaments, menisci, and capsule may also occur in conjunction with the collateral ligament injury.

Clinical Features

The history of the injury is often difficult to reconstruct but will provide clues to the type of force applied to the knee. After the injury, the ability to bear weight on the extremity is often lost. Swelling from an acute ligament or capsular tear is usually immediate due to hemorrhage. A "pop" or tearing sensation may be heard or felt. Incomplete tears or sprains are often more painful than complete ligamentous ruptures.

Patients with chronically unstable knees due to old injuries often complain of the knee going out or giving way and of their not being able to depend on the extremity. These symptoms are always most noticeable during vigorous activities. A chronic effusion is often present.

The examination is of utmost importance in the acute injury. Any swelling or discoloration is noted. The lesion can frequently be localized by palpation alone. Palpation should begin away from the suspected area in order to promote cooperation. A point of maximum tenderness is often present along the course of the collateral ligament or capsule.

The knee should always be tested for stability with the patient relaxed in the supine position. If the examination cannot be adequately performed because of pain or hamstring spasm, it may have to be repeated with the patient under local or general anesthesia. The injured knee is always compared with the opposite, uninvolved knee. The tests are performed in the following sequence:

1. Abduction-adduction stress testing at 30 degrees of knee flexion. With the knee flexed 30 degrees, the cruciate ligaments are relaxed. This

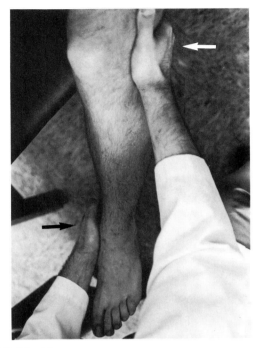

FIG 11–11.
Abduction stress test at 30 degrees. To test the lateral collateral ligament, a varus stress is applied.

prevents them from producing a false negative test result. The medial and lateral ligaments can then be tested by applying valgus and varus stresses to the knee (Fig 11–11). If laxity exists in either direction with testing the test reflects an injury to the collateral ligament.

2. Abduction-adduction stress testing at 0 degrees. Valgus and varus stresses are applied in the same manner as when the knee was tested at 30 degrees of flexion. If the knee was stable at 30 degrees, it will also be stable at 0 degrees because the collateral ligaments are intact. With the knee in extension, however, the cruciate ligaments tighten and by themselves can prevent the joint from opening in spite of a collateral ligament tear. If the knee is unstable in extension, a very serious knee injury has occurred, and a significant cruciate ligament tear is present in addition to the collateral ligament injury.

3. Drawer signs. Anteroposterior and rotatory instability are tested by determining how much abnormal excursion of the tibia is present when anterior and posterior stresses are applied to the tibia with the knee in a flexed position (Fig 11–12). Anterior drawer testing is performed with the foot in external rotation, neutral rotation, and internal rotation. Abnormal forward excursion of the tibia with the foot in either position is highly suggestive of a significant injury to

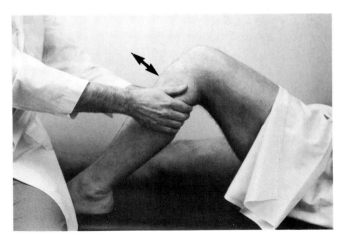

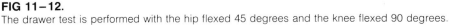

FIG 11–12.
The drawer test is performed with the hip flexed 45 degrees and the knee flexed 90 degrees.

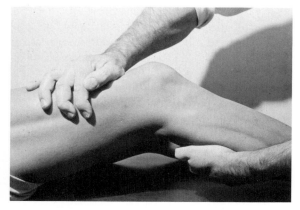

FIG 11–13.
Lachman's test. This is essentially an anterior drawers test performed with the knee in approximately 20 degrees of flexion. The femur is stabilized with one hand, and the tibia is drawn forward with the other. An increase in the forward motion and lack of a definite end point suggests a rupture of the anterior cruciate ligament.

the anterior cruciate ligament and joint capsule. The posterior drawer test is then performed by applying backward pressure against the tibia. Abnormal laxity with this test is present with posterior cruciate and posterior capsular injuries.

4. The anterior cruciate ligament can also be assessed by the Lachman test. This is essentially an anterior drawer test performed with the knee close to full extension. The femur is stabilized with one hand while firm pressure is applied to the proximal portion of the tibia in an attempt to translate it forward (Fig 11–13). A positive test result is one in which there is palpable and visual anterior movement of the tibia with a characteristic soft end point. This test is probably more accurate than the traditional anterior drawer sign and has the other advantage that it can be performed in the position of comfort of the acutely injured knee.

Roentgenographic examination may reveal avulsion fractures pulled off by the injured ligament (Fig 11–14). Stress films may also be helpful in determining whether complete or incomplete ligamentous disruption is present. Roentgenograms should always be obtained especially in the growing child below the age of 15 years with open epiphyses to rule out a fracture of the distal femoral epiphysis that may simulate collateral ligament injury (Fig 11–15). Arthrography may reveal leakage of dye out of the capsule, but

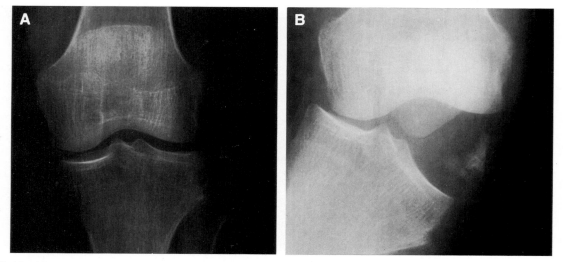

FIG 11–14.
A, anteroposterior roentgenogram of an injured knee. When a stress is applied **(B),** the true significance of the injury becomes apparent.

the test is usually not necessary if a good clinical examination is performed. MRI is helpful in assessing cruciate ligament status.

Treatment

Minor ligament sprains are treated in the same manner as meniscus injuries (Table 11–1). Immobilization in a compression dressing with ice and elevation for 2 to 3 days are followed by exercises to promote absorption of swelling and restoration of motion.

Minor sprains are easily differentiated from complete ruptures, but small partial ruptures are frequently difficult to diagnose. When there is certainty that a complete rupture does not exist, partial tears may be treated by plaster immobilization. The extremity is placed in a long leg cast for 6 weeks with the joint closed on the side of the injury. After removal of the cast, a progressive knee rehabilitation program is begun that consists of range-of-motion and hamstring and quadriceps-strengthening exercises.

Early surgical repair is indicated when the rupture is complete. Restoration of stability can

TABLE 11–1.

Algorithm for Investigation of the Acute Knee Injury

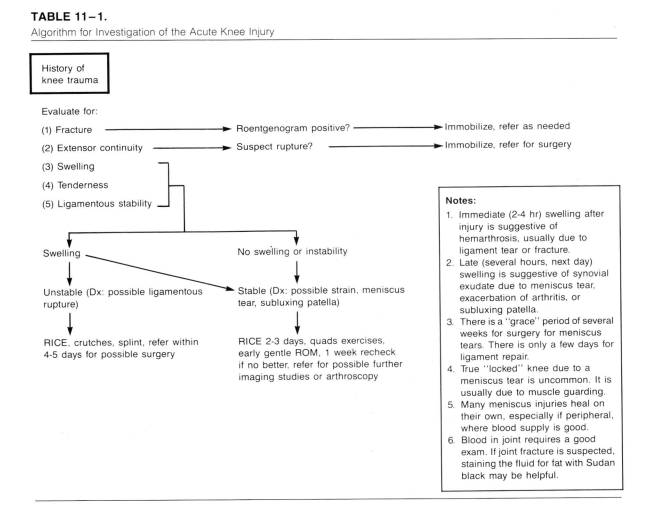

History of knee trauma

Evaluate for:
(1) Fracture ———————→ Roentgenogram positive? ———————→ Immobilize, refer as needed
(2) Extensor continuity ———————→ Suspect rupture? ———————→ Immobilize, refer for surgery
(3) Swelling
(4) Tenderness
(5) Ligamentous stability

Swelling   No swelling or instability

Unstable (Dx: possible ligamentous rupture)   Stable (Dx: possible strain, meniscus tear, subluxing patella)

RICE, crutches, splint, refer within 4-5 days for possible surgery   RICE 2-3 days, quads exercises, early gentle ROM, 1 week recheck if no better, refer for possible further imaging studies or arthroscopy

Notes:
1. Immediate (2-4 hr) swelling after injury is suggestive of hemarthrosis, usually due to ligament tear or fracture.
2. Late (several hours, next day) swelling is suggestive of synovial exudate due to meniscus tear, exacerbation of arthritis, or subluxing patella.
3. There is a "grace" period of several weeks for surgery for meniscus tears. There is only a few days for ligament repair.
4. True "locked" knee due to a meniscus tear is uncommon. It is usually due to muscle guarding.
5. Many meniscus injuries heal on their own, especially if peripheral, where blood supply is good.
6. Blood in joint requires a good exam. If joint fracture is suspected, staining the fluid for fat with Sudan black may be helpful.

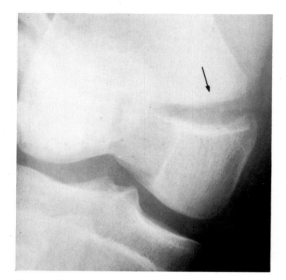

FIG 11–15.
Stress roentgenography of the knee reveals an epiphyseal fracture of the lower portion of the femur that may be misdiagnosed as a ligamentous injury clinically.

only be accomplished by accurate suture of the ruptured ligament followed by casting. Postoperatively, exercises are begun and continued for several months after cast removal. The knee is often protected during this period of time by a specially constructed brace (Fig 11–16).

Chronic ligamentous instability usually requires reconstructive surgery in order to prevent further joint deterioration. A well-constructed brace may provide an alternative to surgery in the active individual.

Anterior Cruciate Deficiency

A common injury that has received special attention in recent years is rupture of the anterior cruciate ligament. Although disability due to injury to the other knee ligaments was well known, rupture of the anterior cruciate was not felt to be very significant. It was often discovered "incidentally" at the time of meniscectomy.

As knowledge advanced, the natural history of this injury became more apparent. While the initial disability might be minimal, especially if the

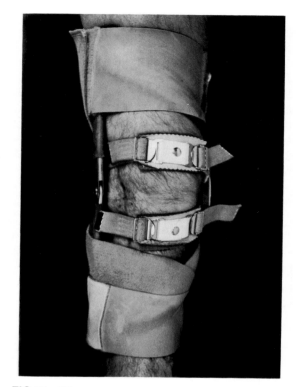

FIG 11–16.
The Lenox Hill brace is made from a cast impression of the injured knee. (Most braces of elastic or leather with hinges are of little value.) Other similar "derotation" braces are also available.

rupture was "isolated," the injury frequently resulted in progressive deterioration with increasing knee laxity, tears in either meniscus, and articular cartilage degeneration. It began to be referred to as "the beginning of the end" of the athlete's knee.

Clinical Features

The acute injury is commonly accompanied by a painful "pop" followed in 1 to 2 hours by swelling (hemarthrosis) that becomes maximal at 8 to 12 hours. If accompanied by other ligament injuries, the laxity is usually evident on examination by drawer or Lachman testing. If isolated, the Lachman test is usually the most sensitive examination to detect weakness.

Older injuries may present with symptoms of instability such as "giving out." This disturbing type of instability is often referred to as the "pivot shift" and usually occurs when the patient comes to a sudden stop or changes directions quickly. The pivot shift is a sign that the tibia is subluxing on the femur. A synovitis is often present. The findings are often suggestive of meniscal injury (which may also be present), but the pivot shift test is usually diagnostic (Fig 11–17).

Treatment

The management of this problem remains a source of controversy. The results of simple repair of the anterior cruciate ligament are poor, primarily because the tissue remaining is usually of poor quality.

The treatment is individualized. The athlete with an acute injury usually needs referral for evaluation (MRI, arthroscopy) followed by surgical reconstruction and augmentation or ligament replacement. This is followed by several months of rehabilitation and exercise.

Treatment of the recreational athlete is often nonsurgical. Exercises, bracing, and occasionally, modification of activities will usually allow a relatively normal life-style. If sufficient symptoms of instability develop later, surgical reconstruction to prevent subluxation is indicated. Surgery in these cases does not relieve pain but may prevent arthritis from developing.

Pellegrini-Stieda Disease

Occasionally, a sprain of the medial collateral ligament is followed by the formation of a calcified mass at the site of the ligament injury (Fig 11–18). This area of dystrophic calcification may remain tender and swollen for an extended period of time. Ossification of the mass may even occur. The symptoms gradually subside, and symptomatic treatment is usually all that is necessary. The mass rarely needs to be removed.

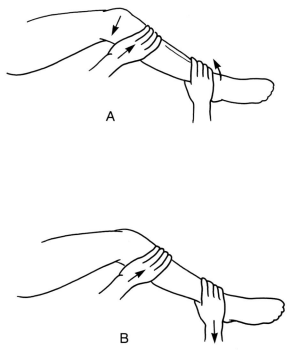

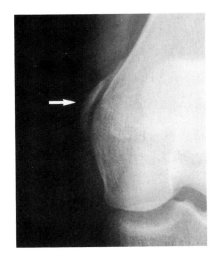

FIG 11–17.
The pivot shift test. **A,** with the knee slightly flexed, the proximal portion of the tibia is lifted forward and internally rotated, and the knee is then extended. (This subluxes the tibia forward, and the femur falls backward.) Valgus force is then applied, and the knee is flexed **(B).** At about 30 degrees, the subluxation will suddenly be reduced with a palpable sensation and reproduce the patient's symptoms of instability.

FIG 11–18.
Pellegrini-Stieda disease.

DISORDERS OF THE EXTENSOR MECHANISM

The extensor mechanism of the knee consists of the quadriceps muscles, the patella, and the patellar tendon. Several painful disorders may alter its function.

Chondromalacia of the Patella

Chondromalacia of the patella is a term that has commonly been used to describe anterior knee pain. Strictly speaking, the term should probably be used to describe only the pathologic lesion of cartilaginous softening and fibrillation that had previously been thought to cause this clinical syndrome. Actually, the anatomic lesion of chondromalacia is a frequent finding in the knee and is usually felt to be asymptomatic. Conversely, the same syndrome of anterior knee pain is frequently present when the articular cartilage is normal. Thus, the term of chondromalacia of the patella is gradually being replaced by a term such as "patellofemoral pain syndrome" or "anterior knee pain syndrome" when it is used to describe the condition of anterior knee pain.

The syndrome is one of the most common causes of pain in adolescents and young adults, but it can occur at any age. Its cause is unknown, but several factors may play a role in its onset.

Any injury or anatomic abnormality that predisposes to an irregular pattern of movement of the patella can lead to this syndrome. Meniscus injuries frequently alter normal tibiofemoral motion, which in turn alters patellofemoral motion and can lead to pain. Recurrent subluxation of the patella, quadriceps imbalance, a high riding patella (patella alta) and angular deformities about the knee may be associated with this syndrome. Direct trauma, such as what occurs with a fall or a dashboard injury to the patella, may also predispose to continued patellofemoral pain.

In some patients, it does appear that the chondromalacia may cause pain. Grossly, the cartilage loses its normal, smooth, glistening appearance and becomes fibrillated and frayed. It may even be completely denuded, thereby exposing the underlying subchondral bone. Fewer than 20% of patients with patellofemoral pain will have gross chondromalacia, however.

Clinical Features

The majority of patients are teenagers or young adults. Pain beneath or near the patella is the most common symptom. It is characteristically aggravated by walking up and down stairs, an activity that puts the patella under the greatest flexion load. Squatting and prolonged sitting with the knee flexed are also uncomfortable. This discomfort is often relieved by extension of the knee. Symptoms of giving way, crepitus, or locking may be present, and a history of previous trauma is common. The disease is frequently bilateral and may be confused with a meniscus injury.

Examination will reveal generalized tenderness around the patella. Direct pressure against the patella may be painful, and contraction of the quadriceps against patellar pressure is often uncomfortable (Fig 11–19). Swelling and crepitus may also be present, although there is no direct correlation between the presence of crepitus and the pain. There may also be findings of malalignment or an unstable patella. Roentgenographic findings are usually normal.

Treatment

Treatment is directed toward the underlying cause, if any is present. "Flexion loads" should be avoided, especially improperly performed quadriceps exercises. Otherwise, aspirin, moist heat, and intensive quadriceps exercises in *extension* are usually helpful. Most cases eventually recover spontaneously. If symptoms persist, surgery may occasionally be indicated. It usually consists of some procedure to realign the patella to prevent abnormal motion or to release abnormal pressure. Shaving or removal of "abnormal" articular cartilage is often only of limited value. Arthroscopy may even trigger a sympathetic dystrophy

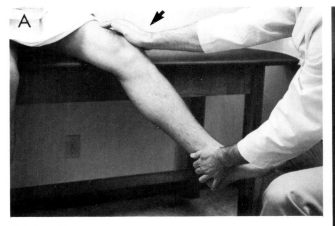

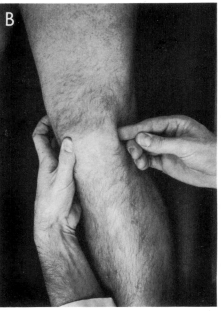

FIG 11–19.
Examination for retropatellar pain. **A,** with the knee slightly flexed, pressure against the patella as the knee is actively extended may produce typical pain. **B,** with the knee extended, the patella is displaced medially or laterally. Pain is reproduced by digital pressure under either the medial or lateral patellar facet.

in some of these cases. Anterior knee pain itself does not appear to lead to patellofemoral arthritis.

Recurrent Subluxation of the Patella

Recurrent subluxation of the patella is a common disorder that is often undiagnosed because the symptoms are similar to other "internal derangements" of the knee. The patella usually subluxes or dislocates laterally. The condition may follow an acute patellar dislocation that fails to heal properly. The disorder is frequently bilateral and is one of the most common causes of internal derangement in the athlete.

Clinical Features

The symptoms are pain, swelling, and a sensation of the knee giving out. Acute dislocation may even occur, but more commonly, the symptoms are due to recurrent subluxation.

Physical examination usually reveals local tenderness over the medial facet of the patella and in the soft tissue medial to the patella. The pa-

tella appears laterally displaced and may also appear higher than normal when the knee is slightly flexed (patella alta). Passive hypermobility with lateral displacement is often noted when pressure is applied against the patella with the knee relaxed (Fig 11–20). A joint effusion and mild quadriceps atrophy may be present.

Roentgenographic studies are frequently helpful. A "sunrise" view taken with the knee relaxed in slight flexion will often reveal lateral displacement (Fig 11–21).

Treatment

Treatment is directed at improving extensor muscle tone. Quadriceps exercises in extension are begun, and aspirin and moist heat are prescribed as necessary. Frequently, the vastus medialis portion of the quadriceps will strengthen enough to prevent further lateral subluxation from occurring.

Surgery may be indicated to reconstruct the extensor mechanism in order to prevent recurrence. A variety of procedures are available. All of them attempt to realign the patella either at

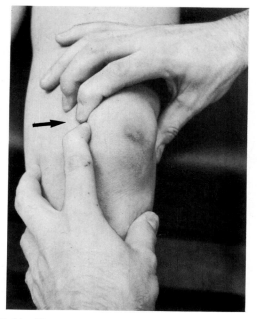

FIG 11–20.
The "apprehension" test. Abnormal lateral hypermobility may be noted when attempting to displace the patella laterally with the knee relaxed and slightly flexed. The patient may even become apprehensive and grab the examiner's arm to prevent further displacement.

the patella itself or distally at the patellar tendon insertion in order to prevent abnormal lateral excursion from occurring.

Acute Dislocation of the Patella

A sudden valgus strain to the knee or a direct blow against the medial aspect of the patella may cause the patella to dislocate laterally. The deformity is usually obvious, with the patella displaced in the lateral position and the knee held in slight flexion. Roentgenographic examination should always be performed in order to rule out any associated osteochondral fracture.

Reduction is easily accomplished by lifting the heel of the extremity off the table. This extends the knee and flexes the hip, thereby relaxing the entire quadriceps mechanism. Gentle pressure against the patella may be necessary to complete the reduction. The knee is immobilized for 2 to 3 weeks by a knee immobilizer. Quadriceps exercises are begun as soon as possible.

Traumatic dislocation is always accompanied by a partial rupture of the medial retinaculum and supporting structures of the patella. This may lead to recurrent episodes of subluxation or dislocation. If it does, surgical reconstruction of the extensor mechanism may be necessary.

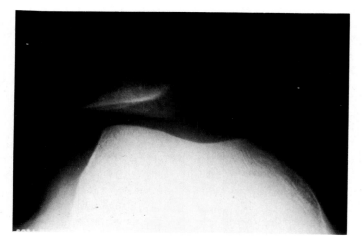
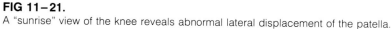

FIG 11–21.
A "sunrise" view of the knee reveals abnormal lateral displacement of the patella.

Ruptures of the Extensor Mechanism

The extensor mechanism is occasionally ruptured as a result of trauma. The rupture may take place in the quadriceps muscle or the patellar tendon. Active extension is immediately lost, but pain may be minimal, especially in an older patient with chronic degeneration of the muscle-tendon unit.

Clinical Features

Clinically, hemorrhage and a palpable sulcus are present in the area of the rupture. Extension of the knee is markedly weakened or even completely absent.

A lateral roentgenogram taken with the knee in 90 degrees of flexion will usually reveal proximal displacement of the patella when the rupture has occurred in the patellar tendon (Fig 11–22). Roentgenograms are usually not helpful when the rupture has occurred proximal to the patella in the quadriceps mechanism.

Treatment

Treatment is immediate surgical repair followed by cast immobilization for 6 to 8 weeks.

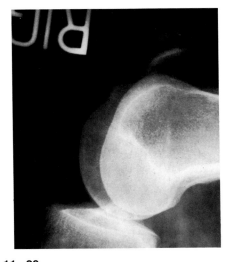

FIG 11–22.
Rupture of the patellar tendon with marked proximal displacement of the patella.

Osgood-Schlatter Disease

Osgood-Schlatter disease is a disorder that involves the growing tibial tuberosity of adolescents. The cause is unknown, but the disorder is generally considered to be a traumatically produced lesion that occurs at the attachment of the patellar tendon to the tibial tuberosity. It is a self-limited condition that ends with closure of the upper tibial epiphyseal plate. The disorder usually becomes evident between the ages of 8 and 15 years and is frequently bilateral. Males are affected three times as often as females.

Clinical Features

Local pain, swelling, and tenderness over the tibial tubercle are characteristic clinical features. The pain is accentuated by activity. Stair walking and squatting on the knees may be especially uncomfortable. The pain is also increased by extension of the knee against resistance.

A lateral roentgenogram of the upper portion of the tibia with the leg slightly internally rotated may reveal variable degrees of separation and fragmentation of the upper tibial epiphysis. Occasionally, the fragmented area fails to unite to the tibia and persists into adulthood (Fig 11–23).

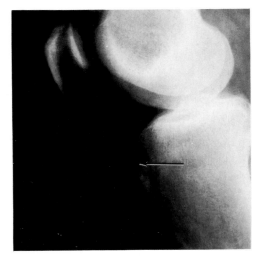

FIG 11–23.
Osgood-Schlatter disease (arrow).

Treatment

Removing the stress on the tendon is usually sufficient treatment. Simple abstinence from physical activity will relieve the symptoms in most cases. Temporary immobilization in a cylinder cast or knee splint for 4 to 6 weeks may be necessary in resistant cases. Surgery is rarely indicated. The prognosis for complete restoration of function and relief from pain is excellent.

OSTEOCHONDRITIS DISSECANS

Osteochondritis dissecans is a condition of unknown cause in which a segment of subchondral bone undergoes avascular necrosis. This segment of bone, with its overlying articular cartilage, may separate or become detached from the joint surface and produce a loose body. The knee is the most common joint affected, and the lateral surface of the medial femoral condyle is the area that is usually involved. The condition is primarily a disorder of young adults, but it may also be seen in children. Males are more commonly affected, and the disorder may be bilateral.

Clinical Features

The symptoms consist of pain, stiffness, and swelling that are worsened with activity. A painful limp is frequently present, and locking may even occur if the fragment has become detached.

Diminished motion, swelling, and medial joint tenderness are usually present. This tenderness may be well localized and is best elicited by deep local pressure over the affected area with the knee flexed 90 degrees.

The roentgenogram is usually diagnostic (Fig 11–24). A fragment of avascular bone is seen that is demarcated from the adjacent femur by a radiolucent line. Occasionally, a loose body may be present.

Treatment

Undisplaced lesions in children are treated conservatively. The joint is protected from weight

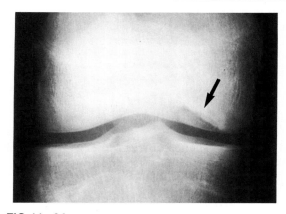

FIG 11–24.
Osteochondritis dissecans of the knee. The "tunnel" view is frequently helpful in visualizing the defect. This fragment may become detached and form a loose body. This area should not be confused with the normal irregularity of the distal femoral epiphysis in young children.

bearing by the use of crutches. A plaster cylinder cast with the knee in slight flexion may also be necessary. Several months are required for complete healing.

In the older child, the lesion is less likely to heal, and surgery is frequently indicated. Simple drilling of the undetached fragment to encourage the ingrowth of blood vessels into the avascular segment is usually all that is necessary. In any age group, detached fragments should be replaced if the weight-bearing surface is involved, but they may be removed if the joint surface is not involved.

LOOSE BODIES

Loose bodies, commonly referred to as "joint mice," are often found in the knee joint. They may be present as the result of osteoarthritis, osteochondral fractures, or osteochondritis dissecans or secondary to primary disease of the synovium.

Clinical Features

Loose bodies may cause swelling and intermittent locking of the joint. There is frequently a feeling of weakness and instability. The loose body is occasionally palpable and freely movable.

The roentgenogram is usually diagnostic (Fig 11–25). A primary lesion such as osteochondritis dissecans may be detected, but frequently no joint abnormality other than the loose body is visualized.

Treatment

Treatment is usually surgical. Because of the mechanical interference with motion and resultant wear on the articular surface, most loose bodies should be removed. Any underlying abnormality is corrected at the same time.

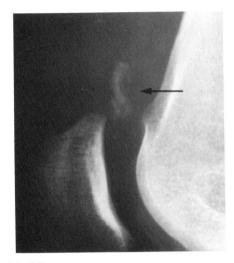

FIG 11–25.
Osteocartilaginous loose body *(arrow)* in the suprapatellar pouch.

DEGENERATIVE ARTHRITIS

The knee is the joint most commonly affected by osteoarthritis. Although the cause is unknown, obesity, trauma, ligamentous instability, and malalignment of the lower extremity all play significant roles. The pathologic features have been described elsewhere (Chapter 10).

Clinical Features

The symptoms are similar to those that occur with osteoarthritis in any other joint. Pain with activity that is relieved by rest is characteristic. Morning stiffness that is relieved by activity is also usually present. A chronic effusion is not uncommon. Crepitus and grating are also frequent complaints. Restriction of motion, joint swelling, local tenderness, and deformity are common clinical findings.

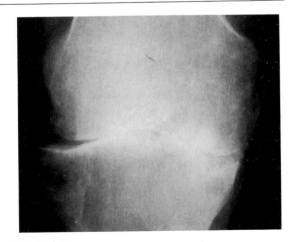

FIG 11–26.
Degenerative arthritis of the knee. The joint space is severely narrowed.

The roentgenographic features consist of joint space narrowing, osteophyte formation, and sclerosis in the subchondral region (Fig 11–26).

Treatment

Symptoms are often relieved by conservative treatment consisting of weight loss, rest, salicylates, and quadriceps exercises. A cane is frequently helpful to relieve the weight-bearing stress. An intra-articular injection of steroid may be indicated in the older patient to relieve the acute inflammatory response. When pain is diminished, gentle range-of-motion exercises are begun in order to overcome contractures.

Surgical treatment involves elimination of the painful weight-bearing articulation. Arthrodesis in the active young adult will eliminate the pain, but the patient may find the permanent stiffness disturbing. Realignment osteotomy and joint replacement are often indicated.

OSTEONECROSIS

Avascular necrosis of bone occurs about many joints and under many conditions. The femoral head, humeral head, and talus are common sites. It may be seen in association with chronic steroid therapy, gout, and chronic alcoholism and even in divers and workers who use compressed air (Caisson disease). Most of the time, the cause is unknown. As in osteochondritis dissecans, the medial femoral condyle is the most common site of involvement in the knee. Secondary osteoarthritis frequently develops.

Clinical Features

The disorder is more common over the age of 50 years. The onset is usually gradual with progressive pain and swelling. The medial femoral condyle may be locally tender.

Roentgenographic findings

Initially, films are usually normal or show minimal degenerative arthritis consistent with the patient's age. An early bone scan may show well-localized increased uptake over the involved area. MRI will also reveal the lesion.

Eventually, radiolucency from a subchondral zone of sclerosis appears. The necrotic area frequently fragments and collapses, and this results in secondary osteoarthritis.

Treatment

Reduction of weight-bearing, strengthening exercises, and salicylates will allow healing within a few months in over half the cases. Surgery is eventually required in the rest, usually in the form of an osteotomy or joint replacement.

BURSITIS

Bursa sacs are present wherever soft tissue, such as muscle or tendon, moves over a bony prominence. One such bursa that is frequently symptomatic in the knee is the *anserine bursa*. This bursa is located deep to the insertions of the semitendinous, gracilis, and sartorius tendons medially (Fig 11–27). Local measures including moist heat, rest, and the injection of a steroid/lidocaine mixture into the tender bursa are usually curative. Salicylates are given to control pain and inflammation.

The *prepatellar bursa* lies between the skin and the patella. It frequently becomes irritated from recurrent trauma, especially kneeling (housemaid's knee). It is also occasionally involved in infection. Chronic traumatic changes may occur with permanent thickening of the bursa, which makes it more prone to recurrent injury.

Acute traumatic prepatellar bursitis usually responds to rest and moist heat. If infection occurs, open drainage followed by the appropriate anti-

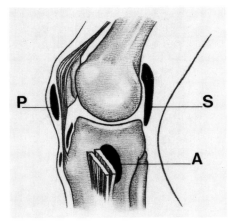

FIG 11–27.
Bursae of the knee: *A* = anserine bursa; *P* = prepatellar bursa; *S* = semimembranous bursa. These may become enlarged and form a Baker's cyst.

biotic coverage is indicated. A chronic, swollen bursa that is vulnerable to repeated injuries should be excised. Complete excision with elimination of all dead space will usually result in a prompt cure.

TENDINITIS

Several tendons adjacent to the knee joint may become chronically inflamed. The patellar tendon, quadriceps tendon, and flexor tendons are the ones most commonly involved. Pain with activity and local point tenderness are characteristic clinical features. As in most cases of tendinitis, the pain is aggravated by passive stretching of the tendon as well as by forceful contraction of the muscle-tendon unit against resistance.

The treatment is symptomatic, with rest, heat, and anti-inflammatory medication. Steroid injections may be helpful, but the patellar tendon should never be injected. Temporary cast immobilization is occasionally necessary in resistant cases.

ARTHROSCOPY

Arthroscopy is a valuable tool in the diagnosis and treatment of many disorders of the knee. The procedure has also been used in the shoulder, elbow, hip, and ankle joint but is most useful in problems of the knee. The procedure is safe and relatively minor with little morbidity. It may be performed on an outpatient basis, with ambulation being possible shortly after the procedure.

Its diagnostic accuracy approaches 100% and by using separate puncture holes of entrance, small instruments may be passed into the knee to perform a variety of functions. The most common are removal or repair of meniscus tears and removal of loose bodies. It is used to evaluate the knee of patients with Baker's cyst to determine whether any intra-articular abnormality is present that may have caused the cyst to develop. In this case, the intra-articular problem might require treatment rather than the Baker's cyst. Arthroscopic surgery is also frequently used to remove damaged articular cartilage from the patella in patients with chondromalacia, but the results in these patients are often inconsistent and unpredictable.

Diagnostic arthroscopy is also helpful in evaluating acute injuries of the knee to determine whether ligamentous repair may be necessary. It is also useful in difficult diagnostic problems in those symptomatic knees with vague symptoms and few physical findings. There is some risk of overuse of the procedure, especially in these patients, and it should be kept in mind that the procedure is still a surgical one that requires an anesthetic and should be undertaken only with proper indications.

Plica Syndrome

The synovial plicae are four (suprapatellar, infrapatellar, medial, and lateral) membranous folds or bands that may be an occasional source of chronic knee pain. They have become items of interest mainly due to the increasing use of arthroscopy. The plica becomes symptomatic only when irritated by direct trauma, overuse, or inflammatory disorders. The most common clinical features are chronic aching, usually medial to the patella, and local tenderness. When the medial plica is visualized arthroscopically, it is released by partial excision. The other folds are not commonly symptomatic.

FRACTURES OF THE KNEE

Many fractures about the knee are intra-articular in nature. They may occur through the femoral condyles or tibial plateaus. Open reduction with internal fixation is usually indicated if any displacement is present that would cause the articular surface to be irregular or lead to instability. Otherwise, traumatic arthritis may develop.

Fractures of the Tibial Plateau

A common fracture in the knee is an injury to the lateral tibial plateau (Fig 11–28). This injury results from a force applied to the lateral aspect of the knee with the leg in the extended weight-bearing position. Undisplaced, impacted fractures are easily treated by a compression dressing and early motion with avoidance of weight bearing for 6 to 8 weeks. Unimpacted fractures in good position are treated by a long leg cast for 6 weeks. Displaced fractures require open reduction and internal fixation with elevation of the depressed plateau fragment.

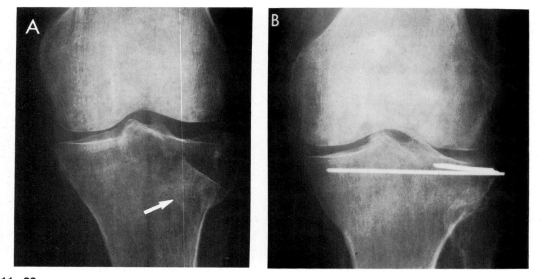

FIG 11–28.
A, depressed fracture *(arrow)* of the lateral tibial plateau. **B,** the fragments have been elevated and internally fixed.

Fractures of the Patella

Fractures of the patella usually result from a direct blow to the knee. They are classified as undisplaced or displaced (Fig 11–29).

Undisplaced fractures are easily treated nonoperatively. A compression dressing followed by a removable splint may be all that is necessary in the conscientious patient. Otherwise, a cylinder cast with the knee flexed approximately 5 degrees is applied and maintained for 5 to 6 weeks. This is followed by an active exercise program to restore strength and mobility.

Displaced fractures usually require surgery. Comminuted fragments are removed, and the patellar fracture and extensor mechanism of the knee are repaired.

Fractures of the Tibial Eminence

Fractures of the intercondylar region of the tibia are more common in children than adults. They usually occur in the area of attachment of the anterior cruciate ligament. If the fragment is only partially displaced, conservative treatment with a long leg cast for 8 weeks is usually sufficient treatment (Fig 11–30). Only the fracture that is

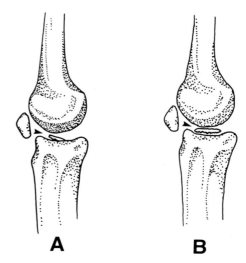

FIG 11–30.
Fractures of the intercondylar eminence of the tibia. **A,** the displaced fracture that is still attached. Conservative treatment is usually adequate. **B,** the avulsed fragment is completely separated from its bed. Surgery is usually necessary for this injury.

completely avulsed and displaced from its bed requires surgical repair (Fig 11–31) in order to restore strength to the cruciate ligament and prevent any mechanical blocking from occurring.

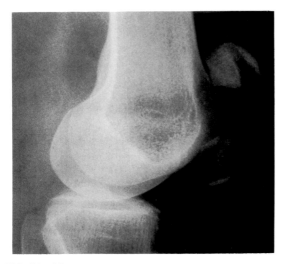

FIG 11–29.
Displaced fracture of the patella.

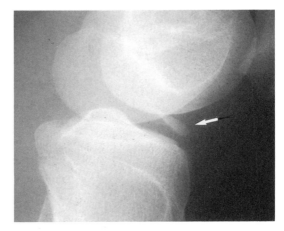

FIG 11–31.
Roentgenogram of completely avulsed intercondylar fracture *(arrow)*.

TRAUMATIC DISLOCATION OF THE KNEE

This is an uncommon injury but one that can be extremely disabling if improperly managed. It usually results from severe trauma. Associated neurovascular injuries are very common, especially peroneal nerve damage. The dislocation is more commonly anterior (Fig 11–32). Some injuries are reduced spontaneously.

Evaluation and Treatment

Occasionally, if the dislocation has spontaneously reduced, there may an absence of obvious gross deformity, except for swelling. Usually, however, there is gross deformity, and there are always signs of severe ligamentous disruption. The neurovascular status of the extremity is always recorded.

The knee should be reduced as soon as possible. The neurovascular status is then re-evaluated. Angiography is indicated if there are any concerns about the vascular status of the limb. Definitive ligament repair is probably helpful in

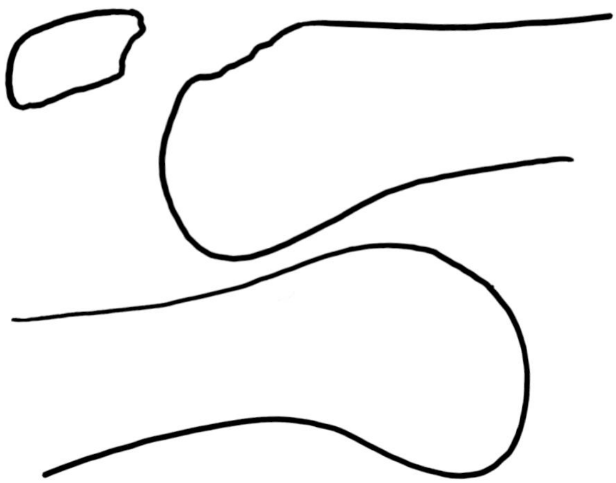

FIG 11–32.
Traumatic dislocation of the knee.

young patients, but older patients may be treated nonsurgically. Nerve repair may be attempted, but the results are poor. Rehabilitation with bracing is helpful in restoring function.

BIBLIOGRAPHY

Abernathy PJ, et al: Is chondromalacia patellae a separate clinical entity? *J Bone Joint Surg [Br]* 1978; 60:205–210.

Aegerter E, Kirkpatrick JA: *Orthopedic Diseases,* ed 3. Philadelphia, WB Saunders Co, 1968.

Aglietti P, et al: Idiopathic osteonecrosis of the knee: Aetiology, prognosis and treatment. *J Bone Joint Surg [Br]* 1983; 65:588.

Ahuja SC, Bullough PG: Osteonecrosis of the knee: A clinicopathological study in twenty-eight patients. *J Bone Joint Surg [Am]* 1978; 60:191.

Allman FL: Clinical diagnosis of anterior cruxiate ligament instability in the athlete. *Am J Sports Med* 1976; 4:84.

Bourne MH, et al: Anterior knee pain. *Mayo Clin Proc* 1988; 63:482.

Brantigan OC, Voshell AF: The mechanics of the ligaments and menisci of the knee joint. *J Bone Joint Surg* 1941; 23:44.

Childress HM: Popliteal cysts associated with undiagnosed posterior lenses of the medial meniscus. *J Bone Joint Surg [Am]* 1970; 52:1487.

Crawford EJ, Emery RJ, Archroth PM: Stable osteochondritis dissecans—does the lesion unite? *J Bone Joint Surg [Br]* 1990; 72:320.

Crosby EB, Insall J: Recurrent dislocation of the patella. *J Bone Joint Surg [Am]* 1976; 58:9.

Dandy DJ, Jackson RW: The impact of arthroscopy on the management of disorders of the knee. *J Bone Joint Surg* 1975; 57:346.

Dinham JM: Popliteal cysts in children. *J Bone Joint Surg [Br]* 1975; 57:69.

Feagin JL: Isolated tear of the anterior cruxiate ligament: Five year follow-up study. *Am J Sports Med* 1976; 4:95.

Ficat RP, Hungerford DS: *Disorders of the Patello-femoral Joint.* Baltimore, Williams & Wilkins, 1977.

Fischer RL: Conservative treatment of patellofemoral pain. *Orthop Clin North Am* 1986; 17:269.

Galway HR, MacIntosh DL: The lateral pivot shift: A

symptom and sign of anterior cruxiate insufficiency. *Clin Orthop* 1980; 147:45.

Goodfellow J, Hungerford DS, Woods C: Patello-femoral joint mechanics and pathology: Chondromalacia patellae. *J Bone Joint Surg [Br]* 1976; 58:291.

Goodfellow J, Hungerford DS, Zindel M: Patello-femoral joint mechanics and pathology: Functional anatomy of the patello-femoral joint. *J Bone Joint Surg [Br]* 1976; 58:287.

Guhl JF: Update in the treatment of osteochondritis dissecans. *Orthopedics* 1984; 7:1744.

Harvell JC, et al: Diagnostic arthroscopy of the knee in children and adolescents. *Orthopedics* 1989; 12:1561.

Hede A, Hempel-Poulson S, Jensen JS: Symptoms and level of sports activity in patients awaiting arthroscopy for meniscal lesions of the knee. *J Bone Joint Surg [Am]* 1990; 72:550.

Helfet AJ: *Disorders of the Knee.* Philadelphia, JB Lippincott, 1974.

Hughston JC, et al: The classification of knee ligament instabilities: I. The medial compartment and cruciate ligaments. *J Bone Joint Surg [Am]* 1976; 58:159.

Hughston JC, et al: The classification of knee ligament instabilities: II. The lateral compartment. *J Bone Joint Surg [Am]* 1976; 58:173.

Insall J: Patellar pain. *J Bone Joint Surg [Am]* 1982; 64:147.

Insall J, Falvo KA, Wise DW: Chondromalacia patellae. *J Bone Joint Surg [Am]* 1976; 58:1.

Jensen DB, et al: Tibial plateau fractures. *J Bone Joint Surg [Br]* 1990; 72:49.

Katz MM, Hungerford DS: Reflex sympathetic dystrophy affecting the knee. *J Bone Joint Surg [Br]* 1987; 69:797.

Kujula UM, et al: Patellofemoral relationships in recurrent patellar dislocation. *J Bone Joint Surg [Br]* 1989; 71:788.

Laurin CA, et al: The abnormal lateral patellofemoral angle: A diagnostic roentgenographic sign of recurrent patellar subluxation. *J Bone Joint Surg [Am]* 1978; 60:55.

Lee JK, et al: Anterior cruciate ligament tears: MR imaging compared with arthroscopy and clinical tests. *Radiology* 1988; 166:861.

Lipscomb PR Jr, Lipscomb PR Sr, Bryan RS: Osteochondritis dissecans of the knee with loose fragments. *J Bone Joint Surg [Am]* 1978; 60:235.

Lossee RE, Johnson TR, Southwick WO: Anterior subluxation of the lateral tibial plateau: A diagnostic test and operative repair. *J Bone Joint Surg [Am]* 1978; 60:1015.

Lotke PA, Ecker ML: Current concepts review. Osteonecrosis of the knee. *J Bone Joint Surg [Br]* 1988; 70:470.

Meyers MH, McKeever FM: Fractures of the intercondylar eminence of the tibia. *J Bone Joint Surg [Am]* 1970; 52:1677.

Mink JH, Levy T, Crues JV III: Tears of the anterior cruciate ligament and menisci of the knee: MR imaging evaluation. *Radiology* 1988; 167:769.

Nicholas JA: The five-one reconstruction for anteromedial instability of the knee. *J Bone Joint Surg [Am]* 1973; 55:899.

Noble J, Erat K: In defence of the meniscus. A prospective study of 200 meniscectomy patients. *J Bone Joint Surg [Br]* 1980; 62:7.

O'Donoghue DH: *Treatment of Injuries to Athletes,* ed 4. Philadelphia, WB Saunders Co, 1984.

Rezing PM, Insall J, Bohne WH: Spontaneous osteonecrosis of the knee. *J Bone Joint Surg [Am]* 1980; 62:2.

Sandberg B, Balkfors B: Partial rupture of the anterior cruciate ligament: Natural course. *Clin Orthop* 1987; 220:176.

Sandow MJ, Goodfellow JW: The natural history of anterior knee pain in adolescents. *J Bone Joint Surg [Br]* 1985; 67:36.

Sherman OH, et al: Arthroscopy—"no-problem surgery": An analysis of complications in two thousand six hundred and forty cases. *J Bone Joint Surg [Am]* 1986; 68:256.

Simonet WT, Sim FH: Current concepts in the treatment of ligamentous instability of the knee. *Mayo Clin Proc* 1984; 59:67.

Sisto DJ, Warren RF: Complete knee dislocation. *Clin Orthop* 1985; 198:94.

Slocum DB, Larson RL: Rotatory instability of the knee: Its pathogenesis and a clinical test to demonstrate its presence. *J Bone Joint Surg [Am]* 1968; 50:211.

Watanabe AT, et al: Common pitfalls in magnetic resonance imaging of the knee. *J Bone Joint Surg [Am]* 1988; 71:857.

Wolfe RD, Colloff B: Popliteal cysts. *J Bone Joint Surg [Am]* 1972; 54:1057.

CHAPTER 12

The Ankle and Foot

The ankle and foot perform two major roles: they support the body and propel it forward. In the process of performing these functions, several painful conditions may develop. Most of these develop in the forefoot, and many of them are caused by poorly fitted shoes.

ANATOMY

The ankle is a hinge joint composed of the articular surfaces of the lower portion of the tibia, talus, and medial and lateral malleoli (Fig 12–1). The stability of this joint or "mortise" is maintained by the malleoli and their ligaments, which grasp the talus and prevent medial and lateral displacement. The talus and socket are both broader in front, an arrangement that provides maximum stability when the ankle is in dorsiflexion or neutral, and this prevents posterior displacement. Only movements of dorsiflexion and plantar flexion occur at the ankle.

The foot is composed of 26 bones, 12 of which are components of the medial and lateral longitudinal arches (Fig 12–2). Strong fascial supports maintain these arches and prevent collapse (Fig 12–3). Eversion and inversion movements of the foot take place in the hindfoot at the subtalar joint. Injury or disease that affects this joint will cause pain in the region of the heel when walking on uneven or irregular surfaces. Abduction and adduction movements occur in the midfoot or midtarsal joints.

FLATFOOT

Flatfoot is a common disorder that is defined as a depression or loss of the medial longitudinal arch of the foot; that is usually combined with valgus or eversion of the heel and abduction of the forefoot. An apparent flatfoot is present in many children up to the age of 2 years. This is due to the presence of a fat pad in the area of the longitudinal arch. As the fat pad atrophies with weight bearing, the normal arch usually becomes visible. Flatfoot is usually one of two types, flex-

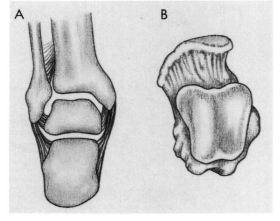

FIG 12–1.
Bones of the ankle and heel. The talus is held in position in the mortise by the malleoli and ankle ligaments **(A).** Its articular surface is wider anteriorly than posteriorly **(B).** The ankle is therefore more stable in neutral or slight dorsiflexion when the wider anterior portion of the talus fits in the mortise. It is unstable in plantar flexion. Wearing high-heeled shoes may therefore lead to chronic ankle and calf pain. Eversion and inversion movements take place in the subtalar (talocalcaneal) joint.

ible or rigid, but it can also be caused by a ruptured posterior tibial tendon.

Flexible Flatfoot

Flexible or hypermobile flatfoot is a disorder frequently seen in both adults and children. The condition is often hereditary and varies in sever-

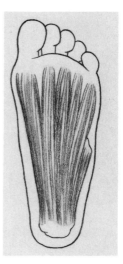

FIG 12–3.
The plantar fascia. It may be affected by Dupuytren's contracture similar to the hand.

ity. It is occasionally associated with a tight Achilles tendon (heel cord). The tight heel cord tends to hold the heel in eversion. With growth, stretching of the medial ligaments of the foot and ankle may then occur.

Clinical Features
Symptoms are rare but may consist of pain, burning, and easy fatigability. With weight bearing, the heels are everted, and the forefoot appears pronated and abducted (Fig 12–4). When it is not

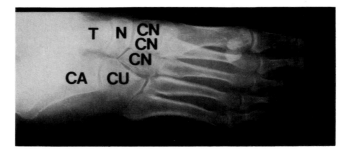

FIG 12–2.
Roentgenogram of the foot: *N* = navicular; *T* = talus; *CA* = calcaneus; *CU* = cuboid; *CN* = cuneiforms, medial, intermediate, and lateral. The foot is divided into the forefoot (phalanges and metatarsals), midfoot (tarsals), and hindfoot (talus and calcaneus).

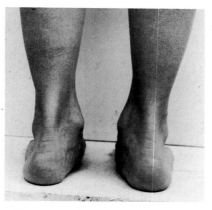

FIG 12–4.
Flatfoot deformity with eversion of the heels and loss of the normal longitudinal arch.

bearing weight, the foot often looks normal. Absence of the medial arch is apparent, and the foot is mobile without any fixed deformity. A mild genu valgum (knock-knee) or internal tibial torsion may be present. With the heel inverted, passive dorsiflexion of the ankle will be limited if the heel cord is tight.

A lateral roentgenogram taken with the foot bearing weight may reveal a loss of the normal arch and plantar flexion of the talus (Fig 12–5). Some secondary bony changes may be present in the adult.

Treatment

The treatment of flexible flatfoot is controversial. Many mild deformities improve spontaneously with maturity as the ligaments tighten. Symptoms are rare during childhood and uncommon even in the adult with moderately severe deformity. Actually, most foot pain in young adults is due to an abnormally high rather than an abnormally low arch. Shoe corrections and orthotics used for this condition have never been scientifically proved to be of benefit. An arch cannot be "created" by supporting it. Exercises are of doubtful value, except for those that stretch the tight heel cords (Fig 12–6). These exercises will cure many cases associated with heel cord contractures. Surgery is reserved for symptomatic cases but is rarely necessary. No treatment is needed in most cases.

Rigid Flatfoot

Rigid or peroneal spastic flatfoot differs from flexible flatfoot in that the deformity is not passively correctable. This condition is usually secondary to a tarsal coalition or arthritis in the hindfoot. Tarsal coalitions are congenital cartilaginous or bony bridges that may be found between the two bones of the hindfoot or between either of these bones and the navicular. The re-

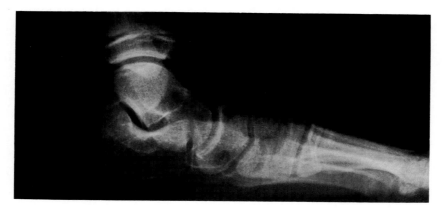

FIG 12–5.
Lateral weight-bearing roentgenogram revealing plantar flexion of the talus.

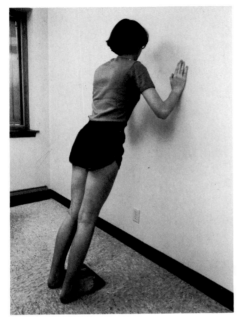

FIG 12–6.
Heel cord stretching exercises. The legs are internally rotated; the forefeet are placed on a 2.5-cm board, and the patient leans forward.

sultant loss of motion in the hindfoot leads to local irritation and protective spasm in the peroneal muscles.

Clinical Features
The onset of the disorder is usually gradual and begins in early adolescence if it is due to a coalition. Stiffness and a painful limp are the most common initial symptoms. Tenderness and pain may be present over the peroneal tendons or in the hindfoot. The heel is frequently everted, and midtarsal and subtalar motions are limited and

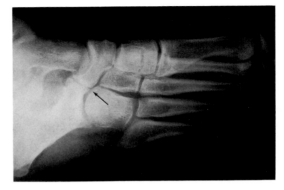

FIG 12–7.
Tarsal coalition. An incomplete calcaneonavicular bar is present *(arrow)*. The anterior process of the calcaneus is abnormally prolonged.

painful. The forefoot may be abducted. Passive stretching of the peroneal tendons by forefoot adduction and inversion frequently reproduces the pain. Swelling will be present if the disorder is secondary to a rheumatoid process.

Roentgenograms may reveal arthritic changes in the hindfoot or the presence of a coalition (Fig 12–7).

Treatment
Symptomatic treatment is indicated in early cases. Rest, heat, and salicylates are usually helpful. A short leg walking cast may be worn intermittently to relieve symptoms. Surgery is frequently necessary, however. If the disorder is secondary to arthritis, arthrodesis of the hindfoot and navicular is indicated. When a tarsal coalition is present, the bony or cartilaginous bar may be resected. If this does not alleviate the symptoms, arthrodesis is usually performed.

CLUBFOOT

Congenital clubfoot, or talipes equinovarus is a fixed deformity that is present at birth. It is frequently bilateral, and a hereditary factor is often present. The cause is unknown.

Clinical Features
The deformity consists of three major components, none of which is passively correctable. This distinguishes clubfoot from other common

foot deformities. The three components are equinus of the ankle and forefoot, varus of the heel, and adduction of the forefoot (Fig 12–8). The medial border of the foot is concave, and the lateral border is convex.

Treatment

Treatment consists of manipulation of the foot in order to stretch the contracted soft tissues, followed by the application of a corrective cast. The cast is changed at weekly intervals, and the foot is further manipulated until complete correction is obtained. Six to 8 weeks are usually required. This method of treatment will frequently succeed if it is begun at an early age.

Approximately 50% of all cases of clubfoot will require some sort of corrective surgery usually within the first year of life. The procedures range from simple heel cord lengthening to wide soft-tissue releases. The most common indication

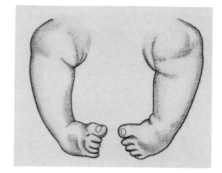

FIG 12–8.
Bilateral clubfeet (talipes equinovarus).

for surgery is resistance to correction by the usual casting methods.

Following full correction, a night brace or splint is worn for 1 to 2 years to maintain the correction and prevent relapse of the deformity. In addition, passive stretching exercises are performed by the patients on a daily basis.

CALCANEOVALGUS

Talipes calcaneovalgus is a common congenital deformity characterized by excessive eversion and dorsiflexion of the foot. The cause is unknown, but positional compression in utero is likely. In contrast to clubfoot, the deformity is not fixed and may be easily overcorrected.

Clinical Features

The deformity is easily diagnosed shortly after birth. Marked laxity of the ligaments of the foot and ankle is obvious, and the foot can often be dorsiflexed so that the toes touch the anterior aspect of the tibia (Fig 12–9). The heel cord may appear to be severely stretched.

Treatment

Mild cases require no treatment. More severe cases respond well to passive stretching exercises. Corrective casts may be necessary for a short period of time. A mild flatfoot deformity may persist.

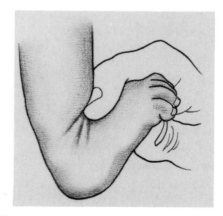

FIG 12–9.
Talipes calcaneovalgus.

KOHLER'S DISEASE

The tarsal navicular may undergo avascular necrosis similar to what occurs in other bones. The cause of all of these disorders is not completely understood, but interference with the circulation to the bone is thought to be the usual cause of the ischemia.

The onset of this disorder is about the age of 5 years. A painful limp is the usual initial complaint. Local pain, tenderness, and swelling over the navicular bone are frequently present.

The roentgenographic appearance is usually characteristic. Flattening, sclerosis, and irregularity of the navicular are usually present (Fig 12–10).

Protection from excessive trauma, usually by the use of a short walking cast for 7 to 8 weeks, is sufficient treatment in most cases. Spontaneous

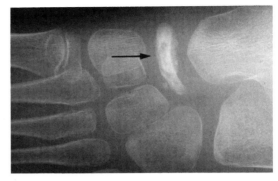

FIG 12–10.
Kohler's disease *(arrow).*

recovery is the rule, and complete reossification of the navicular usually occurs within 2 to 3 years.

ANKLE SPRAINS

The ankle sprain is the most common of all ankle injuries. Most of these injuries occur to the lateral ligaments as the result of an inversion and plantar flexion force that stretch or tear these ligaments (Fig 12–11). Other ligamentous injuries are much less common, but the anterior inferior tibiofibular ligament, deltoid ligament, and interosseus membrane may be injured in eversion injuries. Inversion injuries may also cause severe hemorrhage of the peroneal muscles and even peroneal nerve palsy.

Clinical Features

The symptoms will depend on the severity of the injury. Mild sprains may be associated with only slight loss of function, but in more severe injuries, swelling and pain are significant and prohibit further use of the extremity.

Physical examination reveals hemorrhage and local tenderness at the site of the injury. Motor function should always be evaluated. If the injury is in an adolescent with open growth plates, ten-

derness over the fibular malleolus (even with normal roentgenographic findings) implies the more likely growth plate fracture rather than a sprain, and a cast may be needed.

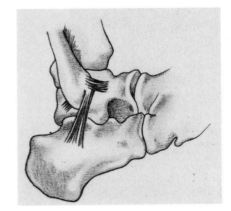

FIG 12–11.
The lateral ankle ligaments, anterior and posterior talofibular and calcaneofibular. Also shown are the anterior tibiofibular ligament and the beginning of the interosseous membrane.

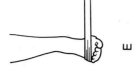

A

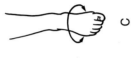

B

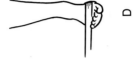

C

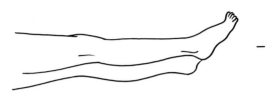

D

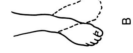

E

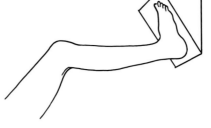

F

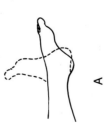

G

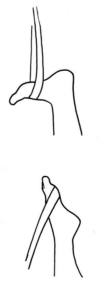

H

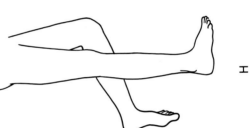

I

J

FIG 12–12.

Ankle exercises. **A–C,** range of motion (dorsiflexion, plantar flexion, circumduction, and "alphabet" writing). **D–G,** strengthening exercises using a rubber strap (invertors, evertors, plantar flexors, dorsiflexors). **H,** static one-leg standing with eyes closed. **I,** toe raises. **J,** heel cord stretches. Each exercise is performed 10 to 15 times. Ice is applied for a few minutes before and after each exercise period, and the exercises are performed 3 times a day.

Treatment

Treatment will depend on the severity of the injury. Although some disagreement exists regarding treatment of a severe injury with complete ligamentous disruption, mild and moderate sprains are always treated nonoperatively.

Initially, all of these injuries are elevated and packed in ice to prevent further swelling. A bulky compression dressing is applied for comfort and to assist in the control of swelling.

Rest, ice, compression, and elevation ("RICE") are continued for 1 to 2 days. Anti-inflammatory medication may be helpful, and crutches are frequently needed for 2 to 3 days. Heat is never used.

Mild to moderate sprains are then treated by

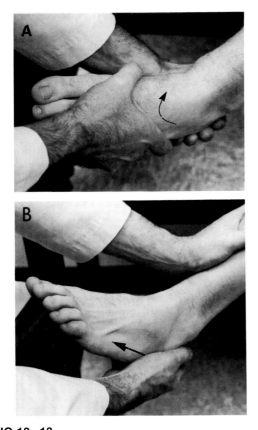

early active range-of-motion exercises (circumduction) and weight bearing as tolerated (Fig 12–12). In 4 to 5 days, exercise against resistance is added. Wrapping or bracing the ankle at this stage may also be helpful. Static bicycling may be added after 1 week along with fast walking. If the pain is particularly severe or the patient requires independence, a short leg walking cast may be applied and maintained for 4 weeks.

Severe sprains with obvious instability may require longer protection. Their treatment remains controversial. Casting and surgical repair have also been advocated. The continuity of the lateral ligament can be determined by observing the amount of displacement or tilting that occurs when an inversion stress is applied to the heel (Fig 12–13). If significant disruption is present, the talus may also sublux anteriorly (anterior drawer test). The instability may be confirmed by stress films (Fig 12–14). Usually, however, even severe sprains are treated in the same manner as less severe injuries, with the same program to control swelling followed by gradual rehabilitation.

Note: Ankle sprains of any severity may also cause lingering symptoms for weeks and months. If healing seems delayed, roentgenograms should be repeated at 6 to 8 weeks to rule out a *talar dome fracture.*

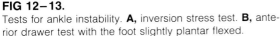

FIG 12–13.
Tests for ankle instability. **A,** inversion stress test. **B,** anterior drawer test with the foot slightly plantar flexed.

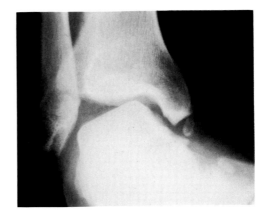

FIG 12–14.
Stress roentgenography of the ankle revealing severe lateral instability.

Ankles that are chronically unstable because of lateral ligamentous laxity may benefit from the application of a 0.3-cm lateral heel and sole wedge to prevent inversion. Taping during vigorous activities is also helpful, as are strengthening exercises. Continuing symptoms require surgical reconstruction of the lateral ligaments to prevent traumatic arthritis from developing and to relieve symptoms of instability.

TARSAL TUNNEL SYNDROME

Nerve entrapment may rarely occur in the foot by compression of the posterior tibial nerve beneath the flexor retinaculum at the ankle. This retinaculum arises from the medial malleolus and inserts into the medial aspect of the calcaneous (Fig 12–15). Space-occupying lesions, traction injuries, fibrosis secondary to fractures, or deformities of the heel and foot can all compromise the tunnel and cause pressure on the posterior tibial nerve.

Clinical Features

The symptoms include a burning pain, numbness, and tingling in the sole of the foot. The exact location of these symptoms is variable. They are frequently worse with activity. The pain may even radiate into the calf. Sensory loss and intrinsic muscle weakness are occasionally present. Tinel's sign may be positive over the tarsal tunnel.

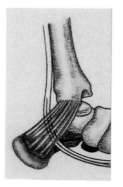

FIG 12–15.
The tarsal tunnel. The posterior tibial nerve runs beneath the flexor retinaculum.

Treatment

The preferred method of treatment is surgical release of the entrapment. A medial heel wedge or heel seat may be used in an attempt to remove traction from the nerve by inverting the heel.

SUBLUXING PERONEAL TENDONS

Sudden, forceful dorsiflexion of the foot accompanied by contraction of the peroneal muscles may cause a tear in the retinaculum that holds these tendons in their groove behind the lateral malleolus. This may allow the tendons to acutely or chronically sublux over the lateral malleolus (Fig 12–16).

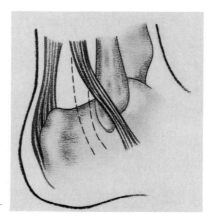

FIG 12–16.
Subluxing peroneal tendons.

Clinical Features

The diagnosis is usually easily made. The tendons are seen or felt to lie over the lateral malleolus. The subluxation can often be reproduced by the patient in chronic cases.

Treatment

Acute cases are treated by reduction and immobilization in a short leg walking cast for 4 weeks or open repair of the retinaculum. Chronic cases are usually treated surgically by reconstruction of the retinaculum.

OSTEOCHONDRITIS DISSECANS OF THE TALUS

This condition is characterized by the formation of a small area of necrotic bone on the articular surface of the talus. The cause is usually traumatic, and the medial aspect of the talus is the area most commonly involved. It is often the lesion causing persistent symptoms following a "sprain" that does not heal.

Clinical Features

The onset is gradual, and a history of the injury is frequently absent. The disorder usually occurs during adolescence or early adulthood. A painful limp and chronic swelling in the ankle with activity are common complaints. Examination of the ankle with the foot in plantar flexion may reveal an area of point tenderness over the articular surface of the talus. Ankle motion is frequently restricted.

Roentgenographic examination usually reveals the characteristic lesion (Fig 12–17). The necrotic fragment may even become detached into the joint cavity.

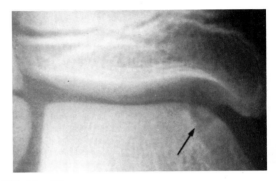

FIG 12–17.
Osteochondritis dissecans of the talus. (Talar dome fracture [arrow]).

Treatment

The undisplaced fragment is treated by prolonged abstinence from weight bearing until the lesion heals. Cast immobilization is frequently indicated. Persistent symptoms or detachment of the fragment require surgical removal of the necrotic piece of bone.

DISORDERS OF THE HINDFOOT

Plantar Fasciitis ("Painful Heel Syndrome")

The plantar fascia extends from the calcaneus to the proximal phalanges of each toe and plays an important role in gait. Inflammation of this fascia is a common occurrence and leads to pain on the plantar aspect of the heel. The pain may be present anywhere along the plantar fascia, but it is frequently found near the heel and along the medial longitudinal arch. It is a nonspecific inflammation that is probably secondary to repetitive strain. Both heels are frequently affected. This bilateral involvement may be an early symptom of other inflammatory disorders, such as ankylosing spondylitis, rheumatoid arthritis, or gouty arthritis. It may be seen in association with tight heel cords.

Clinical Features

The pain is usually felt directly beneath the calcaneus but may be present in the area of the medial arch. The discomfort is usually worse in the morning and after weight-bearing activities.

Examination reveals local point tenderness in the area of involvement. The pain may be aggravated by direct pressure or by maneuvers that place the fascia under a strain, such as dorsiflexing the toes and ankle.

Roentgenographic findings are usually normal but may reveal a traction spur on the os calcis that is directed distally (Fig 12–18). The significance of this spur in the etiology of symptoms is unknown. It may be a response to muscle tension and is frequently found in the asymptomatic foot.

Treatment

Treatment consists of padding the heel of the shoe or placing a relief pad around the area of tenderness (Fig 12–19). The pad is cut out around the tender area. A cup that redistributes the weight bearing on the heel may also be beneficial. Heel cord stretching exercises may help. A

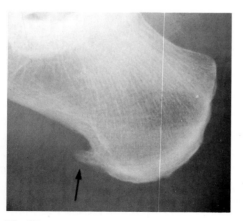

FIG 12–18.
Roentgenography of the os calcis shows the distally directed spur on its inferior aspect *(arrow).*

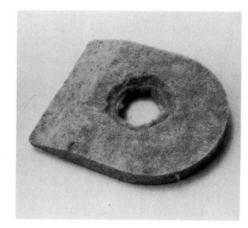

FIG 12–19.
Relief pad used in treatment of the painful heel.

heel lift or high-heeled shoe will often help transfer some of the weight forward, away from the heel to the ball of the foot. Oral anti-inflammatory medication is used as necessary. Many patients will benefit from local infiltration of the tender area with a steroid/lidocaine mixture. The injection may be repeated three to four times. Application of a short leg walking cast for 6 weeks is often very beneficial.

The prognosis is usually good, although healing may be slow (up to 1 to 2 years in some cases). When conservative treatment fails, release of the plantar fascia at its attachment to the os calcis and excision of the bony spur are indicated.

Achilles Tendinitis

Chronic overuse of the calf muscles may result in inflammation of the Achilles tendon. This disorder is frequently seen in the athlete. Pain, swelling, and a dry crepitus may be present. Passive stretching of the tendon by dorsiflexion of the ankle typically aggravates the pain.

Treatment consists of rest, heat, and anti-inflammatory medications. A short leg walking cast may be necessary. Local steroid injections should be avoided because they diminish the normal pain response. In the absence of this response, the patient's return to normal activity may be too rapid, and tendon rupture may result.

Bursitis

Two bursae are consistently present near the insertion of the Achilles tendon (Fig 12–20). The superficial bursa is often irritated by the constant rubbing of the counter of the shoe. The retrocalcaneal bursa may be irritated by a prominent posterosuperior angle of the calcaneus (Haglund's disease).

The treatment of both conditions is similar. Relief pads, heat, and elevation of the heel of the shoe with a soft cushion are usually sufficient. Occasionally, the bursa and any underlying bony prominence may have to be resected.

Calcaneal Apophysitis

A low-grade inflammatory reaction at the insertion of the Achilles tendon is frequently seen in association with irregular ossification and sclerosis of the calcaneal apophysis (Fig 12–21). This disorder, sometimes referred to as *Sever's disease,* usually occurs in boys between the ages of 8 and 14 years. Local pain, tenderness, and swelling that are aggravated by activity are common.

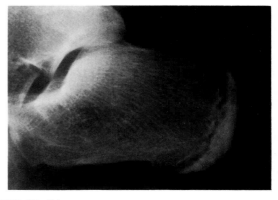

FIG 12–21.
Roentgenogram of the heel in Sever's disease.

Passive stretching of the heel cord may reproduce the pain.

The roentgenographic changes seen in this disorder are probably not related to the presence of pain in the heel because these same findings are frequently found in the normal, asymptomatic foot.

Treatment includes local heat and the avoidance of activity. A 1.25-cm heel lift may diminish the stress on the heel cord. A short leg walking cast applied with the foot in slight equinus may also be necessary in resistant cases. The disease is always self-limited.

Achilles Tendon Rupture

Spontaneous rupture of the heel cord is an uncommon injury that usually results from degeneration of the tendon or excessive force. The rupture usually occurs 2.5 to 5 cm from the insertion of the tendon into the os calcis.

Clinical Features

The injury frequently occurs during an activity that puts great stress on the tendon such as jumping. Following the injury, the patient walks flat-footed and is unable to stand on the ball of the foot. Tenderness and hemorrhage are present, and a sulcus is usually palpable at the site of the rupture. This sulcus may be obscured, however,

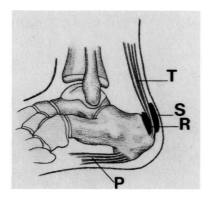

FIG 12–20.
Bursae of the heel: *S* = superficial calcaneal bursa; *R* = retrocalcaneal bursa; *T* = Achilles tendon; *P* = plantar fascia.

by an organizing clot if the examination is delayed. Although active plantar flexion is usually lost, some function occasionally remains because of the activity of the other posterior compartment muscles. Thompson's test is usually positive (Fig 12–22). Excessive passive dorsiflexion of the foot will be present on the injured side.

Treatment

The best results of treatment are obtained by immediate surgical repair. Nonoperative treatment by applying a short leg cast with the foot in equinus will also allow healing in many cases. Recurrence of the rupture is not uncommon regardless of treatment, and protection from excessive activity must be maintained for up to 1 year. Competitive athletes are rarely able to perform as well as before the injury.

Plantaris Tendon Rupture

The plantaris tendon lies medial to the heel cord in the calf. Traditionally, the cause of a sudden sharp pain in the calf with no loss of calf strength was always attributed to rupture of this tendon. Opinions differ as to whether or not the plantaris tendon actually ruptures. This entity may actually be the result of a partial rupture of the gastrocnemius muscle. The injury always occurs with activ-

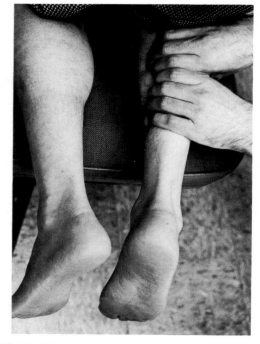

FIG 12–22.
Thompson's test. The normal foot will automatically plantar flex when the calf is squeezed. This movement is absent when the heel cord is ruptured.

ity, treatment is symptomatic, but differentiation from complete Achilles tendon rupture is important.

DISORDERS OF THE FOREFOOT

Morton's Neuroma

A common cause of pain in the forefoot is the interdigital neuroma. This lesion results from perineural fibrosis of the plantar nerve where the medial and lateral plantar branches communicate (Fig 12–23). The condition is probably secondary to repetitive trauma, and the fibrosis results in a painful fusiform swelling of the nerve. Females are more commonly affected.

Clinical Features

The clinical picture is one of severe burning pain in the region of the third web space that is accentuated by activity. The pain may radiate into the third and fourth toes. Tight shoes aggravate the discomfort, and the pain is often relieved by removing the shoe and massaging the foot. Numbness may be present in the affected toes.

The examination is usually unremarkable except for exquisite tenderness on digital pressure

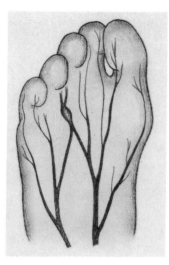

FIG 12–23.
Morton's neuroma.

between the third and fourth metatarsal heads. Compression of the forefoot transversely may also reproduce the pain. Some decrease in sensation may be present on the opposing surfaces of the two affected toes.

Treatment

Surgical removal of the neuroma is usually indicated. A pad that separates the heads of the third and fourth metatarsals may be helpful, but conservative treatment usually does not provide permanent relief. A local injection of a steroid/lidocaine mixture into the tender area and the avoidance of tight-fitting shoes may also give temporary relief.

Metatarsalgia

Pain beneath the metatarsal head is referred to as metatarsalgia. A variety of abnormalities may be responsible for the pain, including an abnormally high arch, improper shoe wear (especially a high-heeled shoe), and a tight Achilles tendon. The disorder is frequently associated with ham-

mertoes, clawed toes, and a hallux valgus deformity.

Clinical Features

The symptoms consist of a typical burning or cramping pain in the region of the metatarsal heads, usually the middle ones. These symptoms are worse with activity and relieved by rest. Tender calluses frequently develop under the metatarsal heads. Variable degrees of dorsal contractures of the metatarsophalangeal joints may be present.

Treatment

The object of treatment is to transfer the weight-bearing pressure away from the affected metatarsal heads onto the metatarsal neck and shaft. The calluses that form secondary to the abnormal pressure will usually disappear with time. Trimming or paring them will only provide temporary relief if the pressures are not removed from the affected metatarsal heads. A low-heeled shoe with sufficient room in the forefoot is worn. A metatarsal bar may be added to transfer the weight behind the metatarsal heads (Fig 12–24). Warm soaks are prescribed as necessary. Surgery

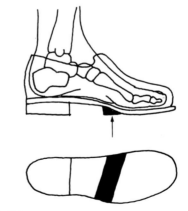

FIG 12–24.
The anterior metatarsal bar (arrow). It is placed behind the metatarsal heads so that weight is transferred to the metatarsal necks.

is reserved for those cases that fail to respond to conservative treatment.

Freiberg's Disease

Freiberg's disease is a disorder of unknown cause in which aseptic necrosis occurs in one of the metatarsal heads, usually the second. The condition is most common in adolescence.

Clinical Features

The disease appears as pain, swelling, and restriction of motion of the metatarsophalangeal joint. The metatarsal head is usually palpably enlarged.

Roentgenographic examination reveals widening and irregularity of the metatarsal head (Fig 12–25). Loose bodies may be present.

Treatment

The inflammation is treated with salicylates, warm soaks, and local steroid injections. An anterior metatarsal bar will frequently relieve pressure on the metatarsal head. Persistent pain necessitates arthroplasty of the involved joint.

Hallux Valgus

Hallux valgus is a lateral deviation of the great toe at the metatarsophalangeal joint. This is usually associated with bony and soft tissue enlargement over the medial aspect of the first metatarsal head that is referred to as the bunion. Females are most commonly affected. The cause is unknown, but heredity and the wearing of tight shoes play important roles.

Clinical Features

Pain and deformity are the main initial symptoms. The soft tissue over the prominence may become inflamed and tender. Painful calluses frequently develop on the second toe, which is forced into hyperextension by the deviated great toe.

Roentgenographic findings include lateral displacement of the proximal phalanx and the pres-

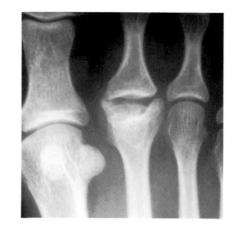

FIG 12–25.
Freiberg's disease, second toe.

ence of a medial exostosis (Fig 12–26). Degenerative changes may also be present in the metatarsophalangeal joint.

Treatment

Conservative treatment is directed at relieving the pressure over the painful bunion prominence. Properly fitted, low-heeled shoes with the

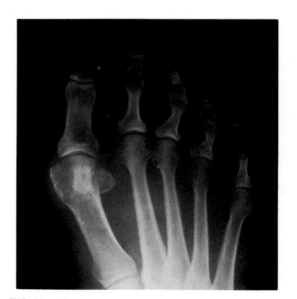

FIG 12–26.
Hallux valgus with bunion exostosis.

toe portion stretched to accommodate the bunion are effective. A splint that separates the first and second toes may also be beneficial. Tight nylons should be avoided. Local measures, such as rest and moist heat are indicated when acute pain is present. Disabling pain and deformity are indications for surgery. Excision of the exostosis and realignment of the great toe are usually performed.

Hallux Rigidus

Hallux rigidus is a painful condition affecting the metatarsophalangeal joint of the great toe and is characterized by restriction of motion. It is usually secondary to traumatic osteoarthritis. The condition may develop at any age but is most common in the third and fourth decades.

Clinical Features

Gradually increasing pain and stiffness are typical. They are often precipitated by a minor injury. The pain occurs with ambulation, especially when the toe is dorsiflexed as the patient comes up on the ball of the foot.

Examination reveals swelling, tenderness, and restricted motion of the metatarsophalangeal joint. Attempts at passive motion, especially dorsiflexion, are painful. The toe is held in a protective position of slight flexion, and as the patient walks, more weight is borne on the outer metatarsal heads and lateral border.

The roentgenogram usually reveals typical findings of degenerative arthritis with joint narrowing and spur formation (Fig 12–27).

Treatment

Symptomatic relief can be obtained by rest, moist heat, and anti-inflammatory medication. An intra-articular injection of steroid may provide additional relief. A shoe with sufficient room in the forefoot is worn, and an anterior metatarsal bar is applied to the shoe. Arthroplasty or arthrodesis of the metatarsophalangeal joint is indicated in resistant cases.

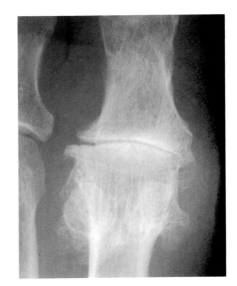

FIG 12–27.
Hallux rigidus. Narrowing and sclerosis are present at the metatarsophalangeal joint of the great toe.

Hallux Varus

Hallux varus is a deformity usually seen in children in which medial angulation of the great toe occurs at the metatarsophalangeal joint. It is usually congenital and associated with other foot deformities, but it may be seen in adults following surgical overcorrection of a hallux valgus deformity.

Mild cases in children may respond to passive stretching exercises and proper shoe wear. More severe cases in both adults and children usually require surgical correction.

Congenital Overlapping Fifth Toe

This is a common familial deformity, frequently bilateral, in which the small toe is dorsiflexed and may come to lie on the top of the fourth toe (Fig 12–28). The capsule and extensor tendon on the dorsum of the metatarsophalangeal joint are shortened and do not allow passive correction of the deformity. Calluses may develop on the dorsum of the toe secondary to chronic irritation by the shoe.

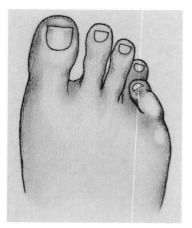

FIG 12–28.
Congenital overlapping fifth toe.

Passive stretching of mild deformities is indicated but usually does not completely correct the problem. Surgical realignment or even amputation may be necessary in symptomatic cases.

Hammertoe

A hammertoe is one in which a flexion deformity develops at the proximal interphalangeal joint and causes the tip of the toe to be depressed downward (Fig 12–29). A mild hyperextension deformity at the metatarsophalangeal joint may be present. Painful calluses develop over the tip of the toe, over the dorsum of the proximal interphalangeal joint, and under the metatarsal heads. The second toe is most commonly affected, and the disorder is frequently seen in as-

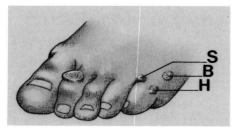

FIG 12–29.
Hammered second toe with a dorsal callus. Also shown are the soft corn *(S)*, bunionette *(B)*, and hard corn *(H)*.

sociation with a hallux valgus deformity of the great toe. The cause is frequently improperly fitted, tight shoes.

Mild flexible deformities may be corrected by stretching exercises and "over-and-under" taping to adjacent toes (Fig 12–30). Toe caps or pads may also be helpful. Properly fitted shoes are a must. Resistant cases usually require surgical correction.

Corns and Calluses

Corns and calluses develop in response to abnormal pressures against the skin of the foot. External pressure due to improper shoe wear combined with internal pressure from abnormal bony protuberances will frequently lead to the production of thickened, painful, hard skin over the bony prominence. In areas where moisture and perspiration collect, the skin becomes macerated, and a *soft corn* (clavus mollis) develops.

Hard corns (clavus durus) are most commonly found on the dorsolateral aspect of the proximal interphalangeal joint of the fifth toe, while soft corns are most common in the fourth web space. The tailor's bunion or bunionette occurs on the dorsolateral aspect of the metatarsophalangeal joint of the fifth toe. Calluses are frequently seen under the weight-bearing portion of the metatarsal heads or sesamoid bones of the great toe.

Removal of the external pressure is essential in the conservative management of all of these soft tissue lesions in the forefoot. A low-heeled shoe with adequate width in the forefoot is worn. Relief pads and metatarsal bars are usually helpful. Warm soaks in soapy water followed by the application of a keratolytic medication such as salicylic acid salve will help eliminate the callus or corn. The normal skin should be avoided when applying the salve. The salve should remain in place for 3 to 5 days and be covered by adhesive tape. After the tape is removed, the hard callus or corn may be shaved in layers. A pumice stone may also be used to pare down the callus. This procedure is frequently helpful, but deep excision of any corn or callus should be avoided

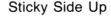

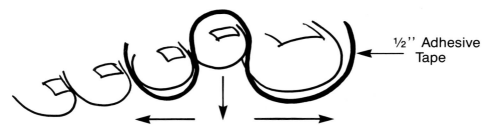

Sticky Side Up

½'' Adhesive Tape

FIG 12–30.
Over-and-under taping for a hammered second toe. The second toe is most often hammered, frequently because it is too long.

because an infected ulcer may result. Soft corns may be eliminated in 1 to 2 weeks, but hard calluses may take longer. A cotton pad may be worn between the toes if a soft corn is present, and a doughnut-shaped pad is always worn around a hard corn or callus. The toes should be kept as dry as possible at all times.

Surgical correction may be advised in resistant cases to eliminate the bony prominence.

Plantar warts also occur near the metatarsal heads but usually not directly on the weight-bearing surface. The wart is generally surrounded by a callus. Characteristic papillary tips are usually present. Paring or curettage of the wart and the use of salicylic acid salve will fre-quently effect a cure. Relief pads are worn as necessary. The lesion has a high incidence of spontaneous disappearance.

Disorders of the Toenail

A common condition that affects mainly the great toe is the ingrown nail. In this disorder, the nail does not actually grow into the soft tissue, but instead, the soft tissue overgrows and obliterates the nail sulcus (Fig 12–31). The nail itself is usually normal, although some older patients have incurved nails. The causes are probably multiple, but incorrect nail trimming, improperly fitted tight shoes and stockings, and bony deformities have all been implicated. Roentgenograms should be obtained to rule out unusual causes

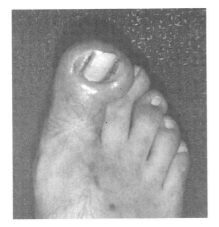

FIG 12–31.
A typical ingrown great toenail.

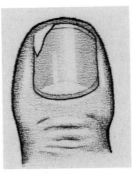

FIG 12–32.
The ingrown toenail frequently results from improper trimming that produces a nail spike. The nail should always be trimmed transversely.

such as subungual exostosis. Because of improper trimming, a small nail spike may be formed that continues to grow and irritate the soft tissue (Fig 12–32). A chronic infection is usually the end result.

In most mild early cases, soaks, antibiotics, and wearing proper shoes and stockings may be curative. The nail edge should be kept elevated with a soft cotton wad or metal shield until it grows out beyond the soft-tissue reaction. Unfortunately, this can be a slow process because the nail takes approximately 3 months to grow 1 cm. Proper transverse trimming of the nail should prevent recurrences.

Surgery may be necessary in resistant cases. Among the procedures used, removal of the central portion of the nail does not seem to allow the lateral margin of the nail to elevate away from the sulcus as theorized. Avulsing the whole nail is usually not effective either. When the nail regrows, it usually runs into the soft tissues again and causes the common recurrence in up to 70%

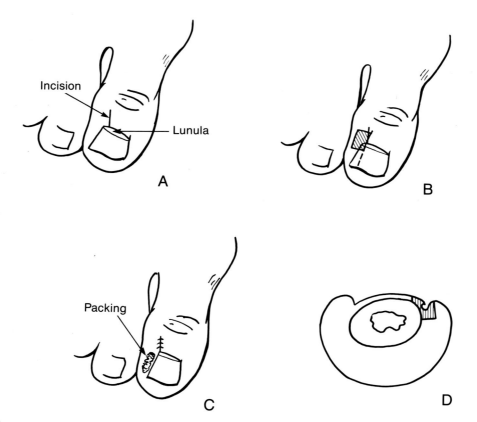

FIG 12–33.
Ingrown toenail removal. **A,** a short, angled skin incision is made in the eponychium down to the nail. **B,** with heavy scissors, the portion of the nail to be excised *(dotted line)* is separated from the remaining nail. (The important area of soft tissue and nail growth matrix to be removed is *crosshatched.*) **C,** a curet is used to remove any granulation tissue and remaining soft tissue in the periosteal area of the phalanx, and the incision is closed. A small pack is left in the gutter. **D,** approximate cross section of a toe showing the area to be removed under the skin. It is not necessary to remove tissue very far beyond the lunula, but be certain to remove all necessary growth matrix to prevent any spikes of nail from regrowing at the margin. (**Note:** The nail grows from a dorsal and deep matrix that envelops the base of the nail and extends just beyond the lunula. This area also extends proximally beneath the eponychium.) Both sides may be done if necessary.

of cases. The surgical procedures most commonly used involve removing (1) only one or both nail margins, (2) the entire nail, or (3) the entire nail plus a tuft of the distal phalanx. Removing one or both nail margins is the most popular. Removing the whole nail sometimes leaves an unsightly nail plate area, and amputating the distal tuft causes some shortening. Soft-tissue procedures are rarely used because of a high recurrence rate.

Surgery for nail margin removal is as follows (Fig 12–33):

1. Local anesthesia and a Penrose drain as a tourniquet are used.

2. A short angled incision is made in the eponychium down to the nail.

3. With heavy scissors, the section of nail to be removed is cut proximally to separate it from the remaining nail.

4. A knife blade is then used to separate the nail and matrix to be removed from the remaining nail and matrix. Along with the nail, the dorsal and inferior matrix is excised from its origin to distal to the edge of the lunula, and the nail margin plus matrix is removed.

5. Curettage is performed on the area to remove any granulation tissue and remaining matrix, and the incision is closed with a single suture.

6. A small pack is left in the sulcus and removed in 2 to 3 days when dressings are changed.

Phenol cauterization and sodium hydroxide have also been used to eliminate the germinal matrix itself. The results are about the same as those obtained with surgical removal.

Surgery for an older, thickened incurved nail usually involves removing the entire nail because, as a rule, the whole nail is involved.

Two other common conditions, the hypertrophied nail and the ram's-horn nail, may result from poor local hygiene. Both are most common in the elderly. A hypertrophied nail is usually caused by a low-grade fungus infection. The affected nail is thickened, and a yellow, powdery substance is present beneath it. A ram's horn nail is characterized by massive overgrowth. The nail may even curl over to the plantar aspect of the toe. Both disorders will usually respond to soaks and proper local care. Removal of the entire nail is occasionally required.

ACCESSORY BONES

Many accessory and sesamoid bones are present in the normal foot (Fig 12–34). Most are asymptomatic. An unusually large accessory navicular bone, however, may cause pain from local pressure. It is frequently associated with weakness in the longitudinal arch and a mild flatfoot deformity. Relief pads may eliminate symptoms, but surgical excision of the accessory bone is sometimes necessary to completely relieve the pain.

FRACTURES OF THE ANKLE

The talus is held in its position by bony and ligamentous structures and occupies a special position in the ankle joint. Any deviation from that position through injury will inevitably result in traumatic arthritis if untreated. Undisplaced fractures of the ankle usually do not disturb the joint or "mortise," but displaced fractures with ligamentous injury frequently do, and surgical repair is often necessary.

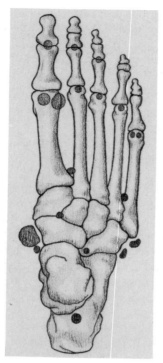

FIG 12–34.
Accessory and sesamoid bones of the foot.

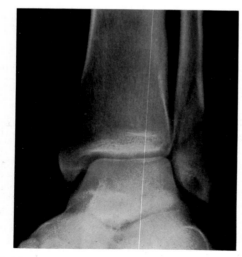

FIG 12–35.
Undisplaced fracture of the lateral malleolus.

Fractures Without Separation

Isolated, undisplaced fractures of either malleolus are usually stable and require only the application of a short leg walking cast with the ankle in the neutral position (Fig 12–35). Immobilization should be continued for 7 to 8 weeks. The fracture line of the lateral malleolus may persist roentgenographically for several months, but immobilization beyond 8 weeks is usually unnecessary.

Undisplaced bimalleolar fractures are treated with a long leg cast to prevent motion and displacement of the fracture fragments. This cast is flexed 30 degrees at the knee in order to prevent rotation of the lower portion of the leg. In 4 weeks, a short leg walking cast may be applied that is maintained for an additional 4 weeks.

The undisplaced fracture of the distal fibular *epiphysis* is diagnosed clinically. There is tenderness over the epiphyseal plate. Roentgenogram findings are usually negative. A short leg walking

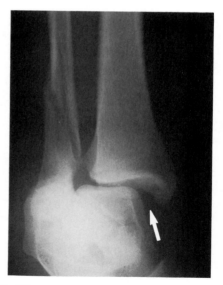

FIG 12–36.
Displaced fracture of the lateral malleolus with widening of the ankle mortise *(arrow)* due to a lateral shift of the talus. (**Note:** A 1-mm shift in the talus changes the contact surface of the ankle joint 40%. Therefore, all ankle fractures need careful evaluation and treatment to avoid traumatic arthritis.)

cast is applied for 4 weeks, and growth disturbance is rare.

Fractures With Separation

Fractures with significant displacement must be reduced, especially if any widening of the ankle joint is present (Fig 12–36). Isolated lateral malleolar fractures can frequently be treated nonoperatively, but bimalleolar and displaced medial malleolar fractures usually require surgery.

Fractures with dislocation of the talus should be reduced as rapidly as possible (Fig 12–37). If the dislocation is not promptly reduced, severe soft-tissue injury with blistering and skin breakdown may result. Definitive surgical treatment of the fractures may also have to be delayed. The dislocation is reduced by traction and manipulation with the patient under local anesthesia. Following the reduction, the ankle is placed in a soft, bulky compression dressing reinforced with plaster splints. Any necessary surgery can then be performed on an elective basis.

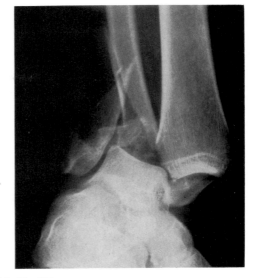

FIG 12–37.
Fracture-dislocation of the ankle.

FRACTURES OF THE FOOT

Fractures of the Calcaneus

A fracture of the calcaneus usually results from a fall on the heel. It is frequently associated with a compression fracture of the lumbar spine. The os calcis is usually crushed, and the fragments are displaced in varying amounts (Fig 12–38).

Fractures of the os calcis are painful injuries characterized by severe swelling. The swelling may be so intense that blistering and even skin necrosis may occur. In order to control the swelling and hemorrhage, all calcaneus fractures are treated initially with a soft compression dressing, ice, and elevation. A cast is never applied immediately after the injury. The pain from the fracture and swelling is only intensified if a constricting circular cast is present over the heel.

Minimally displaced fractures are treated by cast immobilization for 2 to 3 weeks or with crutches and non–weight bearing. The cast is removed as soon as possible in order to begin mobilization of the ankle and heel. Eversion and inversion movements are begun, but weight bearing is not allowed for 6 to 8 weeks until the fracture has healed.

Displaced fractures are treated by either

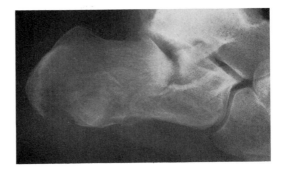

FIG 12–38.
Fracture of the calcaneus with moderate displacement.

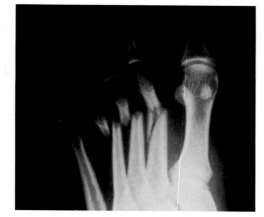

FIG 12–39.
Displaced fractures of the metatarsals.

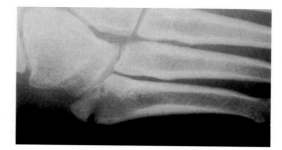

FIG 12–40.
Fracture of the base of the fifth metatarsal.

closed or open reduction. An attempt is made to elevate the depressed central articular fragment and reduce the widening of the heel.

Regardless of treatment, prolonged immobilization is inadvisable. Temporary disability following this injury may persist for 1 to 2 years, and some permanent impairment is common. Early motion without weight bearing appears to be most beneficial. Some restriction of eversion and inversion is usually permanent, which makes walking on rough, irregular surfaces difficult.

Fractures of the Metatarsals

Fractures of the necks or shafts of the metatarsals usually result from compression injuries of the foot. Undisplaced fractures require little treatment other than a compression dressing and crutches for 4 to 6 weeks. A short leg walking cast or hard-soled sandal may be preferable in a few days to allow the patient to discard the crutches.

Displaced fractures of the necks of the metatarsals may need reduction in order to prevent pain from developing under the metatarsal heads (Fig 12–39). Manipulation with the patient under anesthesia is sometimes effective, but maintenance of the reduction is frequently difficult. Open reduction with internal fixation is often necessary.

Fractures of the base of the fifth metatarsal are common and result from an inversion injury to the foot (Fig 12–40). They are usually undisplaced and require little treatment. A light compression dressing and hard-soled sandal are usually sufficient. Crutches may be necessary for 7 to 10 days, and healing is usually complete in 5 to 6 weeks.

Fractures of the *shaft* of the fifth metatarsal heal slowly and may require a short leg walking cast.

Fractures of the Phalanges

Fractures of the toes are common and usually require little treatment. Undisplaced fractures may be treated by taping the injured toe to the adjacent toe for 3 to 4 weeks. Displaced fractures can usually be reduced with the patient under local anesthesia. Open reduction is rarely necessary. Fractures of the proximal phalanx of the great toe, however, should be reduced accurately.

FOOT CARE

Most foot problems develop in the forefoot, and many have been previously discussed. For the treatment of painful conditions of the forefoot, the patient should avoid high heels and keep the foot in a soft shoe with a wide toe box (that portion covering the forefoot). The simple addition of an anterior heel (anterior metatarsal bar) will improve many of the problems that develop under the metatarsal heads.

The diabetic with or without vascular disease has the potential for far more serious problems, and special care must be taken to avoid them. The following general principles are helpful:

1. The feet should be inspected and cleaned daily. The feet should be washed with a bland soap in lukewarm water and patted dry. Overzealous rubbing should always be avoided. The feet are inspected for any cracks or fissures, and a mirror is used if necessary. The shoes should also be inspected for any area that could cause skin irritation.

2. Stockings should fit comfortably and be kept dry at all times to prevent skin maceration. Tight constricting stockings should not be worn, but loose stockings that may wrinkle should also be avoided.

3. Smoking and temperature extremes should be avoided.

4. "Home surgery" should be avoided, especially by the diabetic or the patient with vascular disease. Nails should be left long and cut straight across. A pumice stone may be used on thick calluses in the healthy patient but these same calluses place the diabetic foot at risk for infection because they frequently crack and develop into open sores. Diabetics should not use the pumice stone but should attempt to soften the calluses by changing the weight-bearing stresses on the foot.

5. Diabetics should also avoid applying strong chemical agents to calluses or corns.

6. A bland moisturizing cream should be applied daily, but the web spaces should be kept dry. Powder may be used there, and small pieces of cotton may be placed between the toes if necessary.

7. Shoes should fit comfortably. Soft leather or canvas is preferred because they "breathe" better and cause fewer pressure areas. Foam rubber soles cause fewer plantar calluses. The toe box should be wide and high enough to accommodate any contractures or exostosis. The patient with more severe forefoot deformities may require a specially constructed shoe or an in-depth (extra depth) shoe. This has a wider, deeper toe box that is helpful for hammered or clawed toes.

8. Full-length, soft, molded inlays can be used when pressure sores or painful calluses are present. An in-depth shoe is usually required to provide enough room for the insole, which is usually the full length of the shoe. Insoles reduce and spread the repetitive stress on the foot. Many good over-the-counter materials are available. Excellent materials such as Plastizote can be heat-molded to conform to the individual's foot. Relief areas can then be cut out of the material wherever pressure soles are present on the corresponding part of the foot. These often require an in-depth shoe to allow for the size of the insert. These materials have to be replaced occasionally because they will lose their volume and flatten to some degree.

When ulcers do develop, they are most common on the weight-bearing surface of the foot or on the medial aspect of the great toe. These are often referred to as mal-perforans (Fig 12–41). At this stage vigorous local care, minor debridement, and control of infection are indicated. Excessive heat, which places a great demand on the soft tissue, should be avoided. The previously mentioned metatarsal bars and insoles are used to relieve the pressure on the ulcer. If the foot is

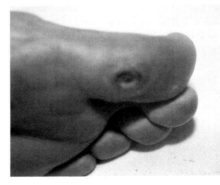

FIG 12–41.
Healing mal-perforans ulcer of the great toe.

warm and has pulses, amputation is usually not necessary, and healing of these ulcers will commonly occur with proper care.

Shoes

Because the majority of foot problems are caused by tight-fitting shoes, the first treatment is addressing the source of the problem. Women's shoes, especially high-heeled ones, are the source of most difficulties. In order for the usual high-heeled shoes or even pumps to stay in place, excessive pressures must be applied to the forefoot. Lowering the heel and widening the forefoot of the shoe could help, but this often results in a shoe that won't stay on because the heel is too wide. The only option is a lace-up shoe. While less attractive, this shoe is more comfortable because more room can be allowed in the toe box for the forefoot and the shoes won't feel loose in the heel. "Orthopedic" prescription shoes are usually unnecessary and expensive. A soft, low-heeled lace shoe of any type will often provide symptomatic relief of many forefoot problems.

The same pragmatic approach may be taken regarding children's shoes. Only rarely are special shoes ever needed, and there are absolutely no advantages for children to wear the traditional, expensive, high-topped leather shoe. Children may outgrow two to four pairs each year, and the total cost of such shoes would be considerable even if they were of some benefit. Children wear shoes to (1) keep the feet warm and (2) prevent harm from sharp objects. Otherwise, they may go barefooted as much as they like or wear any inexpensive brand as long as the shoes are comfortable.

BIBLIOGRAPHY

Anderson IF, et al: Osteochondral fractures of the dome of the talus. *J Bone Joint Surg [Am]* 1989; 71:1143.

Bleck EE: The shoeing of children: Sham or science? *Dev Med Child Neurol* 1971; 13:188.

Bleck EE, Berzins UJ: Conservative management of pes valgus with plantar flexed talus, flexible. *Clin Orthop* 1977; 122:85.

Cass JR, Morrey BF: Ankle instability: Current concepts, diagnosis and treatment. *Mayo Clin Proc* 1984; 59:165.

Cowell HR: Talocalcaneal coalition and new causes of peroneal spastic flat foot. *Clin Orthop* 1972; 85:16.

Downs DM, Jacobs RL: Treatment of resistant ulcers on the plantar surface of the great toe in diabetics. *J Bone Joint Surg [Am]* 1982; 64:930.

DuVries HL: *Surgery of the Foot,* ed 2. St Louis, CV Mosby Co, 1965.

Eckert WR, Davis EA Jr: Acute rupture of the peroneal retinaculum. *J Bone Joint Surg [Am]* 1976; 58:670.

Furey JG: Plantar fasciitis: The painful heel syndrome. *J Bone Joint Surg [Am]* 1975; 57:672.

Greenfield GB: *Radiology of Bone Diseases.* Philadelphia, JB Lippincott, 1969.

Greig JD: Results of surgery for ingrowing toenails. *J Bone Joint Surg [Br]* 1989; 71:859.

Heifitz CJ: Ingrown toenail: A clinical study. *Am J Surg* 1937; 37:298.

Helfet AJ: A new way of treating flat feet in children. *Lancet* 1956; 1:262.

Inglis AE, et al: Ruptures of the tendo Achilles: An objective assessment of surgical and non-surgical treatment. *J Bone Joint Surg [Am]* 1976; 58:990.

Johnson KA: *Surgery of the Foot and Ankle.* New York, Raven Press, 1989.

Keats TE: *An Atlas of Normal Roentgen Variants That May Simulate Disease.* Chicago, Year Book Medical Publishers Inc, 1977.

Korkala O, et al: A prospective study of the treatment of severe tears of the lateral ligament of the ankle. *Int Orthop* 1987; 11:13.

Lea RB, Smith L: Non-surgical treatment of tendon Achilles rupture. *J Bone Joint Surg [Am]* 1972; 54:1398.

Milgram JE: Office measures for relief of the painful foot. *J Bone Joint Surg [Am]* 1964; 46:1095.

Mosier KM, Asher M: Tarsal coalitions and peroneal spastic flat foot. *J Bone Joint Surg [Am]* 1984; 66:976.

Robb JE, Murray WR: Phenol cauterization in the management of ingrowing toenails. *Scott Med J* 1982; 27:236.

Rockwood CA, Green DP: *Fractures in Adults,* ed 2. Philadelphia, JB Lippincott, 1984.

Sarmiento A, Wolf M: Subluxation of peroneal tendons. *J Bone Joint Surg [Am]* 1975; 57:115.

Severance HW Jr, Bassett FH III: Rupture of the plantaris: Does it exist? *J Bone Joint Surg [Am]* 1982; 64:9.

Staheli LT, Chew DE, Corbett M: The longitudinal arch: A survey of eight hundred and eighty-two feet in normal children and adults. *J Bone Joint Surg [Am]* 1987; 69:426.

Staples OS: Ruptures of the fibular collateral ligaments of the ankle: Result study of immediate surgical treatment. *J Bone Joint Surg [Am]* 1975; 57:101.

Sykes PA: Ingrowing toenails: Time for critical appraisal? *J R Coll Surg Edinb* 1986; 31:300.

Tachdjian MO: *Pediatric Orthopedics.* Philadelphia, WB Saunders Co, 1972.

Taylor GS: Prominence of the calcaneus: Is operation justified. *J Bone Joint Surg [Br]* 1986; 68:467.

Thompson TC, Terwilliger C: The terminal Syme operation for ingrown toenail. *Surg Clin North Am* 1951; 31:575.

Turco CJ: Surgical correction of the resistant club foot. *J Bone Joint Surg [Am]* 1971; 53:477.

Wenger DR, et al: Corrective shoes and inserts as treatment for flexible flatfoot in infants and children. *J Bone Joint Surg [Am]* 1989; 71:800.

Zadik FR: Obliteration of the nailbed without shortening of the terminal phalanx. *J Bone Joint Surg [Br]* 1950; 32:66.

Zinman C, Wolfson N, Reis ND: Osteochondritis dissecans of the dome of the talus. Computed tomography scanning in diagnosis and follow-up. *J Bone Joint Surg [Am]* 1988; 70:1017.

CHAPTER 13

Infections of Bone and Joint

Osteomyelitis is defined as an acute or chronic infection of the bone or bone marrow. It is often classified as either acute or chronic. Acute osteomyelitis is usually a disorder of childhood and is less common in the adult. Chronic osteomyelitis, in contrast, is primarily a disease of adult life and usually develops as a result of an open wound, either traumatic or surgical.

OSTEOMYELITIS

Acute

The most common site of involvement in childhood is the metaphyseal end of a single long bone, frequently near the knee joint. The route of infection is usually hematogenous, although local direct extension from a neighboring soft-tissue infection occasionally occurs. A history of trauma may be elicited. A primary site of infection is only rarely found.

The metaphyseal area of growing bone is most frequently involved because as enchondral ossification proceeds, the blood vessels that normally invade the growth zone are looped and, as a result, the circulation is sluggish. This can allow a nidus of infection to become established.

In patients over the age of 50 years, the spine becomes the most common site of infection. Often, these patients have a history of genitourinary disease and/or manipulation, and the onset of the infection may be insidious.

Cause

Most cases of acute hematogenous osteomyelitis are caused by *Staphylococcus aureus,* although the prevalence of *S. aureus* has dropped from approximately 80% to 50%. In infants and children, important causes are nonhemolytic streptococci and *Haemophilus influenzae.* Gram-negative bacilli are particularly important causes of osteomyelitis involving the vertebral bodies in adults. There is a higher incidence of osteomyelitis in socioeconomically deprived individuals that is caused primarily by *Staphylococcus* and tuberculosis. Tuberculous and fungal causes of osteomyelitis can usually be traced to the pulmonary system. Blacks afflicted with sickle-cell disease have a particularly high susceptibility to *Salmonella* osteomyelitis. Osteomyelitis may follow infections of the genitourinary or biliary tracts or any type of surgical manipulation, particularly colorectal surgery.

With the current incidence of intravenous (IV)

drug abuse, there is a much higher rate of osteomyelitis that is predominantly spondylitis or intervertebral disc infection. Involvement of the lumbar vertebrae or sacroiliac joints is peculiar to this type of development of osteomyelitis, and the organism causing the infection is often *Klebsiella aerobacter* or *Pseudomonas aeruginosa,* although the organism may vary from one locale to another.

In general, acute hematogenous staphylococcal osteomyelitis occurs primarily in late infancy and also at puberty. In some of these cases, the source of the infection can be discovered by inspection of the skin, and occasionally, a furuncle is found to be the primary source.

Haemophilus influenzae is particularly virulent as a cause of osteomyelitis from infancy to 6 years of age. In this age group, *H. influenzae* infection can appear as a soft-tissue cellulitis, and this should alert the physician to the possibility of an underlying osteomyelitis. *Haemophilus influenzae* infection is not necessarily a disease only of children because there is also an increased infection rate with this organism in aged individuals as well.

Clinical Features

Acute osteomyelitis is often preceded by signs of systemic disease and/or general sepsis. Anorexia, nausea, malaise, irritability and fever are present, usually during the acute phase. This stage of the disease may last for several days or as long as 1 to 2 weeks before bone pain and local overlying inflammation appear. Fever, chills, and diaphoresis are the usual systemic complaints. Pain, bone tenderness, swelling of the soft tissue, and limitation of joint motion are usually apparent on physical examination.

In infants, the disease may be alarming and life-threatening in its onset and may show overall symptoms of generalized sepsis. The involved area will usually show limitation of motion, and there may be tenderness in the region of the involved bone well before swelling and redness occur. In children, although the usual course is that of high fever, chills, and malaise, an altering

of this presentation may occur, particularly when the underlying infection has been partially treated with antibiotics that were instituted earlier for an upper respiratory tract or skin infection. Only soft-tissue swelling and some limitation of motion of the involved portion of the skeleton or joint may be present with few systemic symptoms.

In the adult, the onset is usually less acute and more insidious. Constitutional symptoms may be considerably less marked or even absent. In the older child and the adult, it is not uncommon for the first symptoms of osteomyelitis to be those of bone involvement. Usually there will be limitation of joint motion, especially if the osteomyelitis involves the spine or if the primary lesions are particularly close to joint spaces where sympathetic effusions may occur in the joint nearest the involved bone.

Tuberculous, fungal, rickettsial, and viral causes of osteomyelitis generally have a chronic, insidious onset. These diseases are more common in patients who are immunologically depressed or who have other underlying diseases such as alcoholism, those of the lower socioeconomic group, or those whose immune systems have been altered by immunosuppressive therapy. As was previously mentioned, the primary source of these infections is often pulmonary, and a low-grade fever, weight loss, anorexia, and chronic cough or sputum production may be present. Tuberculous osteomyelitis may involve the vertebral column with pathologic fractures of the involved vertebrae. This usually results in angular kyphosis of the spine or so-called Pott's disease (Fig 13–1).

In the drug-abusing patient who is afebrile and presents with an onset of back pain that is aggravated by moving, coughing, sneezing, or straining at stool, pyogenic spondylitis and gram-negative osteomyelitis should be suspected.

Roentgenographic Features

The classic roentgenographic finding of acute osteomyelitis in childhood is deep, circumferential soft-tissue swelling with obliteration of muscular

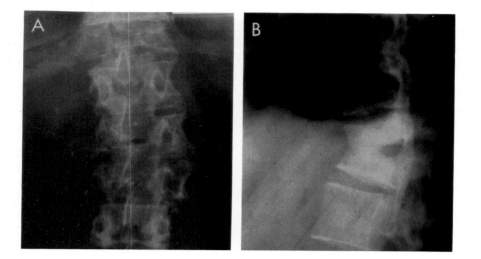

FIG 13–1.
Pott's disease. Angulation is present on both the anteroposterior **(A)** and the lateral **(B)** views.

planes. Spotty rarefactions representing early destruction may appear within 7 to 12 days in the affected bone. Shortly after this, periosteal new bone formation becomes evident and indicates that the infection has spread through the cortex (Fig 13–2).

Roentgenographic changes are of less value in adult osteomyelitis because significant bony changes may not be apparent until at least 50% of bone resorption has occurred, which may be 2 to 4 weeks into the illness. In the spine, infection

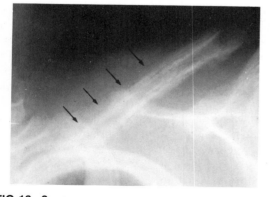

FIG 13–2.
Acute osteomyelitis of the clavicle. Note the periosteal reaction.

can involve the vertebral body or the disc space. Disc space infections are uncommon but do occur occasionally in children and in patients who have undergone surgery on the intervertebral disc. In these cases, the roentgenographic changes are vertebral end-plate irregularities and disc space narrowing. Eventually, new bone proliferation occurs, and frequently, complete fusion of the disc is the result. In osteomyelitis of the vertebral body, the roentgenographic changes are those of bone destruction with loss of vertebral height. Paravertebral swelling and/or paraspinal masses may also be occasionally demonstrated.

Radioisotope bone scans are the mainstay in the early diagnosis of bone infection. The technetium 99 scan is somewhat less expensive than others and requires less radiation than the gallium scan. It is nonspecific, however. An advantage of the technetium scan is that it can be performed within a few hours. Gallium may take 3 days, which is a major drawback. Indium 111 is more specific for infection. It takes 24 hours for completion. Technetium is incorporated directly into bone and therefore depends on the osseous blood flow. Since changes take place in blood flow long before they do in the bone of patients with osteomyelitis, the technetium scan will usually point to the lesion early in the disease.

Magnetic resonance imaging (MRI) and computed tomographic (CT) scanning may also be helpful when there are minor destructive changes present.

Chronic Osteomyelitis

This disorder can occasionally be the end result of an acute hematogenous osteomyelitis, but it is more commonly caused by an open fracture or wound and rarely by a surgical procedure. It is often seen in the lower extremities of the diabetic patient. All forms of chronic osteomyelitis are difficult to eradicate. The cause is often polymicrobial.

Clinical Features

This disorder is characterized by the onset of inflammation and cellulitis following an open fracture or by persistent drainage following an episode of acute osteomyelitis. Occasionally, it develops in the postoperative period following orthopedic procedures.

Fever, pain, and mild systemic symptoms are typical. External physical findings may be minimal, but soft-tissue inflammation and tenderness will usually develop.

Frequently, the infection becomes latent following treatment. The nidus of infection may become surrounded by dense bone and fibrous tissue. This often prevents antibiotic penetration. Later, minor trauma may reactivate the inflammation, cellulitis, and drainage. Repeated hospitalizations and treatment are often necessary, and some chronic wounds drain persistently.

Roentgenographic Findings

Chronic osteomyelitis usually appears as irregular sclerotic bone that may contain several areas of radiolucency. Irregular areas of destruction are commonly present, and there is often periosteal thickening (Fig 13–3).

Small dense areas of dead bone called sequestra may be present. If the acute hematogenous

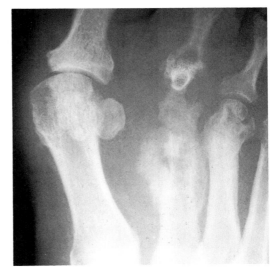

FIG 13–3.
Chronic osteomyelitis of the second toe.

osteomyelitis has been extensive, the entire shaft may become a *sequestrum*. This dead bone is then surrounded by a new shell of bone called the *involucrum*. Fortunately, this extensive involvement is rarely seen in Western society.

Complications

The most common complications of acute osteomyelitis are soft-tissue abscess formation, septic arthritis from extension to the adjacent joints, and metastatic infections from the initial focus. Occasionally, chronic osteomyelitis can be a complication of acute osteomyelitis. This is relatively uncommon in children, however, because the bone of growing children is a more active substance and has the ability to "turn over" and clear itself of infection. Extensive spinal involvement may lead to paraplegia, and pathologic fractures may even occur in weight-bearing bones.

The most common complication of chronic osteomyelitis is repetitive episodes of inflammation and drainage or even simply chronic drainage. If this occurs following the insertion of an orthopedic implant, it is often necessary to remove the orthopedic implant before the infection will subside. In weight-bearing joints, this often results in less-than-optimal function, but removal of the foreign body does increase the chances of curing the infection.

Development of a chronically draining sinus can also be mildly debilitating because of the extensive protein loss. On rare occasions, squamous cell carcinoma can even develop at the drainage site. Amputation is even occasionally necessary in diabetics or other individuals with poor local tissue health. Overgrowth of bone due to stimulation or shortening due to growth plate destruction can also occur in the young.

Diagnosis

Cultures of the blood or of the lesion are essential to determine the exact causative agent and to institute the proper antimicrobial therapy. Blood cultures are positive in the majority of children with acute osteomyelitis but are frequently negative in adults. Every attempt should be made to isolate the organism. Needle aspiration of the site may be attempted, but this is sometimes inadequate. If a primary focus can be identified, a smear, Gram stain, and culture and sensitivity should be taken from this site.

Cultures of the drainage from a chronic sinus tract are also occasionally helpful, but if no drainage is present and a postoperative wound infection is suspected, a deep culture is frequently necessary.

The laboratory workup should include a sedimentation rate determination and a complete blood cell count (CBC) in addition to the above cultures. There is usually a leukocytosis and an elevation of the erythrocyte sedimentation rate (ESR). The ESR is sometimes useful to follow the patient's progress while undergoing treatment.

Differential Diagnosis

The differential diagnosis must include (1) acute suppurative arthritis, (2) rheumatic fever, and (3) cellulitis.

In acute septic arthritis, the most common cause of the disease in young adults is *Neisseria gonorrhoeae,* while *S. aureus* is the major cause of septic arthritis in older adults. Also, in the older population septic arthritis is usually superimposed on some other bone disease, most commonly rheumatoid arthritis. In general, the clinical manifestations of septic arthritis are variable and related to the type of organism causing the underlying infection. Most patients with gonococcal septic arthritis have prominent prodromal symptoms such as fever, chills, headaches, anorexia, and malaise, followed by the development of monoarticular septic arthritis. In gonococcal arthritis, an important portion of the diagnosis lies in the history of a migratory polyarthralgia. A tenosynovitis may be present, but cultures from this involved synovium are usually sterile; however, the skin lesions and small joint effusions are generally positive for the offending organism. The arthritis seen in gonococcal disease is that of involvement of the large joints, primarily the knee, followed by the wrists, ankles, and elbows.

The clinical picture of patients with acute rheumatic fever, gout, and rheumatoid arthritis, or just trauma to a joint, may mimic that seen in acute septic arthritis. Synovial fluid examination is helpful to differentiate these three underlying causes. The diagnosis of acute rheumatic fever is still best obtained by adhering to the Jones' criteria of major and minor manifestations (Table 13–1).

Cellulitis may sometimes be difficult to differentiate from septic arthritis and acute osteomyelitis. In cellulitis, there is no deep soft-tissue swelling on roentgenographic examination. The soft-tissue swelling is primarily superficial. Occasionally, the cellulitis can evoke a sympathetic effusion in an adjacent joint, but passive and active movements of that joint are generally not as painful as they are in acute septic arthritis. In addition, the clinical response to treatment is usually dramatic. If there is a sympathetic effusion in an adjacent joint and there is a problem in differentiation between cellulitis, septic arthritis and

TABLE 13–1.
Modified Jones' Criteria*

Major criteria
  Carditis
  Polyarthritis
  Chorea
  Subcutaneous nodules
  Erythema marginatum
Minor criteria
  Fever
  Arthralgia
  Prolonged PR interval in the ECG
  Increased ESR, white blood cell count, or presence of
  C-reactive protein
  Preceding β-hemolytic streptococcal infection
  Previous rheumatic fever or inactive rheumatic heart
  disease

*The presence of two major or one major and two minor criteria is highly suggestive of rheumatic fever.

acute osteomyelitis, the joint may be aspirated through an area of healthy skin, but great care must be taken to avoid contaminating a normal joint.

Treatment and Prognosis

Acute Osteomyelitis

The treatment of acute osteomyelitis should begin immediately and not be delayed while waiting for the identification of the offending organism. Since the majority of cases are caused by *S. aureus,* it is appropriate to use an IV penicillin-resistant semisynthetic penicillin. Usually, oxacillin or cloxacillin is the drug of choice because these are nearly as active as penicillin G against non–penicillinase-producing *S. aureus* and *Streptococcus pyogenes* group A. These drugs are usually given in daily doses of 8 to 16 g IV in the adult. In addition, antibiotic coverage should be adequate for *H. influenzae,* especially in the infant. Ampicillin is probably the drug of choice for this organism. IV ampicillin would also be the drug of choice in those patients with sickle-cell anemia in whom the incidence of *Salmonella* osteomyelitis is more common.

In addition to the proper antibiotic coverage, the patient should have general supportive measures. Dehydration and anemia should be corrected, and the diet should be high in vitamins and protein. Early surgical decompression is indicated in acute osteomyelitis unless there has been a rapid clinical response within 24 hours. The extremity should be protected postoperatively.

If necessary, changes are made in the antibiotic coverage when the offending organism is identified. The sedimentation rate is followed during treatment. IV antibiotic coverage is usually continued for at least 3 weeks, but each case should be treated individually. If the ESR is nearly normal or falling, the patient has been afebrile for 72 hours, and there is no further clinical evidence of infection, IV treatment does not probably need to continue for longer than 2 weeks. Oral antibiotic coverage should continue for an additional 3 to 4 weeks.

Sometimes, fever may recur following an initially good response to the appropriate antibiotic treatment. At this time, a careful clinical re-evaluation is necessary, and several conditions should be considered: (1) laboratory error in identification of the organism, (2) drug fever (usually due to the cephalosporins or penicillin), (3) superinfection, or (4) abscess formation.

In general, the prognosis for acute osteomyelitis is good, although complications have been reported in as many as 25% of cases. A delay in diagnosis and treatment may lead to chronic osteomyelitis or multiple recurrences. These recurrences can be as long as 30 years later and are usually due to the same organism. They are often reactivated by local trauma.

Chronic Osteomyelitis

The treatment of chronic osteomyelitis is similar to that of the acute form, but prevention remains the most important aspect of this disease. All open fractures are frequently and meticulously debrided, and great care is taken to eliminate contamination. Chronic osteomyelitis may be treated by incision and drainage, sequestrectomy, and appropriate antibiotic coverage, but once it is established, it is difficult to cure. Recurrent drainage and residual deformity both add to the morbidity.

Local infection that develops when a prosthetic device is being used by the patient will usually require removal of the device before the infection can be controlled.

Infections of the bones of the feet are common in diabetics, who often have coincidental peripheral vascular disease. Painless ulcers may develop secondary to diabetic polyneuropathy and diabetic vascular disease. Hyperemia and swelling are frequently noted clinically. If a fracture occurs in the foot of a diabetic, it may be accompanied by a similar redness and swelling and be a source of some confusion. A roentgenogram will usually clarify the diagnosis.

PYOGENIC ARTHRITIS

Septic or pyogenic arthritis may occur in any age group but is more common in the young. It is usually monoarticular, and large peripheral joints are most frequently involved, usually the knee or hip. Polyarticular disease is rare but may occur in patients with pre-existing inflammatory disease or chronic illness. Unusual sites (sacroiliac, sternoclavicular joints, and symphysis pubis) may be involved in IV drug abusers.

Pathogenesis

The offending organism is usually *N. gonorrhoeae* or *S. aureus,* but a variety of other bacteria may be causative. *H. influenzae* is common in children. Gram-negative rods are frequently involved in IV drug users. Entrance to the joint is usually gained by hematogenous seeding, rarely by direct extension from an adjacent infection. In the hip, it may be introduced by an improperly performed venipuncture. The disorder is more common in patients with underlying chronic disease states or those undergoing immunosuppressive therapy.

Upon invasion of the joint by the pathogenic bacteria, the organisms seed the synovial membrane, which becomes swollen and hyperemic. It begins to produce large amounts of fluid that distend the joint capsule. Frank pus eventually accumulates, and destruction of articular cartilage may even occur.

Clinical Features

The onset is usually acute, with pain being the most common early symptom. A history of infection elsewhere is occasionally obtainable. If a weight-bearing joint is involved, ambulation is usually difficult and may become impossible due to the pain. Fever and other signs of systemic infection are usually present.

Examination generally reveals a warm, swollen, diffusely tender joint. The joint is usually held in slight flexion because, in this position, the intracapsular pressure is decreased and discomfort is thereby minimized. Attempts at passive motion tend to be extremely painful.

Special Studies

Roentgenographic findings early in the disease process are usually minimal and consist primarily of distention of the joint capsule. The peripheral white blood cell (WBC) count is markedly elevated as a rule, and blood cultures may be positive. The sedimentation rate is generally high, but the neonate and geriatric patient may show only minimal laboratory abnormalities. Bone scanning and other studies are of limited value but may be very helpful in the evaluation of the patient whose symptoms are of uncertain cause.

Confirmation of the diagnosis is best made by joint aspiration under sterile conditions. Most joints are best aspirated on the extensor side, except the hip, which may be aspirated from the anterior or lateral aspect. Because the joint is usually distended, aspiration is ordinarily not difficult. The fluid is initially cloudy and thin but may be purulent. The joint glucose level is decreased, and the WBC count is markedly increased as a rule. A Gram stain is performed, and cultures are taken. The specimen should always be inspected for crystals.

Treatment

Treatment should begin immediately in order to prevent joint destruction and, in the case of the hip joint, dislocation. Rest, moist heat, and traction will diminish the pain. The definitive antibiotic therapy will depend on Gram stain and culture results. The IV route should always be used. Intra-articular injection is unnecessary because most antibiotics readily pass through the synovial membrane. Direct instillation may even provoke an inflammatory synovitis.

Surgical drainage of the affected joint is usually indicated. This is especially true of the hip. Surgery may be delayed if a dramatic clinical response occurs with conservative treatment, but if such a response is not forthcoming, drainage should be performed immediately. Surgery will diminish the intra-articular pressure, allow evacuation of the thick fibrous exudate, and prevent the articular destruction that may occur in pyarthrosis.

When irreversible joint destruction has occurred, arthrodesis may be necessary. Joint replacement might be attempted, but there is some risk of reactivating the dormant infection.

SPECIAL PROBLEMS

Brodie's Abscess

This is a subacute pyogenic osteomyelitis localized in the metaphysis and appearing on the roentgenogram as a lucent lesion with some surrounding sclerosis. The primary symptom is pain, with fever and leukocytosis being rare. The offending organism is usually *S. aureus* or *S. albus,* but occasionally gram-negative organisms have been identified. This disease is insidious in onset and lacks the systemic symptoms of hematogenous osteomyelitis.

Disc Space Infection

With the increase in drug abuse, disc space infection is not an uncommon cause of *back pain.* The chief complaint is usually localized to the area of the underlying infection, and there is a definite tenderness on palpation of the spine over the infected disc space. Early roentgenograms are usually not beneficial, although occasionally, there may be disc space narrowing. The bone scan is usually positive. There is usually mild leukocytosis and an elevated sedimentation rate. Management is through identification of the inciting bacterial agent and institution of appropriate antibiotic therapy.

Anaerobic Infections

Anaerobes are becoming increasingly recognized as causes of significant clinical infection. The more common organisms involved are *Bacteroides fragilis, Peptococcus, Propionibacterium, Clostridium,* and *Fusobacterium.* They are often mixed with aerobes, and it is often difficult to tell which is the pathogen. These mixed infections are also more difficult to cure.

Anaerobic bone infections are also frequently associated with the presence of a metallic foreign body such as a prosthesis. When they are present in infections in the foot, they are almost always associated with diabetes or vascular insufficiency. Chloramphenicol, clindamycin, moxalactam, and cefotaxime are often used for these infections.

Gas Gangrene

Clostridia organisms are widely distributed in nature, but only a few are severe pathogens. Several species can cause gas gangrene in humans. The most common is *C. perfringens (C. welchii).* Other causes are *C. novyi, C. histolyticum, C. septicum, C. bifermentans,* and *C. fallax.*

Gas gangrene is an uncommon clinical infection in which a severe soft-tissue wound or surgical trauma allows the tissue to become contaminated with the *Clostridium* spore. Local anaerobic conditions (a closed wound) favor conversion from the spore form to the vegetative form, which produces the potent toxins typical of this disorder. These toxins destroy soft tissue and muscle and can cause severe septic shock and death.

Clinical Features

This disease can result from a small innocuous wound but usually results from a severe wound improperly cared for. It may also follow abdominal surgery because clostridia normally inhabit the gastrointestinal tract.

The presentation may vary from a mild local cellulitis to the most lethal myonecrosis. Signs of infection are usually present within 24 hours after the trauma. Pain often precedes local or systemic signs and is frequently out of proportion to the severity of the injury. The wound is usually swollen and red and produces a dark odorous exudate.

The more severe forms are accompanied by chills, fever, tachycardia, delirium, and all of the other signs of a rapidly progressing infection. Renal shutdown and death may even occur. The involved skin and muscle undergo further necrosis, and vesicles appear in the infected area.

Gas may be present in the soft tissue but is not diagnostic of clostridia. It may also be due to mechanical reasons (such as open trauma or pulmonary injuries), or it may be a result of infection by other bacteria such as the coliforms or anaerobic streptococci. The roentgenogram will reveal edema and gas within muscle groups. (In bacterial infections not caused by clostridia, the gas is often in the deeper tissue.)

Treatment

Prevention is accomplished by a thorough debridement of all potentially contaminated cases and by leaving the wound open if necessary. Mild local infection may need only modest debridement and drainage. The more severe forms require early and radical excision of all involved tissue. Amputation may even be necessary.

Penicillin therapy is begun in large doses, and general supportive care is given.

Because moderate levels of oxygen have been shown to suppress bacterial activity, hyperbaric oxygen is often used as an adjunct to surgical debridement. The oxygen is supplied by placing the patient in a special chamber several times a day until the symptoms improve. At this time, these chambers are only available at a modest number of medical facilities.

Septic Bursitis

Infection of superficial bursae is a common occurrence. The bunion, olecranon, and prepatellar bursae are the most commonly affected. In contrast to septic arthritis, this disorder usually occurs in healthy individuals and commonly results from local spread. Occupations that predispose to fluid collection in the bursa (carpet layers, plumbers, etc.) are more prone to sepsis in this area. There may be evidence of a recent local abrasion or break in the skin. *S. aureus* is the most common offending organism.

Clinical Features

A painful localized bursal swelling is usually present. It is frequently accompanied by an intense cellulitis. A partially healed skin abrasion may be seen nearby. Systemic signs of sepsis are commonly present, including regional lymphadenopathy.

A sympathetic joint effusion is fairly common, especially in the knee. The joint itself is not usually tender, and motion is only mildly restricted. The effusion may suggest joint involvement.

Treatment

The bursa is aspirated and the fluid evaluated in the standard manner by Gram stain, culture and sensitivity. Blood cultures, blood counts, and sedimentation rates are also performed as indicated. (**Note:** It is important not to aspirate the joint itself. Passing the needle through the area of cellulitis may spread the infection into the joint.)

A broad-spectrum antibiotic, one that covers *S. aureus,* is begun. Surgical drainage of the bursa may be necessary, but many patients respond well to repeated aspirations.

Prosthetic Joint Infection

Fewer than 1% of joint replacements become infected, but the complication can be disastrous. It may occur at any time following surgery. Early involvement is usually the result of skin contamination, often by *S. epidermidis*. Later, the source is hematogenous, with a variety of pathogens being causative. Joints that have had previous surgery are also more predisposed to infection.

The diagnosis may be difficult. Pain is a common occurrence, but fever and systemic signs may be lacking. Local aspiration is usually necessary. Frequently, in order to cure the infection, all of the hardware must be removed permanently. Arthrodesis is often necessary, but in some cases, the joint is simply left out, and this results in a "resection" arthroplasty. Because of the risk of reactivating the dormant infection, only occasionally is the joint replaced again and, then, only after a long period of antibiotic therapy and local wound care.

Penetrating Wounds

Gunshot Wounds. The amount of damage done to tissues by gunshot wounds is dependent upon the velocity of the weapon. Low-velocity weapons usually cause minimal wound tract injury. Important structures are usually pushed away by the missile. These injuries are best treated on an outpatient basis by minimal local debridement of the entrance (and exit) wound, irrigation, a sterile dressing, and a broad-spectrum antibiotic. Tetanus prophylaxis is administered, and if necessary, delayed closure is performed later. Associated fractures are usually undisplaced and are treated by external immobilization.

Bullet removal or operative exploration is undertaken only if the bullet is superficial or symptomatic or if minor fragment migration could cause damage to major adjacent structures. Missile wounds of the knee joint should be explored surgically and debrided if fragments are present or if the joint was traversed. The missile and osteochondral fragments are removed. It is possible for lead to be dissolved by synovial tissue and lead to arthritis and, rarely, chronic lead intoxication. Elsewhere, the fragments are usually encapsulated by scar tissue; thereby eliminating their exposure to bodily fluids. Fragments near the spine are usually left alone unless a significant or progressive neural loss occurs.

Wounds caused by high-velocity weapons are managed the same way as those caused by low-velocity weapons except that more extensive debridement is usually necessary. Their complication rate is much higher, and delayed closure is the rule.

Shotgun wounds also require more extensive debridement. They are often the most serious of missile wounds. The projectile consists of multiple pellets and a wadding (usually fiber or burlap) that transmits the force. Wounds closer than 20 yd are assumed to contain some of this wadding, and exploration and removal are necessary. If the "scatter pattern" of the shotgun is wide, more damage is assumed, and especially if the shotgun was fired at close range, a small wound can disguise extensive deeper destruction.

Power Gun Nail Wounds. These injuries result from the use, mainly by carpenters, of air power gun systems to drive nails. Occasionally, they are accidentally driven into extremities, often directly into bone. They can usually be simply pulled out of the bone with the patient under local anesthesia. The wound is then treated similarly to any other low-velocity weapon injury. Small pieces that remain embedded in bone are probably best left alone.

Bite Wounds. Over 1% of all emergency room visits are the result of bites, and the majority of these wounds are superficial. Dog bites account for most of these wounds. They usually present as small puncture wounds. The infection rate is low, and closure of any extensive wound is usually acceptable after thorough cleansing, irrigation, and debridement. Small puncture wounds should not be opened. Prophylactic antibiotics, usually an oral cephalosporin, are justified. Rabies prophylaxis is provided when indicated.

Human bites require especially careful evaluation and examination. The most common site of injury is a closed fist that has struck the mouth. The common injury that occurs is a laceration over the metacarpophalangeal joint that may disrupt the extensor tendon and even penetrate into bone (Fig 13–4). The wound may be small, and if the hand is examined with the fingers extended, the true extent of the injury may be overlooked because the injury was sustained with the fingers flexed. If joint involvement is noted, extra care is taken to ensure good cleansing and debridement. The wound should be treated open. Antibiotics are administered, and the wound is followed closely. The most common infecting organisms are *S. aureus,* streptococci, and anaerobes found in the normal flora of the human mouth. (See Chapter 7.)

Puncture Wounds.   The most common site of this wound is the foot. The common clinical picture is that of early improvement followed in 1 to 2 weeks by worsening local signs. A foreign body is sometimes found in the wound, and the most common organism is *Pseudomonas.* Osteomyeli-

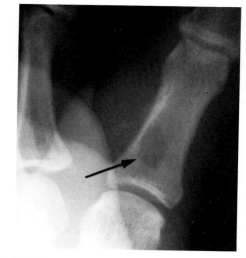

FIG 13–4.
Osteomyelitis of the proximal phalanx secondary to a human bite *(arrow).*

tis and even joint damage can result. Treatment involves drainage, removal of the foreign body (if present), and the appropriate antibiotic.

Local debridement in the emergency room at the time of the original injury may help prevent late infection. Roentgenograms are indicated to rule out foreign bodies. The decision to use antibiotics at the time of initial wound care remains controversial.

ANTIBIOTICS IN ORTHOPEDICS

The initial therapy in severe infections should always be broad enough to cover the most common organisms. More specific therapy will depend upon the proper identification of the offending agent and its sensitivity to the various antimicrobial drugs. With the ever-increasing number of antibiotics becoming available, the physician should become sufficiently familiar with several well-established ones. It is better to become familiar with several good ones than to try every new one that comes on the market. Cost and safety are also important factors to consider.

The duration of antibiotic therapy, especially for bone, joint, and bursa infections, varies depending upon response and the bacteria involved, but in general, antibiotic therapy is usually continued for 4 to 6 weeks. With the availability of home IV therapy, prolonged hospitalization is usually not required.

Penicillins

The penicillins are the most commonly used antibiotics. They are effective and low in toxicity and cost. They are usually classified as natural or semisynthetic (Table 13–2). Penicillins act by interfering with cell wall synthesis. As a group, they share the common structure of a β-lactam ring adjacent to a thiozolidine ring.

Resistance to the penicillins can develop when certain gram-positive and gram-negative organisms produce β-lactamases, which attack the β-lactam ring of the penicillin molecule. Allergic reactions are the most frequent serious problems associated with their use.

Natural Penicillins

Aqueous Crystalline Penicillin G. This is available as either the sodium or potassium salt. The potassium salt is generally preferred except in patients with renal disease who might not tolerate the added potassium. This form of penicillin is used when high serum concentration or rapid effect is needed. Frequent dosing is necessary to maintain serum levels.

Procaine, Benzathine Penicillin G. These drugs are often given intramuscularly. They are absorbed over a period of time and avoid the need for frequent dosing. Detectable levels of procaine penicillin may be present for 24 hours, and benzathine penicillin G may persist in the body for up to 30 days after injection.

Phenoxymethyl Penicillin. Penicillin V is a modification of penicillin G and resists gastric degradation. This allows for oral administration.

Semisynthetic Penicillins

Penicillinase-Resistant Penicillins. These agents resist degradation by pencillinases and are therefore the drugs of choice against *S. aureus.* Oxacillin and nafcillin are the most commonly used.

Aminopenicillins. Ampicillin and amoxicillin are the most frequently used. They have an extended activity against many gram-negative organisms including *Escherichia coli, Proteus, Salmonella, Shigella,* and *H. influenzae.* They are somewhat less active against pneumococci, streptococci, clostridia, and neisseria organisms.

TABLE 13–2.

Commonly Used Penicillins

Penicillins	Comments

Natural
  Penicillin G
    Aqueous
    Procaine
    Benzathine
  Phenoxymethyl (penicillin V)
	Penicillin G can only be given IV or IM because it undergoes degradation by gastric juices when given orally. It is used in the treatment of infections with *Streptococcus, Neisseria, Clostridium,* and *Treponema pallidum.* Very few strains of *S. aureus* are now susceptible to penicillin G

Semisynthetic
  Methicillin
  Oxacillin
  Nafcillin
  Cloxacillin
  Dicloxacillin
	Methicillin may cause interstitial nephritis and is less commonly used. Oxacillin, nafcillin, and methicillin are used parenterally. Oxacillin, cloxacillin, and dicloxacillin can be used orally. These drugs are used mainly for gram-positive penicillinase-producing bacteria. Oxacillin and nafcillin can be used both parenterally and orally

Aminopenicillins
  Ampicillin
  Amoxicillin
	Amoxicillin is only available orally. It is absorbed better than ampicillin and causes less diarrhea but is more expensive

Others
  Carboxypenicillins
  Acylureidopenicillins
	These drugs are generally expensive; they are useful against gram-negative bacilli and many anaerobes

TABLE 13–3.

Cephalosporins

Drugs	Comments

First generation
  Cephalothin
  Cefazolin
  Cephapirin
  Cephradine
	These drugs do well against penicillin-resistant *S. aureus* as well as *E. coli* and *Proteus*. They are excellent for prophylaxis. They may be used against staphylococci and streptococci in the patient who is allergic to penicillin. All of these drugs have about the same spectrum

Second generation
  Cefoxitin
  Cefamandole
  Cefuroxime
  Cefonicid
  Cefotetan
  Ceforanide
	About twice the cost of the first generation. Cefamandole may cause postoperative bleeding (perhaps due to interference with prothrombin synthesis). These drugs offer less staphylococci and streptococci coverage.

Third generation
  Cefotaxime
  Moxalactam
  Cefoperazone
  Ceftazidime
  Cefmenoxime
  Ceftizoxime
  Ceftriaxone
  Cefsulodin
	About four times the cost of the first generation. Lose most of gram-positive coverage, especially against staphylococci. Good in patient with poor renal function instead of aminoglycosides for gram-negative sepsis. May cause bleeding disorders. May be used as single treatment of mixed infections that could otherwise have required two to three antibiotics

Ampicillin is available in both oral and parenteral form.

Carboxypenicillins and Acylureidopenicillins. The major advantage of these drugs is better coverage against *Pseudomonas aeruginosa* and certain *Proteus* and *Enterobacter* species. Otherwise, their range of activity is similar to ampicillin. Carbenicillin, ticarcillin, and indanyl carbenicillin are members of the carboxypenicillins. The acylureidopenicillins are azlopenicillin, mexlocillin, and piperacillin.

Others. Additional advances have led to the combining of a β-lactamase inhibitor (sulbactam or clavulanic acid) with either amoxicillin, ticarcillin, or ampicillin, which form the drugs known by their trade names as Augmentin, Timentin, and Unasyn. This has broadened their antibacterial range.

Cephalosporins

No antibiotic has experienced as much proliferation as have the cephalosporins (Table 13–3). They are usually classified by "generation," which refers to their range of gram-negative activity. Their structure and mechanism of activity are

TABLE 13–4.

Aminoglycosides

Drugs	Comments
Gentamicin Tobramycin Amikacin Streptomycin Kanamycin Netilmicin	Amikacin has broadest spectrum. Gentamicin is cheapest and is usually first choice. These drugs are often used in combination with other drugs. Some resistance to their use may be developing. They are helpful in severe polymicrobial infections. May be necessary to monitor toxicity with audiometer examinations

similar to penicillin, that is, they are also β-lactams that inhibit cell wall synthesis. Cephalosporins are derived from the fungus *Cephalosporium acremonium.* These agents are bactericidal against most clinically significant gram-positive cocci and gram-negative bacilli. They function well alone and are excellent for prophylaxis. The gram-negative activity is greater the higher the generation, but the activity against *S. aureus* and streptococci is less. They are all generally nontoxic. They are contraindicated in patients who have had severe anaphylactoid reactions to penicillin but appear safe when the penicillin reaction (such as skin rash) has been mild and delayed. First-generation drugs should be used whenever possible. Second- and third-generation agents are used if the organism is resistant to first-generation drugs. The second- and third-generation agents are sometimes preferable to the more toxic antibiotics such as the aminoglycosides.

Many oral forms of cephalosporins are avail-

TABLE 13–5.

Antibiotics in Common Adult Infections

Organism	Drugs of Choice	Notes
S. aureus	Oxacillin or nafcillin (2 g IV q4–6h) First-generation cephalosporin Vancomycin (1 g IV q12h)	Nafcillin should not be used in patients with liver disease Vancomycin use should be monitored with peak serum level determinations
S. epidermidis	Variable Methicillin (100–300 mg/kg/day in 4 divided doses up to 12 g) Vancomycin Cephalosporin, first generation	Modern methicillins may be less likely to cause interstitial nephritis
Streptococcus—most varieties	Penicillin G (up to 25 million units/day IV) Cephalosporin Erythromycin (1 g IV q6h)	Erythromycin may cause phlebitis
Pseudomonas aeruginosa	An aminoglycoside (gentamycin, tobramycin, 3–5 mg/kg/day, or amikacin, 15 mg/kg/day in divided doses every 8 hr) *plus* a β-lactam (carbenicillin, ticarcillin)	Monitor serum levels of aminoglycoside and renal function. A third-generation cephalosporin may also be used with the aminoglycoside
Enterococcus	Penicillin G (or ampicillin) with gentamicin	Vancomycin may be substituted for penicillin G
N gonorrhoeae	Penicillin G Ampicillin (500 mg IV q6h) Ceftriaxone	
H. influenza	Cefotaxime Ampicillin Chloramphenicol (500 mg–1 g IV q6h)	Chloramphenicol may cause bone marrow suppression
E. coli	Initial aminoglycoside, then cephalosporin or ampicillin	
K. pneumoniae	Cephalosporin	
P. mirabilis	Ampicillin Cephalosporin	
B. fragilis	Cefoxitin, cefotetan Ampicillin/sulbactam Clindamycin (300–600 mg q6–8 h) Metronidazole	Clindamycin may cause pseudomembranous colitis

able, but they are generally expensive, and other agents are usually equally effective.

Aminoglycosides

These antibiotics are primarily useful in the treatment of serious infections due to gram-negative bacilli (Table 13–4). Their common mechanisms of action is to inhibit protein synthesis. All of these drugs are rapidly excreted by the kidneys. Their most common side effects are nephrotoxicity and ototoxicity. They also have a narrow margin between toxicity and efficacy.

Accordingly, it is usually required that renal function be determined before their use and monitored following initiation of therapy. In addition, aminoglycoside blood levels are obtained frequently and the drug dosage adjusted accordingly.

Other Antibiotics

Vancomycin.   This is a narrow-spectrum bacteriocidal antibiotic used primarily against *S. aureus, S. epidermidis,* and some streptococci. It can only be given by the IV route. It is the drug of choice in resistant *S. aureus* infections. Its main toxicity is neural, usually ototoxicity. Phlebitis at the site of infusion is common.

Carbapenem.   This antibiotic is derived from the fungus *Streptomyces cattleya.* It is also a β-lactam. The only agent currently available from this class is a thienamycin called imipenem. This drug has the broadest spectrum of any antibiotic, but because of renal toxicity and poor urinary concentration, it has been combined with cilastatin, a renal enzyme inhibitor. The combination drug, called Primaxin, provides excellent monotherapy.

Monobactams.   These agents are produced by a chromobacterium. They have a monocyclic β-lactam nucleus. They may challenge the aminoglycosides in the treatment of severe gram-negative infections, especially *Pseudomonas.* Only aztreonam (Azactam) is currently available from this group.

Erythromycin.   This antibiotic is commonly used in patients allergic to penicillins. It acts by inhibiting protein synthesis. It can be given either parenterally or orally, although food in the stomach often reduces its absorption.

Lincosamines.   These drugs (clindamycin, lincomycin) also act by inhibiting bacterial protein synthesis. They are expensive and are primarily used as second-line drugs in the patient who is allergic to penicillin. They are usually employed in the treatment of anaerobic infections, especially infections with *Bacteroides* (Table 13–5).

BIBLIOGRAPHY

Altemeier WA, Fullen WD: Prevention and treatment of gas gangrene. *JAMA* 1971; 217:806.

Ashby M: Low velocity gunshot wounds involving the knee joint: Surgical management. *J Bone Joint Surg [Am]* 1974; 56:1047.

Boll KL, Jurik AG: Sternal osteomyelitis in drug addicts. *J Bone Joint Surg [Br]* 1990; 72:328.

Brettler D, et al: Conservative management of low velocity gunshot wounds. *Clin Orthop* 1979; 140:26.

Brown P: Gas gangrene in a metropolitan community. *J Bone Joint Surg [Am]* 1982; 56:1445.

Chuinard RG, D'Ambrosia RD: Human bite infections of the hand. *J Bone Joint Surg [Am]* 1977; 59: 416.

Eismont FJ, et al: Pyogenic and fungal vertebral osteomyelitis with paralysis. *J Bone Joint Surg [Am]* 1983; 65:19.

Eismont FJ, et al: Vertebral osteomyelitis in infants. *J Bone Joint Surg [Br]* 1982; 64:32.

Emmons CW, Binford CH, Utz JP: *Medical Mycology,* ed 2. Philadelphia, Lea & Febiger, 1970.

Freig BS, et al: Imipenem and cilastatin in acute osteomyelitis and suppurative arthritis. Therapy in infants and children. *Am J Dis Child* 1987; 141:335.

Gentry LO: Overview of osteomyelitis. *Orthop Rev* 1987; 16:255.

Green M, Myhan WL Jr, Fausek MD: Acute hematogenous osteomyelitis. *Pediatrics* 1956; 16:368.

Hart GB, et al: The treatment of clostridial myonecroses with hyperbaric oxygen. *J Trauma* 1974; 14:712.

Hoeprich PD: *Infectious Diseases.* Hagerstown, Md, Harper & Row, 1972.

Holzman RS, Birkko F: Osteomyelitis in heroin addicts. *Ann Intern Med* 1971; 75:693.

Hughes SPF, Fitzgerald RH Jr: *Musculoskeletal Infections.* Chicago, Year Book Medical Publishers Inc, 1986.

LaMont RL, et al: Acute hematogenous osteomyelitis in children. *J Pediatr Orthop* 1987; 7:579.

Lifeso RM, et al: Post-traumatic squamous cell carcinoma. *J Bone Joint Surg [Am]* 1990; 72:12.

May JW, et al: Current concepts review. Clinical classification of post-traumatic osteomyelitis. *J Bone Joint Surg [Am]* 1989; 71:1422.

Rutstein DD, et al: Jones criteria (modified) for guidance in diagnosis of rheumatic fever. *Mod Concepts Cardiovasc Dis* 1955, 24:291.

Schmid FR: Principles of diagnosis and treatment of infectious arthritis, in Hollander JL, McCarty DJ Jr (eds): *Arthritis and Allied Conditions,* ed 8. Philadelphia, Lea & Febiger, 1972.

Smith DL, et al: Septic and nonseptic olecranon bursitis. *Arch Intern Med* 1989; 149:1581.

Thompson RL, Wright AJ: Cephalosporin antibiotics. *Mayo Clin Proc* 1983; 58:79.

Uuzonian TJ, et al: Evaluation of musculoskeletal sepsis with indium-111 white blood cell imaging. *Clin Orthop* 1987; 221:304.

Vu Quoc D, Nelson JD, Holtalin KC: Osteomyelitis in infants and children. *Am J Dis Child* 1975; 129:1273.

Warsman AD, Bryon D, Siemsen JK: Bone scanning in the drug abuse patient: Early detection of hematogenous osteomyelitis. *J Nucl Med* 1973; 14:647.

Wilkowske CJ, Hermans PE: General principles of antimicrobial therapy. *Mayo Clin Proc* 1987; 62:789.

Wright AJ, Wilkowske CJ: The penicillins. *Mayo Clin Proc* 1987; 62:806.

Yuh WTC, et al: Osteomyelitis of the foot in diabetic patients: Evaluation with plain films, 99 Tc-MDP bone scintigraphy and MR imaging. *AJR* 1989; 152:795.

CHAPTER 14

The Arthritides

Disorders of the joints are common and may cause considerable pain and disability. They are frequently classified as either noninflam-matory, inflammatory, or infectious. This chapter will review the more common joint affections.

THE SYNOVIUM

A synovial lining encloses the joint space of all diarthrodial joints. This membrane is also present in bursae and tendon sheaths. It is normally one to three cells thick and is constructed of multiple villi. It will reflect not only local disturbances but also systemic disease and is responsible for the production of joint fluid.

Synovial fluid is a clear, slightly yellow liquid that is present only in small amounts in the normal joint. Its main functions are those of lubrication and nutrition. Its characteristic viscosity is due to the presence of high concentrations of hyaluronic acid, which is produced by the synovial lining cells. This mucopolysaccharide also contributes a portion of the matrix of the synovial lining and is partially responsible for the filtering properties of the synovium.

Joint fluid is a dialysate of blood plasma, that is, crystalloids are present, but colloids are not. Normal joint fluid does not clot because many of the coagulation factors are absent. Glucose is present in concentrations 10 mg/dL lower than serum. This difference increases to 30 mg/dL in rheumatoid and other inflammatory types of arthritis and may approach 70 mg/dL in infectious arthritis. Normal fluid also contains complement, lipids, and proteins in amounts much lower than the serum level. The white blood cell (WBC) count is usually under 200/mm^3, with the majority being mononuclear. Inflammation increases the cell count and the percentage of polymorphonuclear leukocytes.

A great deal of information can be obtained from the examination of a joint aspirate (Table 14–1). This examination is not indicated in every joint effusion, however, and should be limited to those diagnostic problems that are not secondary to trauma. The joint is usually aspirated from the extensor side under sterile conditions. Three test tubes are sufficient for most determinations: (1) a plain tube for gross examination, clotting, and a mucin clot test; (2) one ethylenediamine tetraacetic acid (EDTA)-treated tube for cell and crystal analysis; and (3) one heparinized tube for bacteriologic study. Five milliliters of fluid is placed in each tube.

A quick bedside assessment of the fluid can be made prior to the more extensive laboratory analysis. The color and clarity of the sample are estimated by merely observing the fluid in the sy-

TABLE 14–1.
Synovial Fluid Analysis

Disease	Appearance	Viscosity	Mucin Clot	WBC (%), Polymorphonuclear Leukocytes	Other Findings
			Noninflammatory		
Normal	Clear, yellow	High	Good	Under 200, under 10%	
Traumatic arthritis	Cloudy, straw to red	High	Good	Under 2,000, under 25%	Cartilage debris
Osteoarthritis	Straw, yellow, clear	High	Good	Under 5,000, under 25%	Cartilage debris
			Inflammatory		
Rheumatoid	Cloudy, green/gray	Low	Fair/poor	15,000, 50%–80%	Glucose difference 10–25 mg/dL, rheumatoid arthritis cells
Gout	Coudy, white, flaky	Decreased	Fair/poor	10,000, 25%–75%	Sodium urate crystals
Pseudogout	Cloudy	Decreased	Fair/poor	5–15,000, 25%–75%	Calcium pyrophosphate crystals
Systemic lupus erythematosus	Cloudy, yellow	High	Good/fair	5–10,000, under 25%	Lupus erythematosus cells
			Infectious		
Bacterial	Cloudy, purulent	Low	Poor	50–200,000, over 90%	Glucose difference over 50 mg/dL, culture +

ringe. The viscosity can be roughly determined by the thread test. A drop of the fluid is placed between the apposed thumb and index finger. The fingers are gradually spread apart, and the length of the thread the fluid forms before it breaks is measured. Normal and osteoarthritic fluid may "string" out 2.5 to 5 cm before breaking, but the dilute fluid of inflammation will string very little.

The Mucin Clot Test

This determines the amount of hyaluronate in the fluid. Acetic acid is added to the tube, and the sample is observed for clot formation. A "poor" mucin clot indicates a decrease in hyaluronate. This results from dilution, depolymerization, and loss of filter function from either inflammation or infection. A "good" clot is present in normal fluid and osteoarthritis.

Crystal Analysis

Reliable crystal examination requires the use of polarized light. The sodium urate crystals present in gout are needle shaped and negatively birefringent. The calcium pyrophosphate crystal in pseudogout (chondrocalcinosis) is rhomboid shaped and positively birefringent.

OSTEOARTHRITIS

The most common type of noninflammatory arthritis is degenerative, or osteoarthritis. This condition is characterized by articular cartilage deterioration and bony overgrowth of the joint surface. The cause is unknown, but trauma, heredity, and the normal aging process are all factors. Pathologically, the cartilage loses its normal glistening appearance and becomes roughened and irregular. Eventually, the cartilage becomes completely worn away, thus exposing the subchondral bone. Secondary synovitis and osteophytic spur formation are common. The clinical course is slowly progressive.

Clinical Features

Pain is the most common initial symptom. This frequently occurs with motion or activity and is relieved by rest. Joint stiffness typically occurs with rest and improves with activity.

The physical findings include crepitus, swelling, restriction of motion, and joint enlargement from spur formation. In the hands, these osteophytic overgrowths are termed Heberden's nodes when they are present at the distal interphalangeal joint and Bouchard's nodes when they occur at the proximal interphalangeal joint. Pain is usually present on joint motion. Disuse atrophy of the adjacent musculature may develop rapidly, thus increasing the disability and pain.

The roentgenographic findings consist of joint space narrowing, spur formation, sclerosis, and subchondral cyst formation (Fig 14–1). The laboratory findings and synovial analysis are normal except for occasional flakes of cartilage in the joint fluid.

Treatment

The main objectives of treatment are the relief of pain and prevention of progression. As with any joint disorder, the patient should not be told that arthritis is present unless the physical and laboratory findings are consistent with the diagnosis. The stigma of "arthritis" should not be attached to any condition merely to explain vague or nonspecific symptoms. Once the diagnosis is established, however, the patient should be made to realize that while miracles cannot be expected, there is almost always something that can be done to relieve the pain and deformity, regardless of the cause.

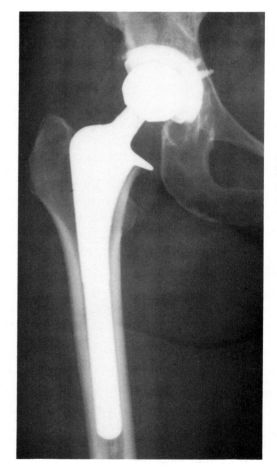

FIG 14–2.
Total hip arthroplasty (uncemented).

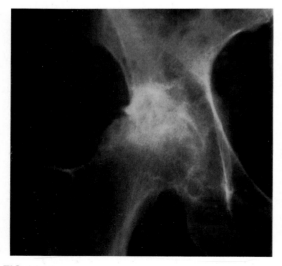

FIG 14–1.
Degenerative arthritis of the hip. Joint space narrowing, sclerosis, and subchondral cyst formation are present.

For osteoarthritis, treatment begins with rest of the involved joint. This will help reduce inflammation and pain. Weight loss and temporary abstinence from weight bearing by the use of a cane or crutch will lessen the pressure on the involved lower extremity. Removable splints or braces are also helpful.

The joint should be passed through a full range of motion several times daily to reduce joint stiffness. The local application of moist heat is beneficial during the acute painful stage and may be especially helpful prior to exercise. Exercises designed to combat stiffness and restore muscle strength are important because the weakness will contribute to joint instability and disability. Anti-inflammatory agents, especially aspirin, in combination with heat and rest are also effective. Intra-articular cortisone injections will frequently relieve a great deal of the pain, but their effect is usually only temporary.

The surgical procedures most commonly employed are arthrodesis and arthroplasty (Fig 14–2). Each is effective in eliminating the painful articulation. Realignment of faulty weight-bearing joints by osteotomy may also be beneficial.

GOUT

Gouty arthritis is an inherited metabolic disease characterized by a disturbance of purine metabolism in which crystals of sodium urate are deposited in various soft tissues. These crystals and the resultant symptoms are due to an increase in the serum uric acid, a normal end product of purine metabolism.

The majority of patients are men in the third and fourth decades. The disorder is uncommon in women and rare before menopause. Secondary gout may follow hyperuricemia from many causes, including leukemia, hemolytic anemia, and other blood dyscrasias.

Clinical Features

The initial attack usually occurs in a single joint in the lower extremity. The metatarsophalangeal joint of the great toe is classically the first site of involvement, although any joint or tendon can be involved. The pain and inflammation are usually severe and may be precipitated by exercise, dietary indiscretion, and physical or emotional stress. The typical attack begins at night.

Swelling, heat, redness, and other signs of inflammation are usually present. The physical findings may even simulate cellulitis. The area is often tender to even the slightest touch. Fever, tachycardia, and other constitutional symptoms may accompany the attack. The initial episode may be followed by polyarticular involvement.

Eventually, deposits of urate crystals, termed *tophi,* may form in the subcutaneous tissue.

Early in the disease, roentgenogram findings are normal. Later, erosive changes appear that have a characteristic punched-out appearance (Fig 14–3). Destruction and degeneration of the articular cartilage frequently follows.

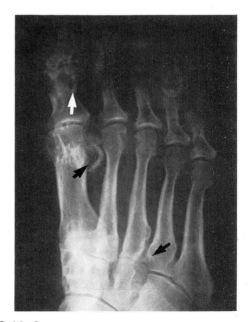

FIG 14–3.
Gouty arthritis. Multiple punched-out lesions are present *(arrows).*

Laboratory findings include a mild leukocytosis, elevated sedimentation rate, and hyperuricemia. The synovial aspirate is usually cloudy and mildly inflammatory in nature. Urate crystals are usually demonstrable.

Treatment

The treatment will depend on the stage of the disease. The objectives in management are to terminate or prevent the acute attack, encourage mobilization of tophaceous deposits, and reduce the level of serum uric acid.

Patients with asymptomatic hyperuricemia (over 9 mg/dL) should probably be treated to prevent the acute attack and complications of elevated uric acid levels. For the initial acute episode, colchicine is the drug of choice. Two 0.5-mg tablets are given initially, followed by 1 tablet every hour up to 12 tablets until the symptoms subside or diarrhea ensues. This is accompanied by rest, elevation, and moist heat. Disappearance of symptoms with the colchicine therapy also helps to confirm the diagnosis. Future acute attacks are treated with phenylbutazone.

Between attacks, prophylaxis is maintained by one of two agents, probenecid or allopurinol. Probenecid is a uricosuric agent, that is, it increases the renal excretion of uric acid. It should not be used in the presence of renal disease. Probenecid is also effective in reducing the size of the tophaceous deposits. Allopurinol is a xanthine oxidase inhibitor that prevents the formation of uric acid from xanthine and hypoxanthine. It is especially valuable in the patient who forms urate stones because it directly decreases the production of uric acid.

Surgery is usually limited to excision of large tophi and, occasionally, arthroplasty.

PSEUDOGOUT (CHONDROCALCINOSIS)

Pseudogout is a condition that resembles gout in its clinical manifestations except that large rather than small joints are more commonly involved. It is characterized by the deposition of crystals of calcium pyrophosphate in the joint cartilage and capsule.

Clinical Features

The symptoms are similar to those of chronic gouty arthritis. Intermittent acute episodes occur, but the joint most commonly involved is the knee rather than the great toe. The condition is frequently familial and is occasionally associated with diabetes, renal disease, and other systemic conditions.

In addition to the gout-like symptoms, calcification of the cartilage of the knee, especially the meniscus, is common (Fig 14–4). Calcification of the anulus fibrosus, radioulnar disc, and symphysis pubis may also be seen. Synovial fluid analysis reveals typical rhomboid-shaped crystals that exhibit positive birefringence under polarized light. There are no specific changes in blood or urine.

Treatment

Aspiration and cortisone injections are often effective in the acute phase. A short course of phenylbutazone or indomethacin may also be beneficial.

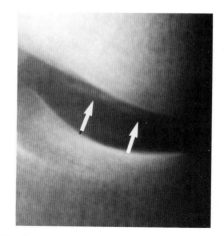

FIG 14–4.
Calcification of the meniscus *(arrows)*.

RHEUMATOID ARTHRITIS

Rheumatoid arthritis is a systemic disorder of unknown cause characterized by joint inflammation. In contrast to many of the other arthritides, it is a potentially crippling disease. The condition is most common in women between the ages of 25 and 45 years.

Pathologically, the synovium becomes thickened, inflamed, and hypertrophic. Infiltrating granulation tissue from the synovium (pannus) typically spreads over the joint cartilage. Eventually, erosion and destruction of the articular surface result from the chronic inflammatory process.

Clinical Features

The onset is usually gradual. Weakness, fatigue, and anorexia are common prodromal symptoms. Eventually joint involvement becomes apparent, with stiffness, swelling, heat, and redness. Most cases initially present with multiple symmetric joint involvement, most often in the hands and feet (Table 14–2). Remissions and exacerbations are common, but the condition is chronically progressive in the majority of cases.

The physical signs are due to the inflammation of the synovial membrane. Joint effusions, tenderness, and restriction of motion are usually present early in the disease. Eventually, characteristic deformities appear that consist of subluxations, dislocations, and joint contractures.

In addition to the joint manifestations, extra-articular findings are common. Tendon sheaths and bursae are frequently affected by the chronic inflammation. Tendon rupture may even occur. Rheumatoid nodules are present in 25% of cases and are most common over bony prominences such as the elbow and shaft of the ulna. Splenomegaly, pericarditis, and vasculitis may also occur.

The roentgenogram usually reveals soft-tissue swelling and osteoporosis early in the disease. Eventually, joint space narrowing, erosion, and deformity become visible as the result of continued inflammation and cartilage destruction (Fig 14–5).

The laboratory findings consist of a mild anemia, leukocytosis, and elevated sedimentation rate. The rheumatoid factor is positive in approximately 75% of cases. The joint fluid is usually turbid and forms a poor mucin clot. The cell count is elevated, with an increase in polymorphonuclear leukocytes.

Treatment

Proper management requires close cooperation among primary physician, therapist, and orthopedist. Rest is beneficial in reducing inflammation. When combined with an exercise program, moist heat, and splinting, joint deformities can frequently be prevented or corrected.

Aspirin remains the drug of choice for most

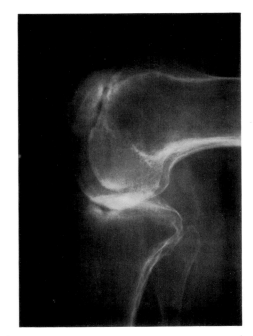

FIG 14–5.
Rheumatoid arthritis of the knee. Osteoporosis and severe joint space narrowing are present. Hypertrophic spurring is typically absent.

TABLE 14–2.

Joint Swelling—Differential Diagnosis*

Disorder	Symptoms/History	Findings
Pyogenic arthritis	Usually painful but sometimes low grade. Fever, acute onset. Usually monoarticular	Febrile, increase heat, painful movement. Systemic signs of illness. Joint fluid positive for bacteria
Gouty arthritis	Knee, great toe, or generalized foot pain. Symptoms may be initiated by physical stress such as surgery. May be extremely painful but usually low grade. Usually monoarticular. Previous episodes?	Redness, increased heat. Crystals in joint fluid. Elevated serum uric acid. Fluid often cloudy
Osteoarthritis	Chronic, gradual. Monoarticular. May have history of mechanical injury. Stiffness after rest, pain after prolonged activity	Restricted movement but pain usually only at the extremes of movement. Fluid is clear, only excessive amounts
Pseudogout	Middle age to elderly. Usually monoarticular. Previous episodes?	Crystals in cloudy fluid (calcium pyrophosphate)
Rheumatoid arthritis	Multiple joints may be involved. Females most commonly affected. Usually subacute or insidous in onset but occasionally acute. Often symmetric. Metacarpophalangeal, proximal interphalangeal joints usually involved	Subcutaneous nodules in late cases. Laboratory studies may show positive rheumatoid test and increased ESR
Others	History may reflect skin rash or other skin changes. Note other system involvement (complete history, especially GI, and pulmonary system)	FANA, ESR may be abnormal. Many collagen disorders have polyarticular symptoms and act like rheumatoid arthritis

*Notes: The workup should include (1) aspiration of joint fluid. Fluid is observed for color, and the string test is performed. The fluid is analyzed for cell count, Gram stain, crystal analysis, and culture and sensitivity. (2) The blood work should include complete blood cell count, uric acid, blood cultures if indicated, sedimentation rate, fluorescent antinuclear antibody (FANA), and rheumatoid factor. Blood cultures should include aerobic and anaerobic cultures. (3) Roentgenographic evaluation is always performed to evaluate for osteoarthritis and calcific changes in soft tissues.

patients. The usual dose is 2 to 3 tablets every 3 to 4 hours. Although it is not curative, it will suppress the symptoms and many of the objective signs of articular inflammation. When salicylates fail to alleviate the symptoms, several other drugs, including gold, steroids, antimalarial and other anti-inflammatory agents, have been used with varying success.

Among the surgical procedures that are helpful are synovectomy, soft-tissue releases, arthroplasty, and arthrodesis. The soft-tissue procedures are most beneficial early in the disease before significant fixed deformity or subluxation appears. The results of synovectomy in particular are better when it is performed before irreversible articular damage occurs.

Juvenile Rheumatoid Arthritis (Still's Disease)

The rheumatoid arthritis that occurs in youth differs in many respects from what occurs in the adult. The main differences are the systemic toxicity that occurs in children and the tendency for fewer joints to be involved. The juvenile variety is frequently difficult to differentiate from other childhood diseases, especially rheumatic fever.

Clinical Features

Juvenile rheumatoid arthritis is usually one of three types: (1) systemic (20%), (2) pauciarticular (30%), or (3) polyarticular (50%). *Systemic* or acute febrile juvenile rheumatoid arthritis is characterized by extra-articular manifestations, especially spiking fevers and a typical rash. The rash frequently appears in the evening and may be elicited by gently scratching the skin in susceptible areas (Koebner's phenomenon). Splenomegaly, generalized lymphadenopathy, pericarditis, and myocarditis may also occur. The articular findings are often minimal and are usually overshadowed by the systemic symptoms. The morbidity from this form is usually from chronic arthritis, however.

The *pauciarticular* or *oligoarticular* form usually involves the larger joints, such as the knees, elbows, and ankles. Systemic features are often minimal, and only one to three joints are usually involved. The joint disease rarely causes impairment, but iridocyclitis develops in approximately 30% of cases with this form, and permanent loss of vision will develop in a high percentage of these patients. Frequent ocular examinations, early detection, and treatment are therefore indicated. In this form of juvenile rheumatoid arthritis, accelerated growth of the affected limb from chronic hyperemia may result in a temporary leg length discrepancy that is eventually equalized in most cases on control of the inflammation.

Polyarticular juvenile rheumatoid arthritis resembles the adult rheumatoid disease in its symmetric involvement of the small joints of the hands and feet. Cervical spine involvement is not uncommon and may produce marked restriction of motion. Early closure of the ossification centers of the mandible may produce a markedly receding chin, a characteristic of this form. Systemic manifestations are similar to the febrile variety but are not as dramatic.

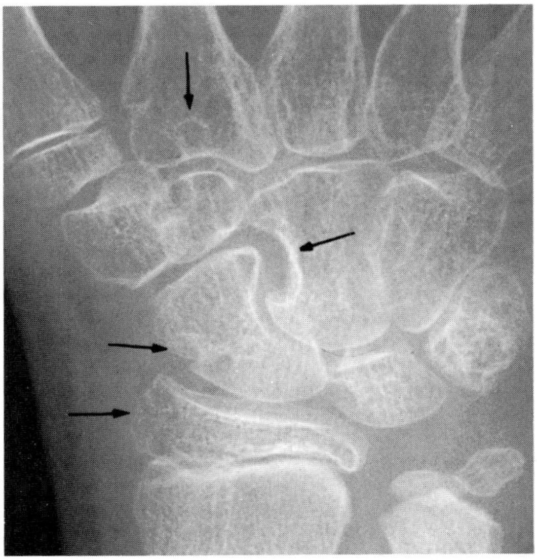

FIG 14-6.
Juvenile rheumatoid arthritis. Osteoporosis is present, but joint destruction is minimal. Multiple erosions and cysts *(arrows)* are present due to synovial hypertrophy.

The roentgenographic findings in juvenile rheumatoid arthritis are the same as those in the adult, except that joint destruction is less frequent (Fig 14-6). The laboratory findings are also similar, except that the peripheral WBC count may be very high and the rheumatoid factor is rarely demonstrable in the serum of children.

Treatment

The treatment is similar to that given the adult except that phenylbutazone and indomethacin should not be used.

NEUROARTHROPATHY

The neuropathic or Charcot's joint is one that results from a disturbance in the sensation to the joint. It is usually associated with central or peripheral nerve lesions. The most common causes are tabes dorsalis, diabetic neuropathy, and syringomyelia. The loss of sensation leads to extreme destruction, new bone formation, and instability of the joint.

Clinical Features

The foot is usually involved in diabetes, the shoulder and elbow joint in syringomyelia, and the vertebrae and lower extremities in tabes dorsalis. Gradual enlargement and instability of the affected joint are common complaints. Pain is usually present but tends to be relatively mild when compared with the severity of the joint destruction.

The examination is characterized by swelling and hypermobility. Palpation frequently reveals overgrowth of bone, crepitus, and loose bodies.

Variable degrees of joint destruction and disintegration with exuberant osteophyte formation are usually present on roentgenographic examination. Later, subluxation and deformity may be seen (Fig 14–7).

Treatment

Ordinarily, conservative and surgical treatment, including arthrodesis, is usually unsuccessful. Immobilization and protection of the affected joint with braces is sometimes effective.

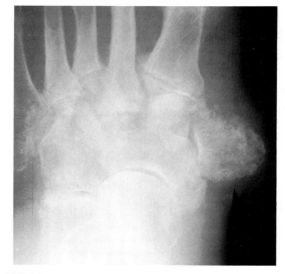

FIG 14–7.
Diabetic neuroarthropathy of the midfoot. Destruction, debris, dislocation, and density (4 D's) are usually present in neuropathic joints. The medial cuneiform is dislocated.

SYSTEMIC LUPUS ERYTHEMATOSUS

Systemic lupus erythematosus is an inflammatory disease that affects the vascular and connective tissue of many organ systems but commonly appears with joint pain and swelling similar to that seen in rheumatoid arthritis. It should always be considered in the differential diagnosis of systemic arthritis. It is most common in women in the third and fourth decades and affects the joints in 90% of patients. The joint involvement is usually accompanied by the other characteristic features of the disease, namely, a butterfly rash on the face and hematopoietic, renal, and cardiac involvement. Lupus erythematosus cells and antinuclear antibodies are usually present in the serum.

OCHRONOSIS

Alkaptonuria is an uncommon inherited disorder that results from a failure to properly synthesize homogentisic acid oxidase. Homogentisic acid is thus excreted in the urine, which causes it to turn black on oxidation. Ochronosis is the result of alkaptonuria and is characterized by the deposition in the soft tissue and cartilage of a pigment derived from homogentisic acid.

The arthropathy of ochronosis primarily involves the spine, hips, knees, and shoulders. Typical calcifications appear in the intervertebral discs and menisci. Eventually, the peripheral joint changes become indistinguishable from osteoarthritis while the spine involvement resembles ankylosing spondylitis.

No specific treatment is available. The peripheral arthritis is treated as osteoarthritis.

REITER'S SYNDROME

Reiter's syndrome is characterized by (1) urethritis, (2) conjunctivitis, and (3) arthritis. The cause is unknown, but the disorder is probably transmitted by sexual contact.

The arthritis is usually polyarticular. Large joints are most commonly affected, with joint involvement occurring 2 to 3 weeks after the urethritis. The patient may be febrile, and the joint is often warm and tender.

The disorder is self-limited. Symptoms usually resolve in 6 to 8 weeks, and complete recovery is the rule. No treatment is available, but because of the similarity of the disorder to gonococcal arthritis, penicillin should probably be administered until the diagnosis is clarified.

PSORIATIC ARTHRITIS

Psoriasis may occasionally be accompanied by a form of arthritis that is clinically similar to adult rheumatoid arthritis. The skin disorder usually precedes the arthritis by several years.

The arthritis is usually progressive and initially involves the distal interphalangeal joints of the fingers and toes. Its activity tends to parallel the activity of the skin disease. Severe bone destruction and ankylosis are not uncommon, especially in the hands.

PALINDROMIC RHEUMATISM

Palindromic rheumatism is an uncommon benign condition characterized by episodic attacks of arthritis. The small joints of the hands are typically involved. The attacks may last only a few hours or days and are usually followed by complete remission. The condition is believed by many to represent an atypical form of rheumatoid arthritis.

SJÖGREN'S SYNDROME

Sjögren's syndrome is a fairly common disorder characterized by (1) dry eyes (keratoconjunctivitis sicca), (2) dry mouth (xerostomia), and (3) chronic arthritis. The chronic arthritis is usually polyarticular in nature and occurs in two thirds of cases. The patients typically are middle-aged women.

The joint involvement resembles rheumatoid arthritis in its pathologic, clinical, and roentgenographic appearance. It commonly precedes and may be accompanied by rheumatoid nodules. The rheumatoid factor is positive in almost 100% of patients. Treatment of the arthritis is the same as for rheumatoid arthritis.

POLYMYALGIA RHEUMATICA

This is a disorder of unknown cause affecting older adults. It is characterized by chronic inflammation that causes stiffness and aching of the shoulder and hip regions. Constitutional symptoms such as malaise, anorexia, and headache may also be present. It may be accompanied by temporal arteritis. An elevated erythrocyte sedi- mentation rate is the only laboratory abnormality.

The diagnosis is difficult to make because there are no diagnostic criteria for this disorder. Low doses of prednisone have traditionally been used in its treatment, and the response is usually rapid.

MYOFASCIAL PAIN SYNDROME

This is a term given to a controversial clinical syndrome characterized by multiple trigger points and referred pain. Similar disorders have been called fibrositis, fibromyalgia, and psychogenic rheumatism.

Many physicians doubt the existence of such syndromes. No inflammatory changes have ever been demonstrated. The diagnosis is often used in patients with vague aching near joints for which no other obvious cause can be found. Chronic increased muscle tension may play a role.

Clinical Features

The patient is frequently anxious and depressed. There may have been some recent trauma, especially to the neck or lower portion of the back. The patient may occasionally present with a list of other vague symptoms such as headache, stiffness, sleep disorders, and fatigue. Tender "nodules" and trigger points may be present, and when palpated, regional referral of the pain may occur. There are never any objective findings. The usual roentgenographic and laboratory assessments are always normal.

Treatment

Before making this diagnosis, rule out other, more likely causes for the pain. Then, the treatment is mainly empiric and symptomatic. Physical therapy, nonsteroidal anti-inflammatory drugs (NSAIDs), acupuncture, transcutaneous nerve stimulation, sympathetic blockade, muscle relaxants, trigger point injections, and anti-depressants are among the many treatments used, all with varying success.

HYPERTROPHIC OSTEOARTHROPATHY

This syndrome is characterized by (1) clubbing of the fingers and toes, (2) periosteal new bone formation, and (3) osteoarthritis. The periosteal reaction is usually associated with pulmonary neoplasm or long-standing suppurative disease of the lung.

Clinical Features

The findings are usually bilateral and symmetric. A typical clubbing of the fingers and toes usually develops first, although early pain over the shafts of the bones of the extremities is common. Joint stiffness, swelling, and pain are usually later in onset and may simulate rheumatoid arthritis.

Roentgenographic Findings

Periosteal new bone formation is usually present. The long bones of the extremities are most often involved.

Treatment

Treatment is strictly symptomatic. The signs and symptoms usually subside when the underlying pulmonary disease is successfully treated.

LYME ARTHRITIS

Lyme disease is a spirochetal infection transmitted by ticks. It is characterized by an acute phase manifested by fever, myalgia, and other constitutional symptoms followed weeks to months later by recurrent skin lesions, neurologic and cardiac abnormalities, and intermittent bouts of arthritis.

Joint involvement occurs in over half the cases, and usually less than two or three joints are involved. Five percent to 10% of patients may develop chronic arthritis, most commonly involving the knees. Erosion and cartilage destruction may even occur.

Treatment

Antibiotics (usually penicillin or tetracycline) given for the disease can prevent the chronic arthritis. Even after the arthritis is established, antibiotic therapy is helpful. Chronic cases may require surgery.

ANTI-INFLAMMATORY MEDICATION

Throughout this text, salicylates have been recommended for their anti-inflammatory effect. Like all other NSAIDs, they probably act by blocking the synthesis of prostaglandins. Salicylates are effective, inexpensive, and generally well tolerated. For best results, 8 to 12 tablets (5-grain) should be taken daily. If tinnitus develops, the dose should be decreased, but aspirin treatment should not be discontinued. If stomach intolerance is a problem, enteric-coated or buffered products are available that lessen the gastric distress. The only disadvantage of aspirin as compared with other products is the frequent dosing interval.

If salicylates are ineffective, inconvenient, or not tolerated, a number of other drugs may be tried (Table 14–3). These drugs are categorized into several classes, and when switching from one to another, it is best to select from a different class. Patients must also be reminded that all of these drugs are most effective when taken routinely, not "as needed." Physicians should also be reminded that prescription NSAIDs are expensive and should not be used casually.

Side Effects

Because of their common mechanism of activity, many of these agents have similar side effects. Most of them are reversible when the drug therapy is discontinued.

Central Nervous System. All of these drugs can cause CNS symptoms, most of them minor. Dizziness, drowsiness, and confusion may occur. Tolmetin, sulindac, and especially indomethacin frequently cause such unpleasant symptoms such as depression, headache, and nausea.

Renal and Hepatic. Ibuprofen, fenoprofen, and meclofenamate are most likely to cause renal problems, and all of the drugs can cause some loss of hepatic function. The symptoms resolve in most cases when treatment with the drug is stopped. Patients with impaired function should probably avoid the drugs.

Fluid Retention. Salt and water retention are fairly common. Salt retention may even effect the lens and cornea and lead to blurred vision.

Gastrointestinal. Gastric irritation is common to all of these drugs. In most cases, the discomfort can be minimized by giving the drug with food. Ulcers that may develop are usually gastric, and as many as 60% of patients taking NSAIDs will develop gastric erosions. Many are asymptomatic, however. While these drugs may have detrimental gastrointestinal side effects, they are all that is available for the treatment of many inflammatory conditions. For those patients at greater risk of gastric ulceration, misoprostol (Cytotec)

TABLE 14–3.

Frequently used NSAIDs*

NSAID	Usual Dose	Comments
Salicylates		
Aspirin (acetylsalicylic acid)	3000 mg daily	All salicylates should be given in divided doses following meals
Choline magnesium trisalicylate (Trilisate)	3000 mg daily	
Salicylsalicylic acid (Disalcid, Monogesic)	3000 mg daily	
Diflunisal (Dolobid)	500 mg BID	May cause marrow depression
Proprionic or arylacetic acids		
Ibuprofen (Motrin, Rufen)	600–800 mg TID	Use carefully in patients with renal dysfunction. Occasional photosensitivity
Fenoprofen (Nalfon)	600 mg TID	
Ketoprofen (Orudis)	75 mg TID	
Flurbiprofen (Ansaid)	100 mg TID	
Naproxen (Naprosyn)	500 mg BID	
Indole and indene acetic acids		
Sulindac (Clinoril)	150–200 mg BID	Both may cause CNS side effects. Indocin also available in time release capsule (75 mg once daily)
Indomethecin (Indocin)	25–50 mg TID	
Pyrazole derivatives		
Phenylbutazone (Butazolidin, Azolid)	100 mg TID	May cause marrow depression, salt retention
Oxyphenbutazone (Tandearil, Oxalid)	100 mg TID	
Others (each chemically different from all other NSAIDs)		
Tolmetin (Tolectin)—a pyrole acetate	600 mg BID	May cause CNS side effects
Diclofenac sodium (Voltaren)—a phenylacetate	50 mg TID	
Piroxicam (Feldene)—an oxicam	10–20 mg once a day	Occasional photosensitivity
Meclofenamate sodium (Meclomen)—a fenamate	100 mg TID	

*Notes: The following side effects are common to most NSAIDs: (1) gastric irritation, (2) interference with platelet function, (3) salt and water retention, and (4) visual disturbances. These drugs should not be used in combination. When changing drugs, change from one class to a separate class. Aspirin, the most commonly used NSAID, is also available under the trade name of Zorprin. This drug is released in the small intestine rather than the stomach. The usual dose is two 800-mg tablets twice a day.

may be helpful. An analogue of prostaglandin, misoprostol is effective in the *prevention* of gastric (not duodenal) ulcers caused by NSAIDs. It is recommended for use in those patients more likely to develop ulceration: (1) older (over 60 years) or debilitated patients, (2) those with a known ulceration or previous gastrointestinal bleed, or (3) patients taking oral steroids.

Cotreatment with misoprostol (200 mg four times a day) has been shown to be effective during NSAID use. Not everyone taking NSAIDs should be treated with it, however, because the cost of the two drugs together would be prohibitive. Other drugs such as H_2 antagonists and antacids produced inferior results to misoprostol in preventing gastric ulceration.

BIBLIOGRAPHY

Aegerter E, Kirkpatrick JA: *Orthopedic Diseases,* ed. 3. Philadelphia, WB Saunders Co, 1968.

Bjelle A, Sunden G: Pyrophosphate arthropathy: A clinical study of 50 cases. *J Bone Joint Surg [Br]* 1974; 56:246.

Bloom BS: Risk and cost of gastrointestinal side effects associated with nonsteroidal anti-inflammatory drugs. *Gastroenterology* 1989; 149:1019.

Chuang T, et al: Polymyalgia rheumatica: A 10-year epidemiologic and clinical study. *Ann Intern Med* 1982; 97:672.

Decker JL (ed): Primer on the rheumatic diseases. *JAMA* 1964; 190:127–140, 425–444, 509–530, 741–751.

Flatt AE: *The Care of the Rheumatoid Hand,* ed 2. St. Louis, CV Mosby Co, 1968.

Gatter RA: *A Practical Handbook of Joint Fluid Analysis.* Philadelphia, Lea & Febiger, 1984.

Graham DY: Prevention of gastroduodenal injury induced by chronic nonsteroidal anti-inflammatory drug therapy. *Gastroenterology* 1989; 96:675.

Gutman AB: Views on the pathogenesis and management of primary gout—1971. *J Bone Joint Surg [Am]* 1972; 54:357.

Hollander JL, McCarty DJ (eds): *Arthritis and Allied Conditions,* ed 8. Philadelphia, Lea & Febiger, 1972.

Jaffe HL: *Metabolic, Degenerative, and Inflammatory Diseases of Bones and Joints.* Philadelphia, Lea & Febiger, 1972.

Katz WA: *Rheumatoid Diseases, Diagnosis, and Management.* Philadelphia, JB Lippincott, 1977.

King BG, Jr, Galveston SN, Evans EB: Palindromic rheumatism: An unusual cause of the inflammatory joint. *J Bone Joint Surg [Am]* 1974; 56:142.

Laskar FH, Sargison KD: Ochronotic arthropathy. *J Bone Joint Surg [Br]* 1970; 52:653.

Laurin CA, et al: Long-term results of synovectomy of the knee in rheumatoid patients. *J Bone Joint Surg [Am]* 1974; 56:521.

McLaughlin TP, et al: Chronic arthritis of the knee in Lyme disease. *J Bone Joint Surg [AM]* 1986; 68:1057.

Reynolds JC: Famotidine therapy for active duodenal ulcers. *Ann Intern Med* 1989; 111:7.

Steere AC, et al: Successful parenteral penicillin therapy of established Lyme arthritis. *N Engl J Med* 1985; 312:869.

CHAPTER 15

Sports Medicine

Participation in athletics is both enjoyable and a part of keeping physically and mentally fit. Some individuals may only be interested in general conditioning and weight loss (Table 15-1). Others may want specific exercises for certain events. Regardless of the activity, risks are always involved, and today's physician must not only be able to treat the various injuries that arise but also to offer counsel on a wide range of other interrelated subjects such as technique, training, and injury prevention.

If the participants are children, other responsibilities are necessary. The physician should help make certain that realistic goals are set and that the activity is enjoyed by those who take part in it. Parents and coaches should be reminded that success is measured not necessarily just by winning but by the enjoyment and the amount of effort put forth. Whenever team sports are involved, all members should be allowed to play, and attempts should be made to match size and physical maturity as closely as possible. Children should learn how to play the various games as well as their rules. They should be properly supervised and not be encouraged to play with pain. The role of the coach should be to instruct and supervise and not to give medical treatment or advice.

Treating athletes is also somewhat different than treating other patients in that many of them, whether young or adult, are unwilling to simply "give it up" when injuries arise. Many of them may accept a more physically tolerable substitute activity, however.

PREVENTION OF INJURIES

The most effective means of minimizing the complications of sports injuries is by prevention, and the first step in that prevention begins with a complete physical examination. This is especially important in the youth and should take place even before conditioning is begun. Special attention should be paid to those areas that will be most involved in the athletic activity, and all musculotendinous disorders or abnormalities should be noted and evaluated. The frequency and severity of many injuries may then be lessened by proper conditioning and preparation.

TABLE 15–1.

Calories Expended in Common Activities*

Activity	Calories per Hour
Light housework	120
Walking	250–300
Golf	300
Singles tennis	480
Bicycling	450–500
Jogging	600
Swimming	650–700

*To be effective, an exercise should be performed three to five times per week for at least 30 to 60 minutes each time.

Conditioning

Proper conditioning means the development of strength, endurance, cardiovascular fitness, power, and flexibility. It also includes the development of proper body mechanics, form, and agility. The exact skill training will depend upon the specific sport involved, but lower extremity injuries can generally be lessened by strengthening exercises for individuals with loose joints to protect against ligament damage and stretching exercises for individuals with tight joints to avoid muscular strains. Staying in shape during the off-season may involve running the stairs and jogging in place at home.

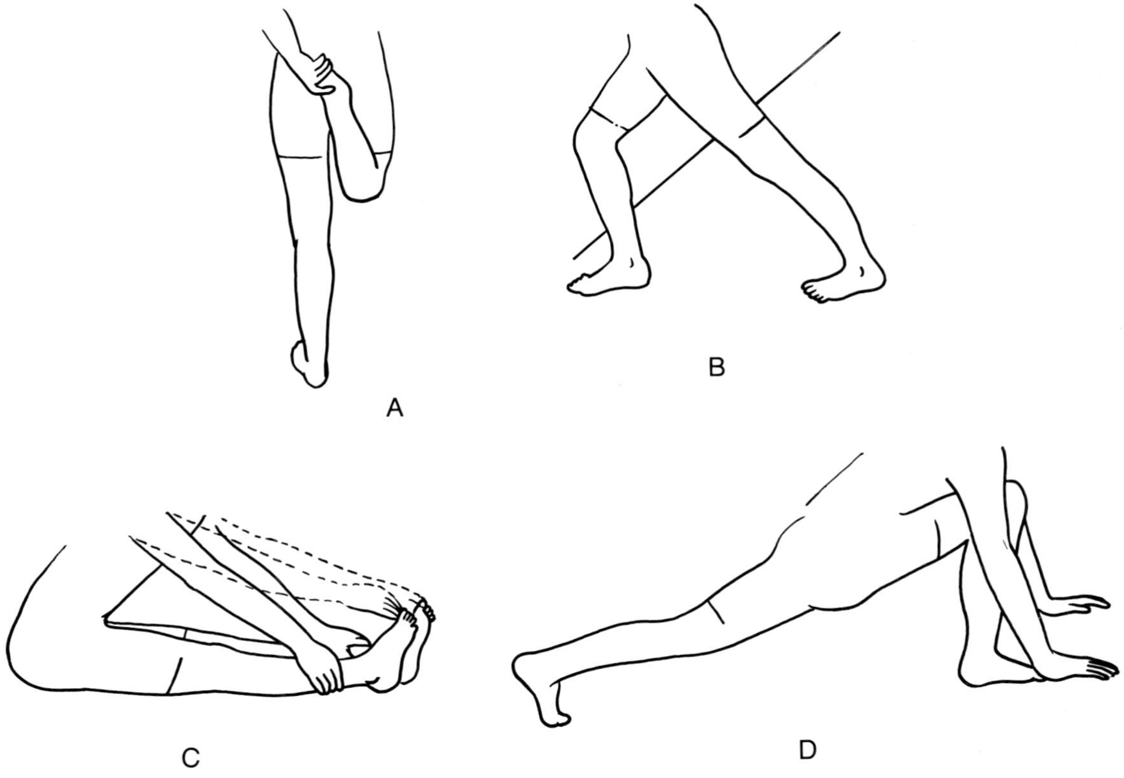

FIG 15–1.
Stretching exercises. These should be performed before vigorous exercise and after warming up for a few minutes by walking. The patient should be instructed not to "bounce" or cause strain. The stretch is held for several seconds and repeated several times, and then the legs are reversed. **A,** quadriceps stretch. **B,** heel cord stretch. **C,** hamstring stretch. **D,** hamstring and quadriceps stretch.

Warming Up

Beginning any activity gradually will reduce the incidence of injury, especially injury to the muscle-tendon unit. Stretching is especially important to avoid strain. Flexibility is often diminished after a long period of inactivity, and stretching is particularly important when resuming a sport. The heel cord, hamstrings, and quadriceps should have special attention. (Fig 15–1).

Tissue stretches better when warm. Therefore, stretching is best performed following slow jogging or walking for 5 minutes. Two types of stretching exercises may be performed. Static stretching is a slow, gradual stretching through full movement, and holding at the position of maximum stretch for 10 to 20 seconds before re-laxing. A pulling sensation should be felt but no pain. Ballistic stretching, which involves rapid, repetitive movements, is also occasionally used but is generally less effective and may even cause minor muscular tears. It is usually not recommended.

Cooling Off

Proper habits after rigorous exercise permit muscles to cool off adequately and to dissipate heat. Following running, it is usually advised not to simply stand still or lie supine but to walk for 5 to 10 minutes and then rest in a sitting position. This may be especially important for the cardiac status of the individual.

INJURIES TO MUSCLES

Strains

Vigorous muscular activity can lead to three common problems: (1) muscular tears, (2) cramping during exercise, and (3) soreness following exercise.

Muscular Tears

Pain that develops acutely from violent activity is usually the result of a muscle tear. This may be partial or complete and even involve the fascia. Muscles that cross two joints, such as the hamstrings, seem to be the most vulnerable.

The diagnosis is usually not difficult, although it may not be easy to differentiate complete from incomplete ruptures. Sudden onset of pain, swelling, and marked local tenderness are characteristic. Pain is increased by stretching the affected muscle unit. Complete rupture may reveal a palpable defect on examination but muscle spasm and swelling often make it difficult to diagnose a complete tear.

Ice (30 minutes every hour) should be applied immediately and the injured area elevated. There is probably little to be gained by attempt-ing to aspirate the hematoma. A pressure bandage is always applied, and complete bed rest may even be necessary. After 24 to 48 hours, very gentle, active contraction of the muscle may be started. Ice should be continued when the exercises have begun. Heat and massage should be avoided, and the extremity should be protected against further injury. Weight bearing, passive stretching, or excessive muscular activity should also be avoided until swelling is under control and the limb can be actively moved through a full range with little pain. Cool whirlpool baths are often helpful at this stage. Gradually, a return to activity is allowed when motion is painless.

Although complete tears should theoretically be surgically repaired, many (if not most) surgeons do not support this concept. Immediate repair is often difficult because of the poor texture of the muscle and the difficulty in holding the sutures. The results are often poor. Late repair may occasionally be indicated, but the overall results are only fair. Therefore, unless surgery is contemplated, all acute muscular strains should be treated essentially the same.

Rehabilitation is often slow, and the functional

capacity of the athlete occasionally may never return to normal. Stretching exercises should be continued as strength returns. An elastic wrap is occasionally helpful when activity is resumed. If the injury has been to a hamstring muscle, strains can often be prevented by being certain that the hamstrings are at least 60% to 70% as strong as the quadriceps. This 60:40 ratio of quadriceps to hamstring strength is important to prevent hamstring strain due to their relative weakness as compared with the quadriceps. Athletes may return to regular activity when full, pain-free motion is present, muscle strength is restored, and tenderness and swelling have subsided.

Muscle Cramps And Soreness

Muscle cramps are common during exercise and are of unknown cause. They usually occur during the latter part of exercise and may be a result of the accumulation of waste products or electrolyte imbalance. Any muscle may be affected, but the most common are the thigh, calf, and foot.

Treatment is primarily by static stretching through a full range of motion and local massage. Cramps may be prevented by proper stretching exercises and warm-up and by the maintenance of adequate oral fluid and electrolyte intake. It is inappropriate to ever have an athlete "run it out."

Muscle soreness may also develop 24 to 48 hours after exertion. The etiology of this type of muscle pain is also not completely understood but may be due to localized muscular spasm and ischemia. It is treated by stretching exercises and heat to increase the circulation.

Nocturnal muscle cramps are also common in both adults and children. In adults, they are usually not in the athletic individual, whereas they are common in the physically active child. In the adult, these cramps may be quite severe and cause the development of a palpable muscular knot. The acute spasm is treated by static stretching and massage. Stretching exercises may prevent their development. Frequent changes in foot position by sleeping with the feet over the edge of the bed and avoiding heavy blankets over the ankles that keep them in the plantar-flexed position may also be helpful. Quinine tablets taken before retiring may occasionally be of benefit by an unknown mechanism.

Children's night cramps are usually not as severe and do not cause acute contractions. They are treated symptomatically by heat and massage and may be prevented by not allowing the child to become fatigued during play.

Contusions

Muscular bruises are common in all athletic events, even in the so-called noncontact sports. They are differentiated from ruptures and strains because function remains following the injury and the contusion usually results from direct trauma. The thigh and upper portion of the arm are most commonly involved. The diagnosis is usually not difficult. Tenderness is present at the site of injury, and there is usually ecchymosis, although it may not appear until later.

Treatment is directed at avoiding the complications of myositis ossificans and contractures and returning the athlete to full, pain-free competitive activity. This is accomplished by the rapid application of ice to the affected area to control bleeding and the removal of the athlete from further competition. Crutches may be necessary for the lower extremity injury, and complete bed rest with elevation of the extremity may even be indicated to control swelling and pain. A compression wrapping is sometimes helpful in early stages. After 24 to 48 hours, gentle isometric muscle contractions may be started, and active gentle range of motion is gradually added at the patient's tolerance. Passive range of motion should be avoided. Any increase in pain or swelling is an indication to resume complete bed rest and application of ice. Full strength and complete flexibility are gradually restored by exercise. Reinjury is avoided by allowing complete healing to occur before returning to activities and by appropriately protecting the injured site. A return to athletics should only follow complete recovery.

Myositis Ossificans

This is a condition characterized by the formation of heterotopic bone in the soft tissues. It usually develops in muscle as the result of trauma (myositis ossificans circumscripta). It also occurs in the lower extremities in conjunction with severe brain injuries. A rare congenital form (myositis ossificans progressiva) may begin without trauma or shortly after birth.

The common traumatic form usually follows a single injury. The mechanism of bone formation is unknown, but interstitial hemorrhage is thought to play a role. Eventually, the hematoma becomes calcified and ossified.

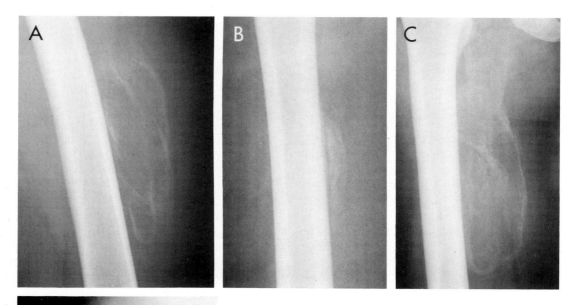

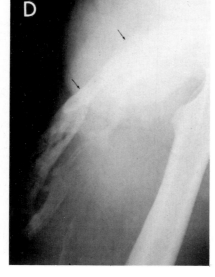

FIG 15-2.
Examples of myositis ossificans (ossifying hematoma). **A,** the typical early (2½ weeks) roentgenographic appearance. **B,** a more broad-based variety. **C,** massive involvement of the hamstring area. **D,** the same case, after maturity. These injuries can occasionally be confused with malignant bone lesions, but in contrast to tumors, there is no involvement of the adjacent bone.

The favorite sites of development are the quadriceps, brachialis, deltoid, and hamstrings. After the injury, a large hematoma forms. The area becomes swollen and tender, and motion is restricted. Increased heat may even be present locally, and some patients have a mild febrile episode. The tenderness and heat tend to persist. The erythrocyte sedimentation rate (ESR) is sometimes increased. As the swelling, pain, and heat subside, a firm mass becomes palpable in the involved area. Motion may continue to be restricted because of obstruction by the mass or from inelasticity of the muscle.

The roentgenographic diagnosis can usually be made 2 to 4 weeks after the contusion. The initial appearance is that of a poorly defined opaque mass in the soft tissue adjacent to the bone (Fig 15–2). As the mass matures, it becomes more clearly outlined and dense. The lesion usually stabilizes in 3 to 6 months and begins to resorb slowly, often without any disability. Eventually, it transforms itself into mature bone and is partially resorbed.

Ice, elevation, and rest will control swelling. Although usually not practical, early aspiration of large, well-localized hematomas could prevent heterotopic bone formation. Once bone formation has developed, rest of the affected part is indicated. Moist heat and gentle exercise may be helpful to prevent stiffness, but physical therapy will only lead to more disability. If the heterotopic bone is locally painful or disabling, it may be removed, but excision is absolutely contraindicated until complete maturity of the bony mass is reached. This may take several months. Premature removal could result in a recurrence more extensive than the original mass. It is generally recommended that athletes not resume their physical activity until the bone has completely matured, which may take 3 to 6 months. The

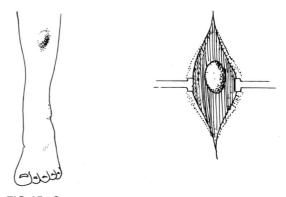

FIG 15–3.
Fascial hernia. **A,** the clinical appearance. **B,** the lesion at surgery.

injured area should then be protected by padding.

Fascial Hernias

These often develop as a result of a contusion or small puncture wound that causes a rent to develop in the fascia and aponeurosis that envelops all muscle. The defect may vary from 1 cm to any size. Hernias may also develop in weak fascial areas in patients with chronic compartmental syndromes as a result of increased pressure in the compartment. They are also seen where nerves emerge from the fascia.

Examination will reveal a palpable "tumor" mass, especially when the muscle is relaxed (Fig 15–3). Muscle contraction may cause the mass to disappear.

Treatment is usually unnecessary. If pain is present, surgical closure or enlargement of the hole is indicated. Closure of the defect in a compartmental syndrome, however, is contraindicated because this could cause a further increase in the pressure inside the compartment.

INJURIES TO RUNNERS

Millions of Americans enjoy running, and each year, over half of them will sustain injuries. Many physicians from whom they seek advice are unfamiliar with their particular injuries and may simply prescribe medication and suggest that they give up running for a while. Although these are good recommendations, many runners will seek more specific advice. It is important, therefore, that physicians treating these patients have at least some understanding of the special problems that develop in these athletes.

Biomechanics

The running gait pattern is a repetitive movement that consists of a support phase, when the foot is on the ground, and a nonsupport phase. It is during the support phase that most injuries develop. Distance runners usually begin this phase by landing on the heel (sprinters usually land on the forefoot). As weight is taken on the heel, the calcaneus will begin to roll laterally (pronate, evert) under the talus at the subtalar joint (Fig 15–4). This allows the heel to absorb shock and adapt to the underlying surface. The forefoot will follow this motion by pronating, and at the same time, the tibia begins to rotate internally in proportion to the amount of heel pronation. As the weight moves forward, the calcaneus begins to supinate (invert) or roll back medially under the talus, and the tibia will begin to externally rotate. This allows the foot to become more rigid and gives the heel cord a strong lever upon which to act and transfer power. There are also a number of other coordinated motions that occur in the pelvis, hip, and other joints throughout the gait

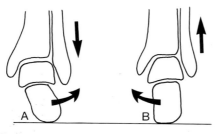

FIG 15–4.
Movements of the subtalar joint. **A,** eversion (pronation) allows for shock absorption upon impact. **B,** inversion (supination) converts the hindfoot to a more powerful lever for push-off.

cycle, but understanding the subtalar joint mechanics is the most important.

History

An accurate history, especially of the training program, is extremely important in evaluating injuries to runners because only 40% will actually have an anatomic problem causing their disorder (James, 1978). The remaining 60% can usually be traced to errors in training. The history begins by determining whether the individual was ever treated for any childhood malalignment problem. It should be ascertained whether the individual has had any other significant past musculoskeletal diseases. An accurate running history is then taken: (1) How often does the patient run and how many miles? (2) Has there been any recent change in the running pattern? (3) When does the pain occur? (4) What effect does running have on the pain? (5) On what sort of surface and terrain does the running take place? (6) Does the runner do stretching or other exercises to warm up? (7) What kind of shoe is used, and what is its wear pattern?

Examination

The examination should consist of a complete evaluation of the lower extremities to determine whether any anatomic problems of extremity alignment are present as well as a local examination of the injured part. There is obviously a proper position or alignment for the foot and leg in which it functions most efficiently. This is the neutral or straightforward position. Minor deviations from this alignment may not cause problems with normal walking or running, but because of the great accumulation of repetitive stresses applied to the lower extremities in long distance running, subtle malalignment problems may translate into major disturbances for the runner. This may even cause abnormal compensatory motions to develop in other joints and cause them to break down. To determine whether a problem with alignment exists, a complete examination of the lower extremities is necessary. The most important aspects of the examination can be ascertained with the patient standing, supine, and kneeling.

With the patient standing, any gross abnormalities such as torsion, varus, or valgus of the legs, laterally directed patellae, or obvious foot deformities such as high or low arches should be noted. Any eversion of the heels as visualized from behind is especially important.

In the supine position, the true leg lengths are measured between the anterior superior iliac spines and the medial malleoli. Discrepancies of 0.5 to 1.0 cm may be significant in the runner and require correction by a shoe lift. The range of motion of the hips is then determined. Internal and external rotation should be within 30 degrees of each other. Marked external rotation may cause an out-toed gait. The knee is closely examined, especially if patellar pain is present, and the Q-angle is determined (Fig 15−5). Pa-

tients with high Q-angles may develop knee pain with running. The range of motion of the ankle is then determined with the knee extended. Fifteen degrees of dorsiflexion is normal. Any tightness of the heel cord is noted.

The patient then kneels on the examining table, and leg-heel and heel-forefoot alignments are determined. First, the neutral position of the subtalar joint is found by everting and inverting the foot and finding the point where the head of the talus is placed in the navicular and is no longer palpable (Fig 15−6). This may require a little practice and is often only a rough estimate. Next, leg-heel alignment is determined by drawing lines posteriorly that bisect the lower portion of the leg and calcaneus (Fig 15−7). The lines should be parallel or have no more than 2 to 3 degrees of varus. Heel-forefoot alignment is estimated by observing the relationship of the calcaneal line to the plane of the metatarsal heads. Normally, these lines should be perpendicular.

If the alignment of the leg is not satisfactory, the knee and the foot are the most commonly affected areas. The foot may be adversely affected by too little pronation or a heel that is in too much inversion. This will not allow force to be absorbed during weight bearing. Excessive pronation may lead to strain on the medial side of the foot and ankle. This also prevents the heel from completely returning to the stable position before push-off.

The knee may also be secondarily affected because as the heel pronates, the tibia normally internally rotates and the femur externally rotates.

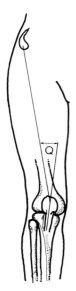

FIG 15−5.
The Q-angle, formed by the intersection of a line from the anterior superior iliac spine (ASIS) through the midpatella and a line from the midpatella to the tibial tubercle. The normal angle is 15 to 20 degrees. Higher angles, by causing a bowstringing effect and lateral tracking, may cause peripatellar pain.

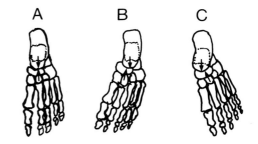

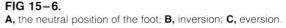

FIG 15−6.
A, the neutral position of the foot; **B,** inversion; **C,** eversion.

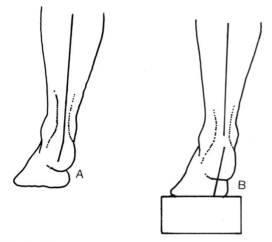

FIG 15–7.
Leg-heel **(A)** and heel-forefoot **(B)** alignment. The foot and
subtalar joint are held in the neutral position.

If heel pronation is excessive, internal tibial rotation may increase, and require that the knee absorb more rotation during this support phase.
This may lead to strain or inflammation.

A common example of a malalignment problem is what James calls "malicious malalignment
syndrome." The patient with this disorder usually
has a broad pelvis, femoral anteversion, genu valgum, a high Q-angle, external tibial torsion, and
pronated feet.

Back, Hip, and Thigh Pain

Back, hip, and thigh pain are relatively uncommon in long-distance runners. Back pain is especially rare but may be caused by disc disease
with or without radicular symptoms. Congenital
or developmental problems such as spondylolisthesis may also become symptomatic under the
conditions of long-distance running. The usual
early course of treatment is symptomatic, but
long-distance running may aggravate the condition under treatment, and a decision may have to
be made not to return to the sport.

Trochanteric bursitis is occasionally seen in
runners and may be associated with tendinitis of
the gluteus medius. The pain often radiates down
the iliotibial band of the lateral aspect of the
thigh and, thus, may be confused with disc herniation. Point tenderness is usually present. The
condition may develop when running on banked
surfaces or in association with a leg length inequality. The treatment is heat, anti-inflammatory
medication, and a local cortisone injection. A lift
may be tried in the running shoe if a leg length
inequality is present.

Stress fractures occasionally occur in the pelvis and femur of the distance runner (Fig 15–8).
They should be ruled out in all cases of chronic
pain that fail to respond to routine symptomatic
management. The appropriate roentgenographic
study should include a bone scan. As with other
stress fractures, reduction of activity is usually
curative, but fractures of the femoral neck may
require internal fixation.

Hamstring strains are a less common cause of
disability in the distance runner than in the
sprinter. They are treated as previously described. Stretching exercises are important not
only for prevention of local injury but because
tight hamstrings may cause excessive lumbar lordosis that adds strain to the back when running.

Contractures of the hip joint also add strain to
the back and should be treated by static stretching exercises. Inflammation may also develop in
the piriformis, adductor, and iliopsoas tendons
and in the ischial and iliopsoas bursae. Inflammation of the symphysis pubis (osteitis pubis) and
sacroiliac joints may also develop because of the
repetitive shearing forces applied to these areas.
The treatment for these disorders is also symptomatic.

Knee Pain

Overuse Syndromes
Major injuries of the meniscus or ligaments are
uncommon in the knees of runners. More frequent are "overuse" injuries that develop because of the repetitive nature of the running activity (Fig 15–9). Several areas are commonly affected: (1) tenosynovitis of the popliteus tendon
may develop near its insertion just above the lat-

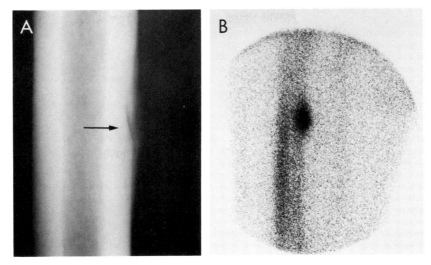

FIG 15–8.
Stress fracture of the femur. **A,** plain anteroposterior (AP) roentgenogram; **B,** bone scan.

eral joint line and anterior to the lateral collateral ligament. This insertion is deep to the iliotibial band. The inflammation may be caused by excessive downhill running. (2) The iliotibial band friction syndrome is an inflammation of the band as it rubs over the lateral femoral condyle. A snapping sensation may be present during flexion and extension. (3) Anserine bursitis causes pain beneath the anserine tendons over the medial flare of the tibia. A stress fracture of the upper portion of the tibia should be ruled out in resistant cases. (4) "Jumper's knee" is a tendinitis of the patellar tendon, usually where it attaches to the patella. As the name implies, it is also seen in athletes whose events require jumping. (5) Tendinitis of the quadriceps mechanism may also

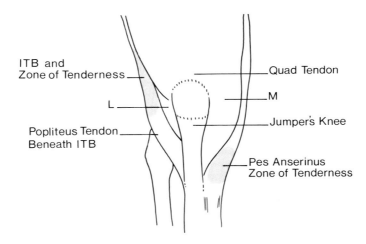

FIG 15–9.
Common areas of tendinitis of the knee. The most common areas of involvement are the quadriceps tendon and its medial *(M)* and lateral *(L)* expansions.

occur over its wide insertion or over the medial or lateral retinaculum that helps support the patella.

Synovitis

Chronic inflammation of the joint may also develop from overuse. An effusion is usually the only physical finding, and a history will not reveal any apparent cause for the swelling, except occasionally a history of increased mileage. Oral anti-inflammatory medication and a period of decreased mileage may be curative, but complete rest for 6 to 8 weeks may be necessary. An occasional steroid injection may be tried if all other treatments fail, but repeated injections are probably not advisable.

Chondromalacia Patella ("Anterior Knee Pain Syndrome")

This is a condition in which pain develops beneath the patella, sometimes in conjunction with varying amounts of fibrillation and degeneration of its articular cartilage (see Chapter 11). Anything that adversely affects the normal "tracking" of the patella in its femoral groove may lead to pain, usually on the lateral side. The causes are often those of malalignment: (1) an increased Q-angle with a bowstringing effect; (2) tightness of the lateral retinaculum with relative weakness of the vastus medialis muscle; (3) subluxing patella; (4) direct trauma; and (5) genu valgum, excessive heel pronation, and/or external tibial torsion (Fig 15–10).

Clinically, patellar or peripatellar pain and discomfort are present and are usually aggravated when stress is applied to the extensor mechanism by stair walking or running up and down hilly terrain. Sitting with the knee flexed for any excessive period of time may cause a stiff feeling to develop that is usually relieved by knee extension. An effusion is occasionally present, and palpation of the undersurface of the patella is often painful. A Q-angle of more than 20 degrees or other physical findings of malalignment may be present. Roentgenograms are usually not helpful unless subluxation is present.

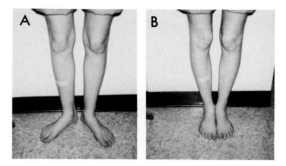

FIG 15–10.
External tibial torsion. **A,** with the patella pointing straight forward, the feet are externally rotated. This may cause peripatellar pain with excessive use because of abnormal pressure. Note the high Q-angles. **B,** the knees face inward with the feet pointing straight ahead.

The wide variety of treatments used to manage this condition attests to the difficulty in curing it. Conservative measures such as rest, anti-inflammatory medication, local heat, quadriceps exercises in extension, and avoiding the offending activity are useful. Patellar straps or braces seem to be of only limited benefit. Theoretically, removal of the damaged articular cartilage by shaving could relieve the symptoms. This can easily be done arthroscopically, but the results are often inconsistent. If a distal malalignment problem is present, an orthotic device in the shoe may occasionally be beneficial to help correct the tracking problem. As a last resort, a surgical procedure to realign the patella could eliminate the symptoms, but it would seem difficult to justify such a major operation simply to allow continued running.

Lower Leg Pain

Posterior Tibial Tendinitis

A common cause of leg pain is what is sometimes referred to as the "shin splint." This is a specific overuse syndrome involving the origin of the tibialis posterior muscle and causing pain along the deep midthird of the medial border of the tibia (Fig 15–11). It often develops in poorly conditioned athletes or runners who run on hard surfaces. There is usually tenderness to palpation

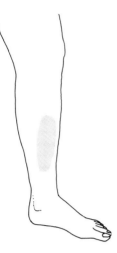

FIG 15–11.
The area of tenderness and pain with posterior tibial tendinitis.

along the posteromedial border of the midtibia. The roentgenogram may show some late periosteal reaction or cortical thickening in this area.

The treatment is by modification of the running schedule or complete rest. A change to a softer running surface may be helpful. The condition does not usually become chronic.

Compartmental Syndromes

Vigorous exercise may lead to swelling and mild ischemia in any of the four natural compartments in the calf (Fig 15–12). The anterior and lateral

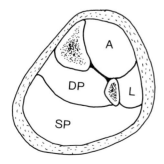

FIG 15–12.
A cross section of the lower portion of the leg shows its four compartments; *A* = anterior; *L* = lateral; *DP* = deep posterior, and *SP* = superficial posterior.

compartments are the most commonly affected in runners, and the condition is usually chronic or recurrent rather than acute. The disorder develops either from local arterial spasm or swelling that increases the pressure in the unyielding compartment. This compromises the local blood flow and leads to muscle ischemia and pain. Permanent muscle and nerve damage may result, but this is rare in the common chronic type seen in runners. More frequently, the only symptom is cramping pain during exercise that is relieved by rest and recurs after resumption of activity. Physical findings are minimal, but tenderness may be present in the affected compartment as well as slight weakness of the involved muscles. Mild paresthesias are occasionally noted.

Treatment for the rare acute case is usually by surgical release of the affected compartment. The more common recurrent type seen in runners is treated by rest and modification of training techniques and mileage. Conservative treatment is often unsuccessful, and individuals who wish to continue competitive long-distance running may require fasciotomy to decompress the affected compartment.

Stress Fractures

These are common injuries of the lower portion of leg and must always be ruled out in the evaluation of pain. They usually develop in response to a sudden increase in the stress applied to a weight-bearing bone. Thus, they are more likely to occur in the novice who is just beginning running or in the individual who suddenly increases mileage. Any weight-bearing bone may be affected. The proximal medial tibial border and the lower portion of the fibula are the most commonly affected areas in the lower part of the leg.

The only physical findings are local tenderness and edema. The roentgenograms are usually negative initially and begin to show healing changes in 2 to 4 weeks. The bone scan is often more sensitive.

The treatment is symptomatic by modification of activities. Casts are usually not necessary. Activity is resumed as symptoms subside. Swimming may be substituted during the healing phase to allow the runner to maintain fitness.

Ankle and Foot Pain

Several overuse syndromes may affect the ankle and foot. They are all treated in the same manner by rest (or modification of activities), anti-inflammatory medication, and local heat. An occasional local steroid injection may also be helpful, but the Achilles tendon should not be injected. Rupture of this tendon is always a concern, and it is possible that this event may be hastened by local injections.

Stress fractures also occur in the foot, and the most common areas of involvement are the metatarsals, navicular, or calcaneus (Fig 15–13). They are treated by protection.

The Pump Bump

This is a painful thickening that develops over the lateral attachment of the tendo Achillis (Fig 15–14). It is usually the result of irritation from a poorly padded heel counter. Conservative measures including proper shoes are usually cura-

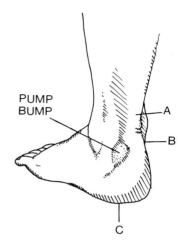

FIG 15–14.
The "pump bump" and common areas of inflammation around the heel. A = Achilles tendon; B = retrocalcaneal bursa; C = plantar fascia.

tive. The back of the shoe may have to be cut out for a period of time. A heel lift may also be helpful. In resistant cases, the small bump must be removed surgically.

Blisters

Blisters are common in runners and are best treated by the following preventive means: (1) begin workouts gradually and increase the mileage as tolerated, (2) make certain shoes are well ventilated and socks are clean and dry, (3) apply powder or petroleum jelly to the feet prior to long runs, and (4) use tincture of benzoin to toughen the skin before running. Once a blister does form, it should be drained with a sterile needle. The dead skin should be left intact and a bandage applied. Broken blisters should be trimmed and kept clean and dry.

Another common condition that develops in runners is the black toe or subungual hematoma. This often develops in a shoe that lacks sufficient room to accommodate the forefoot. It is usually asymptomatic, but the occasional painful tense hematoma may be evacuated by penetrating the nail with a heated paper clip.

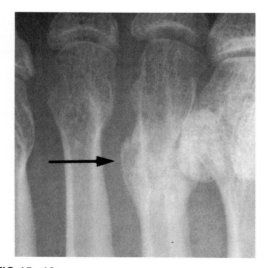

FIG 15–13.
Stress fracture of the second metatarsal *(arrow).*

Running Shoes

A properly constructed shoe is an absolute necessity for the runner (Fig 15–15). There is no single perfect shoe but a good shoe should have the following: (1) a long, firm heel counter to control the hind foot, with a soft Achilles pad to prevent heel cord irritation; (2) a beveled heel that is flared for stability; (3) a cushioned heel lift 1.5 cm thick and a cushioned sole; (4) a high and rounded toe box and a well-padded tongue; (5) a last that is straight rather than adducted, with the shoes balanced, that is, not leaning to one side; and (6) a midsole that is flexible and contains a soft arch support. Shoes should be kept in good repair and replaced or resoled once they become badly worn.

Orthotics

From the previous discussion, the importance of the position and movements of the subtalar joint is apparent. The ability of this joint to absorb shock and function normally is greatest when the center of gravity passes through the joint in the neutral position. The subtalar joint absorbs shock by pronation, but excessive pronation can, at least theoretically, lead to some of the overuse syndromes that are seen in runners not only in the foot and ankle but in the knee. This excessive pronation is one of the most common "malalignment" problems seen in runners and is the usual reason orthotic appliances are prescribed. Orthotics can be used in an attempt to support the foot, especially the heel, more near its neutral position. They are used more or less on an empiric basis as a last resort. There are no conclusive studies that show that these devices actually perform as expected, but some patients seem to benefit from their use, and they continue to be prescribed. They can be expensive, however, and are best used only when more simple treatment modalities have failed.

Orthotics may be soft, semirigid, or hard; several materials can be used. Simple supports are available in sporting goods stores and are usually made from rubber. Other soft orthotics can be made from materials that are heated and applied to the individual's foot while the heel is held in a neutral position (Fig 15–16). "Posts" may be added for additional support. Custom-fabricated rigid orthotics can also be made from plaster molds of the feet by laboratories that specialize in their preparation.

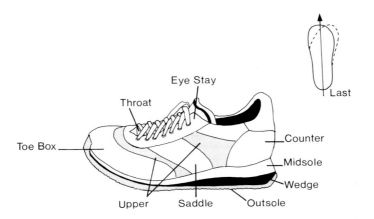

Eye Stay

Throat

Toe Box

Last

Counter

Midsole

Wedge

Upper   Saddle   Outsole

FIG 15–15.
The properly constructed running shoe. Good heel fit is particularly important. The last or form from which the shoe is made should be straight and not 6 to 7 degrees inward as it is in many manufactured shoes. It should be unnecessary to "break in" good running shoes.

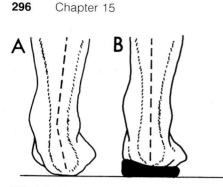

FIG 15–16.
The "neutral" orthotic device. Excessive hindfoot pronation **(A)** may occasionally be corrected by the use of an orthotic device **(B)**.

Treatment Summary

The general care of runners involves the following: (1) accurate diagnosis, (2) evaluation for alignment problems, and (3) assessment for training errors. It has been found that the majority of injuries are related to training errors and that excessive mileage accounts for many of these. In addition to excessive mileage, other causes of training problems are running on improper surfaces or terrain and abrupt increases in the runner's routine. It can therefore be seen that minor modifications in the runner's schedule may be helpful. Complete rest is occasionally the only acceptable treatment, however, and a rest of 4 to 6 weeks is often necessary to allow for complete recovery. The following recommendations are often helpful:

1. Heavy workouts should alternate daily with light workouts.
2. Rest or at least reduce mileage until symptoms subside. Substitute bicycle riding or swimming temporarily.
3. Gradually return to running the previous mileage following the injury.
4. Static stretching exercises for 10 to 15 minutes should precede each workout. This should be particularly directed to the hamstrings and calf muscles.
5. Proper shoes should be worn at all times and should be changed as necessary.
6. Runners who use roads should alternate sides because the crown of the road may create uneven stress. Training should take place on as flat a surface as possible, and slopes should be avoided.
7. Complete rest may be necessary for 6 weeks in some cases. It should also be remembered that not all individuals are able to run long distances any more than they are able to run fast. Biking, swimming, and rowing may be better activities for some.

INJURIES TO THE UPPER EXTREMITY

The Shoulder

Disorders of the Rotator Cuff

The overarm throwing motion may rank second only to running as a common factor in athletic events. The range of motion of the shoulder is the greatest of all joints and is made possible because of the relatively minimal amount of bony contact between the humeral head and the glenoid. Thus, stability is sacrificed for flexibility, and this places a great burden on the capsule and rotator cuff musculature for joint stability. As a result, the soft tissue may develop overuse injuries because of repetitive strains placed on it during exercise. These strains may lead to overuse changes ranging from simple tendinitis or bursitis to rotator cuff rupture. Tissue calcification may even occur. Swelling of the rotator cuff and subacromial bursa then develops, which narrows the space between the head of the humerus and the overlying acromion and coracoacromial ligament. This may lead to the development of crepitus and impingement when the shoulder is abducted. Abduction further narrows the subacromial space and can result in a painful catching sensation, thus, the term "impingement syndrome" (see Chapter 5).

Clinically, shoulder pain is present during and

after use. The pain may radiate down the deltoid muscle because of the common innervation of the deltoid and supraspinatus muscle. Crepitus is common, and there is tenderness to palpation over the rotator cuff, usually the supraspinatus tendon. Shoulder arthrography is usually negative unless a complete tear of the cuff has developed.

The treatment of rotator cuff tendinitis is usually conservative. Rest and avoiding the offending activity are most important. Push-ups should be avoided. Local steroid injections may relieve pain but should be used cautiously. Their use may shrink the swollen, inflamed tissues enough to diminish the impingement, but tendon rupture has been reported following (although not necessarily as a result of) their use. Repetitive injections should certainly be avoided (especially in the young), and vigorous use of the shoulder following injections should not be allowed. Rest, stretching and strengthening exercises, and proper throwing or swimming mechanics should be stressed.

Surgery is occasionally helpful in resistant cases. A complete rotator cuff rupture may sometimes benefit from repair. In addition, removal of the bursa and the underneath surface of the acromion and release of the coracoacromial ligament may eliminate much of the impingement. Surgery is somewhat unpredictable, however, and it may not always allow full return to the athletes' previous competitive status.

"Little League shoulder" is a condition previously thought to be similar to overuse tendinitis only seen in adolescence. The presenting complaints were similar. This is now considered to be a traction irritation of the upper humeral epiphysis that causes a stress reaction around the epiphysis. Roentgenography may reveal widening of the epiphyseal plate. The disorder usually heals with rest and leaves no residuals.

Injuries to the Acromioclavicular Joint

The acromioclavicular joint sustains a wide range of injuries. The most minor is the so-called "shoulder pointer," which is a contusion of the deltoid, trapezius, and acromioclavicular joint. It usually heals with rest and protection.

More common is acromioclavicular separation or dislocation (see Chapter 5). The lesion is often divided according to severity into first-, second-, and third-degree injuries. A grade 1 injury is simply a minor strain of the acromioclavicular ligaments. A grade 2 injury involves rupture of the acromioclavicular ligaments but preservation of the coracoclavicular ligaments. In a grade 3 injury, there is complete rupture of all supports with upward displacement of the clavicle.

Grade 1 and 2 incomplete injuries are usually treated symptomatically. The treatment for grade 3 injuries remains unsettled. If the injury involves the dominant shoulder of an athlete who throws, surgical repair is probably indicated. Except for the cosmetic deformity, however, most individuals with chronic acromioclavicular separations are asymptomatic. Even at a later date, however, the individual with a chronic acromioclavicular separation will benefit from simple removal of the lateral 1.5 cm of the clavicle or reconstruction surgery.

Dislocation of the Glenohumeral Joint

Most shoulder dislocations are anterior in direction and result from trauma (see Chapter 5). The usual cause is a fall on the outstretched arm. The diagnosis is suspected when there is an absence of the normal fullness beneath the deltoid. If the dislocation is anterior, the humeral head is palpable anteriorly, the arm is held externally rotated, and internal rotation is painful. Posterior dislocations characteristically have pain on external rotation, the arm is held in internal rotation, and there is flatness of the anterior shoulder contour. Both types often become recurrent.

The treatment is reduction, and this should be accomplished as soon as reasonable. Roentgenograms should always be taken before reduction to rule out other bony injury. Epiphyseal fracture of the upper portion of the humerus should especially be ruled out.

Following reduction, the shoulder should be immobilized 3 weeks if the dislocation was the initial one. Recurrences do not benefit from immobilization. General strengthening exercises are begun, although there is little evidence that they prevent recurrence. Surgery is often necessary for the recurrence and is usually successful in preventing dislocation, but the throwing abilities of the athlete may never return to their previous status.

Shoulder instability may also manifest itself by subluxation rather than dislocation. This is sometimes termed "anterior capsular insufficiency." In this disorder, the anterior capsule and cartilaginous rim of the glenoid become weak from repetitive stretching. The shoulder may not completely dislocate but slips slightly forward and downward. This causes a feeling of weakness, pain, and apprehension, especially when the arm is externally rotated and abducted. Surgery is often necesssary to restore strength to the anterior shoulder capsule.

The Elbow

Tennis Elbow

Inflammation of the tendinous origin of the forearm muscles is a common disorder. The extensor origin is more commonly involved than the flexor side. The disorder is not restricted to tennis players but may be caused by any activity that involves repeated forceful gripping. Tennis players who use both hands for backhand strokes do not develop this condition as often as those who use the one-handed grip.

Physical examination will reveal point tenderness over the affected side, with the pain being aggravated by gripping against resistance.

The treatment includes rest, anti-inflammatory medication, local heat, ice, or ultrasound and local steroid injections. A tennis-elbow brace may help relieve the strain, and a gradual, progressive, controlled stretching and strengthening exercise program for the forearm and hand muscles may be helpful (Fig 15–17). Tennis players can prevent recurrences by using proper techniques. The handle of the tennis racquet should be the proper size, and the ball should be struck

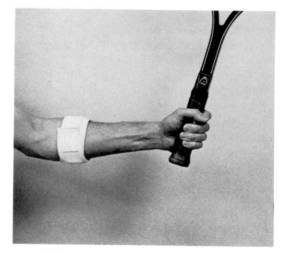

FIG 15–17.
Tennis-elbow dressing. The dressing should be applied approximately 2.5 cm below the epicondyle and fit snugly enough to partially relieve the strain on the affected muscles. A variety of other devices are available.

in the center of the racquet face. The body rather than the arm should be used for power. In addition, a good ball should always be used, and there should be less tension on the strings for the average player. Oversized racquets seem to help by providing a larger "sweet spot."

Little League Elbow

Little League elbow is a term that has been used for a variety of lesions in immature athletes. All of them are related to the repetitive act of throwing, an act that places unusual stress on the elbow. Osteochondritis, avulsion fractures, loose bodies, and a variety of other bony and soft-tissue disorders have been reported.

The symptoms may be of acute or gradual onset. When the onset is sudden, the symptoms are usually secondary to an avulsion injury of either the lateral or the medial epicondyle (Fig 15–18). More commonly, the process is chronic, and the symptoms are usually those of persistent discomfort and stiffness that are aggravated by use of the extremity.

The physical findings are dependent on the

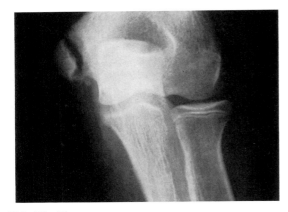

FIG 15−18.
Avulsion of the medial epicondyle in association with a throwing injury in an adolescent.

specific lesion. There is usually point tenderness to palpation over the affected area. The range of motion may be restricted, and a chronic joint effusion is not uncommon.

Treatment is usually conservative, with rest and the elimination of the offending activity all that is necessary. If osteochondritis dissecans is present, the joint may have to be protected for several months in order to allow healing to occur and to prevent the formation of a loose body. If a loose body is present, surgical removal is usually indicated.

In order to protect the elbow from developing these disorders, most authorities believe that no more than six innings of baseball should be pitched per week by the immature player. In addition, at least 3 to 4 days of rest should be al-lowed between games. If enough irritation and swelling are present that a flexion contracture of 20 to 30 degrees exists, the adolescent should not be allowed to pitch again until normal motion has returned.

The Hand

The anatomy of the hand and finger is complex, and injuries to the bones and soft tissues are common in sports (Fig 15−19). The joint may simply be referred to as "jammed," and the injury is therefore frequently not fully appreciated or properly treated. Permanent loss of function may be the end result.

Mallet Finger (Baseball Finger)

Avulsion of the insertion of the extensor tendon at the base of the distal phalanx is a common injury. It occurs secondary to sudden forceful flexion of the distal phalanx, often from a blow to the tip of the extended finger. A fragment of bone may be avulsed along with the tendon.

Active extension of the distal phalanx is lost. Tenderness and swelling are noted on the dorsum of the distal interphalangeal joint, and the distal phalanx rests in the position of moderate flexion. Long-standing cases occasionally develop a mild hyperextension deformity of the proximal interphalangeal joint (Fig 15−20). Roentgenographic examination may reveal an avulsion fracture of the distal phalanx.

If no fracture is present or if the fracture is small, the joint is immobilized in hyperextension

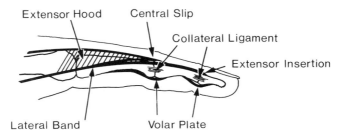

FIG 15−19.
Structures frequently involved in soft-tissue injuries to the finger. Local tenderness or instability will usually assist in establishing the diagnosis.

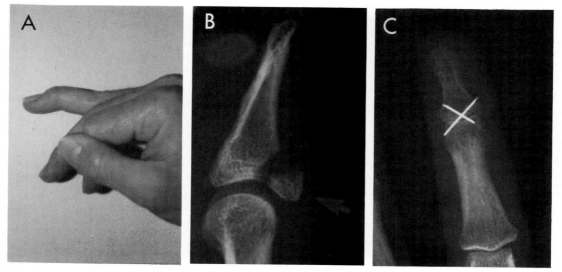

FIG 15–20.
A, mallet finger. A mild hyperextension deformity is present at the proximal interphalangeal joint. **B,** roentgenogram of a mallet finger with an avulsion fracture that required open reduction with internal fixation **(C).**

for 5 weeks (Fig 15–21). Vigilance is the key. The splint should not be removed by the patient until the treatment is complete. If the fracture fragment is large (over 25% of the joint surface) and displaced, the joint should be tested for stability (Fig 15–22). If the joint is stable, the same treatment is recommended, that is, treatment in hyperextension. If the joint is unstable or the fragment is quite large, surgical repair may be necessary.

Some lack of extension may persist regardless of treatment, but the functional result is usually satisfactory. Cases diagnosed after 4 to 6 weeks do not respond well to splinting. If a major fragment has been avulsed, surgical repair is often beneficial. If no fracture is present, the amount of actual functional loss that the injury represents to the patient should be assessed. If the impairment is minimal, which is often the case, then no treatment is indicated. Otherwise, surgical reconstruction is necessary.

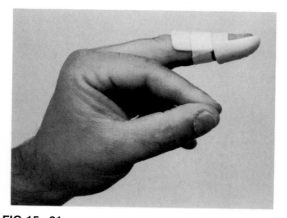

FIG 15–21.
Mallet finger splint maintaining the distal interphalangeal joint in hyperextension.

Flexor Digitorum Profundus Avulsion

The deep flexor may be avulsed from its attachment by sudden distal interphalangeal (DIP) hyperextension. The injury commonly occurs in football when a tackler grabs the jersey of the opponent. The tendon eventually retracts proximally into its sheath (Fig 15–23). If bone is avulsed, it may be evident, but otherwise, roentgenograms are not revealing.

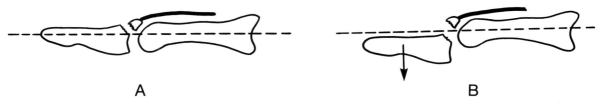

FIG 15–22.
Testing for subluxation of the distal phalanx. The phalanx is grasped, and volar pressure is applied **(A)**. If instability is present, the distal phalanx will sublux **(B)**.

Clinically, the volar aspect of the DIP joint is tender, and the patient is unable to flex the distal phalanx. The end of the tendon with its bony fragment may be palpable.

Treatment is by surgical repair. Early recognition is important because direct repair produces the best clinical results. Late cases may require tendon-grafting procedures.

PIP Joint Injuries

This joint is one of the most commonly called "jammed." Several different areas may be injured. A careful physical examination should always be performed in order to establish the diagnosis.

Central Slip Injuries

Damage to the central slip attachment to the middle phalanx is easily missed. The PIP joint is usually swollen, and if injury to the slip is present, there will be point tenderness on the dorsum of the joint. If the slip is completely avulsed, Elson's test is usually positive (Fig 15–24).

The diagnosis may be difficult. If untreated, the lateral bands gradually migrate into a volar position, anterior to the axis of rotation of the proximal interphalangeal (PIP) joint. The lateral

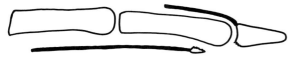

FIG 15–23.
Flexor digitorum profundus avulsion.

bands then become flexors of the PIP joint and hyperextend the DIP joint to produce the typical boutonniere deformity. Late loss of DIP flexion is the most disabling problem.

Roentgenograms are usually normal, although on rare occasions a fragment of bone may be avulsed (Fig 15–25).

Treatment. Whenever this injury is suspected, the PIP joint must be splinted for 4 to 6 weeks to allow healing. The PIP joint is placed in full extension, and the DIP joint is allowed movement. Chronic injuries may require reconstructive surgery, but the results are never as good as with acute care.

Volar Plate Injuries

The volar plate normally acts to protect the PIP joint and prevent hyperextension. It can be avulsed (with or without a bony fragment) by a forced hyperextension to the joint (Fig 15–26).

Clinically, there is usually local volar tenderness, and passive joint extension is painful. If untreated, hyperextension of the PIP joint may occur and produce a "swan-neck" deformity.

The injury is treated by splinting both interphalangeal (IP) joints in 20 degrees of flexion for 4 to 5 weeks.

Collateral Ligament Injuries

Rupture of either collateral ligament is usually the result of a dislocation but may occur with other injuries. Stress testing usually reveals the

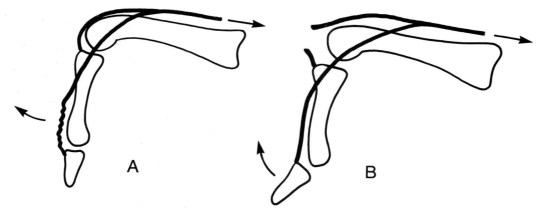

FIG 15–24.
Elson's test. The PIP joint is held firmly flexed over the edge of a table, and the patient is asked to extend the finger. If the central slip is intact, pressure will be felt against the middle phalanx, and the distal phalanx will remain flail **(A).** If the central slip is ruptured **(B),** the pressure will be felt at the distal phalanx, which will extend via the lateral bands.

diagnosis. Incomplete ruptures are treated by buddy-taping to the adjacent finger for 3 to 4 weeks. Complete ruptures are sometimes treated surgically, but good results are also obtained by splinting at 30 degrees for 5 to 6 weeks.

Interphalangeal Dislocations

These are common injuries and are almost always dorsal in direction (Fig 15–27). They are usually easily reduced. If they are stable following reduction, they may be treated by taping the finger to the adjacent finger in slight flexion for 3 to 4 weeks. Collateral ligament stability should always be evaluated.

Proximal Interphalangeal Fracture-Dislocations

Many minor IP joint injuries are accompanied by small "chip fractures." If the joint is stable, the fracture can usually be ignored and the joint injury treated conservatively by splinting for 4 to 5 weeks. A more serious injury is the fracture-dislocation or subluxation of the PIP joint (Fig 15–28). This injury should be suspected if any volar instability is present when the finger is tested in extension. Special splinting is usually necessary, and surgery may even be indicated.

Metacarpophalangeal Dislocations

These injuries are sometimes difficult to recognize. The index finger and thumb are more com-

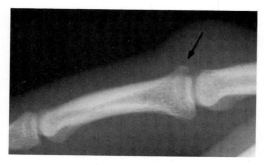

FIG 15–25.
Avulsion fracture of the central slip (arrow). Also note the dorsal soft-tissue swelling.

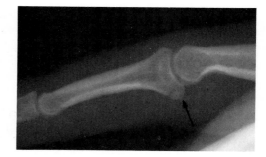

FIG 15–26.
Avulsion fracture of the volar plate (arrow).

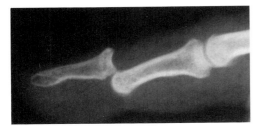

FIG 15–27.
Distal IP dislocation. Simple traction will usually reduce most IP dislocations. Occasionally, the joint must be hyperextended and the reduction accomplished by digital pressure.

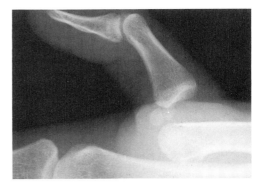

FIG 15–29.
Metacarpophalangeal dislocation of the thumb.

monly involved. The proximal phalanx is displaced dorsally (Fig 15–29). This injury often requires surgical reduction because the metacarpal head may buttonhole through the volar soft tissue. The more vigorous the attempt at reduction, the more the tissue tightens around the metacarpal neck. Closed reduction should be attempted, however. As after any reduction, the joint should "feel" reduced, and motion should be free. If the joint does feel reduced, soft-tissue interposition or an incomplete reduction should be suspected. Open reduction is then required.

Bowler's Thumb

This is a traumatic digital neuroma that develops from the irritation of the bowling ball against the digital nerve on the web side of the thumb. Pain and tenderness are present over the affected

nerve, and paresthesias may be present along the course of the nerve. A tender mass is usually present, and Tinel's sign may be positive. Rest and avoiding the offending activity are often curative. Changing the grip on the ball may also help, and protective devices are available to prevent recurrent irritation.

Gamekeeper's Thumb, "Skier's Thumb" (Ruptured Ulnar Collateral Ligament)

The radial and ulnar collateral ligaments of the metacarpophalangeal joint of the thumb prevent subluxation of the proximal phalanx and provide the stability that is necessary for normal pinch and grip (Fig 15–30). Either ligament may be chronically or acutely injured, but injury to the ulnar collateral ligament is more common and of more importance.

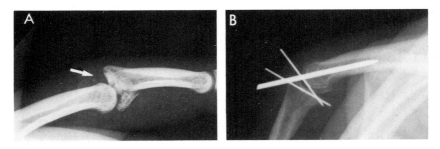

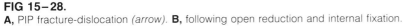

FIG 15–28.
A, PIP fracture-dislocation *(arrow).* **B,** following open reduction and internal fixation.

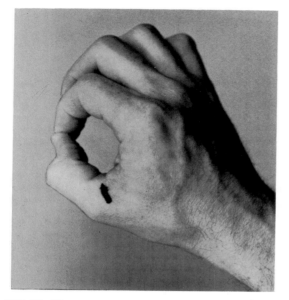

FIG 15–30.
The ulnar collateral ligament *(marked)* maintains stability of the thumb when pinching. Injury to this ligament may cause significant loss of strength of the thumb.

The patient usually has a history of a "sprained thumb," often from a fall on the hand. Chronic cases may have a history of instability, weakness with pinch, and recurrent effusions of the metacarpophalangeal joint. Local tenderness over the ligament and a joint effusion are usually present on physical examination. The ligamentous laxity is usually manifested clinically and may be confirmed by stress roentgenograms (Fig 15–31).

Surgical repair is indicated in acute cases. Partial ruptures are treated by immobilization for 5 weeks in a cast that includes the thumb. Chronic cases without traumatic arthritis are treated by ligamentous reconstruction. If the disorder has progressed to the point where degenerative arthritis is present, arthrodesis of the metacarpophalangeal joint is usually necessary.

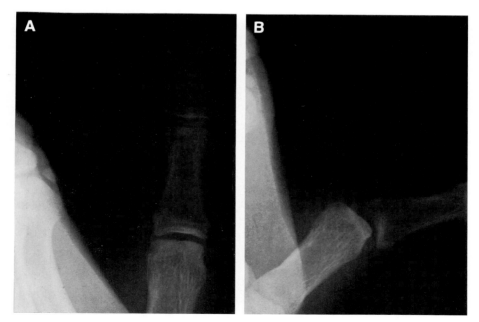

FIG 15–31.
Normal **(A)** and stress **(B)** roentgenograms of the thumb with complete rupture of the ulnar collateral ligament.

INJURIES TO THE LOWER EXTREMITY

The Knee

Injuries to Ligaments

Along with fractures, these are the most important injuries to diagnose immediately. The first individual on the sideline has the best chance to evaluate the knee before spasm and swelling develop. As previously described (see Chapter 11), the knee should first be palpated for specific areas of tenderness. With the knee flexed 30 degrees, the collateral ligaments are evaluated, and Lachman's test is performed. If possible, the cruciate ligaments are then tested with the knee flexed 90 degrees. Any acute rapid swelling suggests an anterior cruciate ligament rupture, especially if a "pop" is felt at the time of injury.

If only a minor strain is present, it may be possible for the athlete to return to activity, but any more severe injury should have a compression dressing and ice applied, and the activity should be ceased pending further evaluation.

Plain roentgenograms should always be performed. Stress films may be especially helpful in the adolescent with open growth plates. In this age group, epiphyseal fractures are more common than ligamentous injuries because the growth plate is weaker than the ligaments (Fig 15–32).

Injuries to the Meniscus

These are the most common of all knee injuries. They usually result from a twisting force applied to the knee with the extremity bearing weight. The athlete will experience sudden pain and is usually unable to continue playing. Swelling develops gradually in contrast to ligament injury. The pain may be localized to one joint line. The knee may actually lock if the meniscus is sufficiently torn and catches across the joint surface.

Suspected meniscus injuries are initially treated conservatively with a Robert Jones dressing, ice, quadriceps exercises, and elevation. Over the next several weeks, the response to rest and time will determine whether or not surgery will be necessary to remove the torn meniscus.

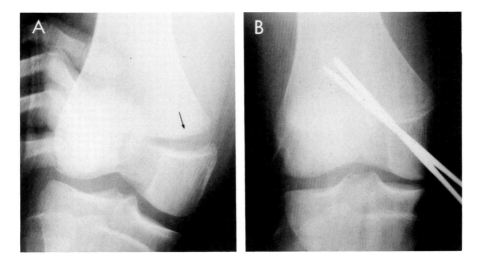

FIG 15–32.
A, stress roentgenogram of an epiphyseal fracture of the lower portion of the femur that easily simulates ligamentous disruption *(arrow)*. **B,** the same injury reduced and pinned.

The Role of Arthroscopy

Arthroscopy is a helpful adjunct in evaluation of the athletic knee. It is especially helpful in assessing two situations: (1) acute hemarthrosis and (2) chronic knee effusion. If acute joint swelling develops within 1 to 2 hours following injury, rupture to the anterior cruciate ligament must be suspected. This may be present in the absence of any clinical instability, although the usual tests for anterior cruciate laxity will usually show some abnormality. If an acute hemarthrosis is present and the individual is involved in more than simple recreational athletics, consideration should be given to arthroscopic evaluation of the anterior cruciate ligament. It is important to establish this diagnosis relatively soon so that the appropriate surgical repair and reconstruction may be undertaken. If the patient is only a recreational athlete, such major surgery is often not recommended, and therefore, arthroscopy is generally not indicated.

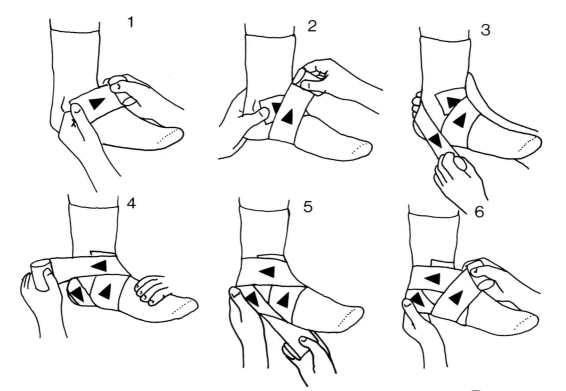

FIG 15–33.
The "Louisiana" ankle wrap. Approximately 100 in. of webbed bandage is used. The patient sits on the table holding the ankle at 90 degrees. The wrap may be applied over a stocking. Steps 1 and 2 secure the wrap; steps 3, 4, and 5 are the lateral and medial "heel locks" that prevent eversion and inversion, respectively. Following step 6, the procedure is repeated. The wrap is then spiraled up over the ankle, as shown in step 7, and secured with tape. This technique may prevent needless ankle taping.

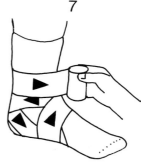

If a chronic effusion develops in the knee, it is important to determine the cause of swelling. The athlete should not be allowed to participate until the problem is resolved. There is little place for aspiration or steroid injection under these circumstances and certainly not until the cause of the effusion has been determined and appropriately treated. The most common cause of a chronic effusion in the knee is a torn meniscus, and arthroscopy may confirm the diagnosis. By special triangulation techniques, the torn piece of meniscus can usually be removed at the same time or repair performed.

Rehabilitation

A program of progressively increasing exercises to improve strength and endurance is begun on

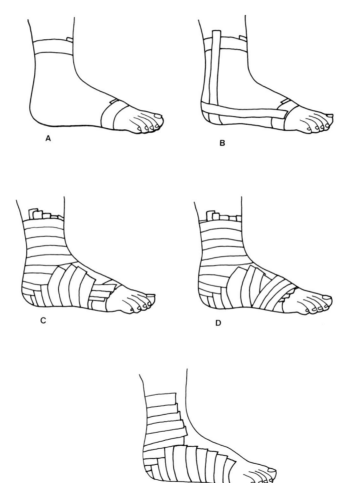

FIG 15–34.
The closed basket weave taping technique. **A,** two anchor strips are applied, one at the base of the gastrocnemius and one below the midfoot. **B,** the first stirrup and horizontal strips are applied. **C,** the finished weave. Close the strapping by alternating strips with stirrups. Overlap half the width of the tape. **D,** apply three circular anchoring strips distally and add a set of medial and lateral heel locks (not shown). **E,** the open Gibney method. No heel lock system is used. Whatever method is used, avoid taping too low, and avoid wrinkles.

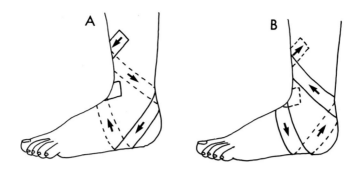

FIG 15–35.
The heel lock system. **A,** the lateral heel lock that prevents eversion. **B,** the medial heel lock that prevents inversion. Both may be applied together in a continuous wrap.

all athletes with injured knees as soon as tolerated (see Chapter 11). Specific exercises to strengthen the quadriceps, hamstrings, and calf muscles are begun. Progressive range-of-motion exercises are added as tolerated, and the athlete is allowed to return to activities only when the effusion and pain have completely subsided and strength, range of motion, and thigh circumference have returned to normal.

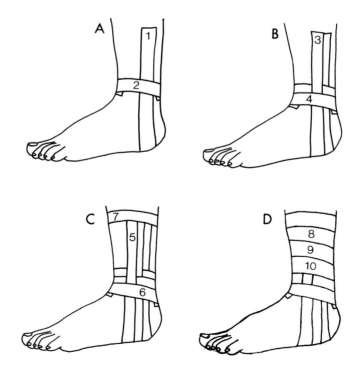

FIG 15–36.
The modified Gibney technique. **A,** the circular strip completely encircles the leg, and the vertical strips may extend as high as necessary. **B,** additional vertical and circular strips are added. **C,** a top circular strip *(7)* anchors the vertical strips. After the rest of the circular strips have been applied **(D),** heel locks should be added.

The Ankle and Foot

Ankle Sprains

The ankle sprain may be the most common of all athletic injuries. The lateral ligaments are the most frequently involved as a result of an inversion force (see Chapter 12). Mild to moderate sprains are best treated by early gentle motion (avoiding inversion) and exercise the day after the injury when pain begins to subside. Ice should be continued. Heat is never used. Peroneal muscle exercises are added and progressed against resistance as tolerated. More strenuous activity is allowed when the athlete is able to perform more vigorous activities such as hopping. Limited workouts may be resumed at this stage, but the ankle should always be taped. Return to full activity should not be allowed until there is full, pain-free motion and equal strength and the athlete is able to change direction quickly and jump without discomfort.

Treatment of severe sprains remains controversial. Surgery, casting, and simple symptomatic treatment have all been recommended with varying results. Recent studies have suggested improved results, in the athlete at least, following surgery. Casting may even prolong disability in the athlete, although applying a cast to the nonathlete makes activity more comfortable.

Wrapping And Taping

In order to prevent ankle injury, many physicians and trainers advise wrapping the normal ankle (Fig 15–33). A reusable dressing may be applied by the athlete over a sock.

Even though half of the support of tape loosens in 10 minutes, the athlete who has had previous injury will benefit from taping when activity

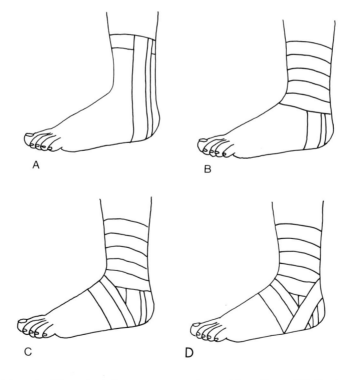

FIG 15–37.
A slightly quicker method than the Gibney technique uses an anchor and two stirrups **(A),** five to six circular strips **(B),** two to three arch strips **(C),** and a heel lock system **(D).**

is resumed. For this individual, wrapping is probably not adequate, and applying adhesive tape is necessary to prevent reinjury. Adhesive taping is more beneficial because it can be applied tighter and extended as high on the leg as necessary for protection.

Several taping techniques are commonly used. Each physician should become familiar with a single method and learn to apply it easily. The closed basket weave described by Gibney is the most commonly used (Fig 15–34). The open basket weave is the same except that the tape does not overlap in front. The open method may be used in acute sprains with excessive swelling because the tape is not circumferential and allows for swelling and ankle motion. An elastic wrap is applied over the open taping method.

The closed basket weave may be supplemented by a heel lock taping system for added medial or lateral support (Fig 15–35). With any method, the ankle is first prepared by shaving and spraying with adhesive spray or tincture of benzoin. Either 1- or 1½-inch tape is normally used. Many modifications of these techniques are used (Figs 15–36 and 15–37). Always be alert to a possible sensitivity to benzoin.

Athlete's Foot

Many varieties of fungus affect the foot. The most common areas of involvement are between the toes and under the arch. Moisture predisposes to their development. Allergy to stockings or shoe materials should be ruled out.

Treatment is with one of the many commercial medicated powders available. The foot should be kept dry, and stockings may need to be changed frequently.

MISCELLANEOUS PROBLEMS

Avulsion Fractures

Avulsions of the bony origin of muscles are common injuries in young athletes. The areas most commonly affected are (1) the coracoid process, (2) the greater tuberosity of the humerus, (3) the lesser and greater trochanters, (4) the iliac apophysis, (5) the ischial tuberosity, (6) the anterior superior iliac spine, and (7) the transverse and spinous processes of the vertebrae (Fig 15–38).

These injuries usually result from sudden muscular contraction or strain that causes the muscle to pull a portion of its bony attachment away from the main body of the bone. This causes sudden pain, and roentgenography usually reveals the injury.

Treatment will depend on the athlete and the area involved. The professional athlete may require open reduction and reattachment of the avulsed tendon. The recreational athlete is usually treated nonsurgically. Enough soft-tissue healing will occur to restore function. In spite of surgical repair, the skills of the professional athlete are sometimes diminished.

Brachial Plexus Injuries

An injury that is unique to American football players is sometimes referred to as the "burner" or "stinger." This is a bruise or stretching injury, usually of the upper brachial plexus, that often results from sudden depression of the shoulder with extension or lateral deviation of the neck to the opposite side. It is characterized by sudden unilateral burning pain originating in the neck and radiating to the shoulder, arm, and hand. It may be accompanied by weakness of the affected area. The injury is sometimes graded according to resolution of symptoms. Grade I injuries are most common. Typically, there is transient pain and motor loss that resolves within minutes or hours without any anatomic damage. Grade II and III are more severe, with evidence of nerve

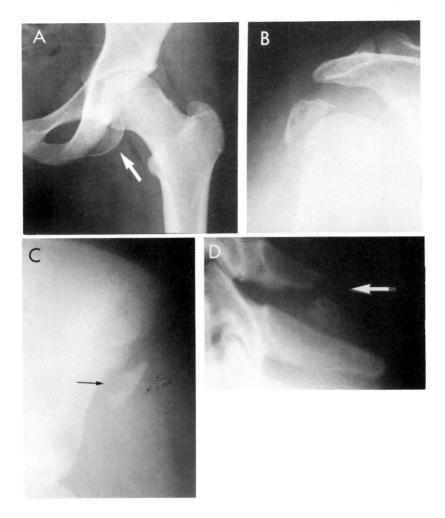

FIG 15–38.
Avulsion fractures. **A,** the ischial tuberosity. **B,** the greater tuberosity of the humerus. **C,** the anterior superior iliac spine. **D,** the spinous process of C6 ("clay-shoveler's" fracture).

injury lasting for weeks or months. These symptoms are usually *unilateral.* (Bilateral symptoms should cause concern for a *neck* injury.)

Evaluation

Any patient with neck pain with or without burning should not be moved until a complete medical evaluation is performed. It is important to determine whether the injury is *outside* or *inside* the cervical spine. On-the-field screening should

include an evaluation of (1) the location of pain and tenderness; (2) the amount of pain with isometric contraction of neck muscles; (3) deltoid, biceps, and triceps strength; and (4) range of neck motion. The latter should be evaluated very carefully.

Treatment

If the neck examination is negative and complete recovery (full strength and motion with no pain or tenderness) occurs in 1 to 2 minutes, the athlete may return to play. In most cases, the symptoms subside quickly. A protective collar worn inside the shoulder pads may prevent further injury. Repeated episodes, however, may be accompanied by demonstrable motor weakness, and this athlete should stop sports and undergo a complete evaluation.

If there are any signs of acute *neck* involvement (pain on neck movement, etc.) or transient cord symptoms, the player is not allowed to return to play. The neck is immobilized, and full neurologic and roentgenographic examinations are performed.

Prognosis

Most brachial plexus injuries are minor and recover in a short time without residuals. Prevention of neck injuries involves a good helmet and proper technique. Isotonic strengthening exercises for the neck by using a halter and weight system may also be beneficial. The athlete should break the habit of using the head as a ram in tackling or blocking.

Athletes with cervical spine instability, disc degeneration, or stenosis are at greater risk of serious neurologic injury and should be precluded from further participation in contact sports.

Turf Toe

This is a sprain of the metatarsophalangeal joint (MPJ) of the great toe that is often caused by hyperextension. The incidence has increased with greater use of artificial playing surfaces. The capsular structures are stretched and cause painful swelling. The injury may take several weeks to heal. The disorder is initially treated by ice and rest. A stiffer solid shoe that inhibits movement of the forefoot may be tried, and figure-of-8 taping to limit motion is usually helpful.

The "Loose-Jointed" Athlete

During the physical examination of the athlete, especially the adolescent one, it is important to note any characteristics or physical problems that might predispose the individual to injury. One determination that should always be made is whether the athlete is vulnerable to ligamentous or musculotendinous injury. It is possible to make some predictions in this regard if the athlete has loose or tight ligaments. The value of this determination is that the loose-jointed athlete is at higher risk for ligamentous injuries. The "tight-jointed" athlete is more vulnerable to muscular injuries. Some of the criteria used to determine whether an athlete is loose-jointed are as follows: (1) greater than 100 degrees of MP joint hyperextension, (2) greater than 30 degrees of ankle dorsiflexion with the knees straight, (3) the ability to touch the thumb to the forearm, (4) greater than 15 to 20 degrees of knee or elbow hyperextension, (5) the ability to touch the palms flat to the floor with the knees locked, and (6) the ability to stand with the feet turned out 180 degrees (Fig 15–39).

Loose-jointedness is often familial and affects the female athlete more often than the male. Laxity often diminishes during the late teenage

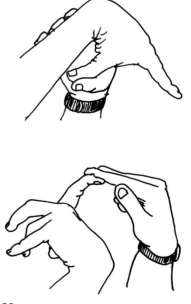

FIG 15–39.
Tests for loose-jointedness.

years, but before that time is reached, this athlete is vulnerable to injury, especially at the knee. This is commonly due to a subluxing patella or ligament damage.

The goal of treatment is prevention. Tight joints withstand stress better but often suffer more severe muscular injuries. These athletes require stretching exercises to increase flexibility and avoid muscular strain. The athlete with loose joints needs strengthening exercises to avoid ligamentous injury and sprain.

The Hip Pointer

This injury is a contusion of the iliac crest and is often seen in football players. It can be extremely painful, and a large hematoma frequently develops. Activities are allowed as tolerated, and a protective pad should be worn over the involved iliac crest for the remainder of the season.

BIBLIOGRAPHY

Adams JE: Bone injuries in very young athletes. *Clin Orthop* 1969; 58:129.

Albright JP, et al: Nonfatal cervical spine injuries in interscholastic football. *JAMA* 1976; 236:1243.

Cofield RH, Simonet WT: The shoulder in sports. *Mayo Clin Proc* 1984; 59:157–164.

Dobyns JH, et al: Bowler's thumb: Diagnosis and treatment. *J Bone Joint Surg [AM]* 1972; 54:751–755.

Elson RA: Rupture of the central slip of the extensor tendon of the finger. A test for early diagnosis. *J Bone Joint Surg [Br]* 1986; 68:229.

Jackson DW, Feagin JA: Quadriceps contusions in young athletes. *J Bone Joint Surg [Am]* 1973; 55:95–105.

James SL, Bates BT, Osternig LR: Injuries to runners. *Am J Sports Med* 1978; 6:40–50.

Light TR: Buttress pinning techniques. *Orthop Rev* 1981; 10:49–55.

Mannarino F, Sexson S: The significance of intracompartmental pressures in the diagnosis of chronic exertional compartment syndrome. *Orthopedics* 1989; 12:1415.

O'Donoghue DH: *Treatment of Injuries of Athletes,* ed 3. Philadelphia, WB Saunders Co, 1976.

Torg JS, et al: Neuropraxia of the cervical spinal cord with transient quadriplegia. *J Bone Joint Surg [Am]* 1986; 68:1354.

Tullos HS, King JW: Lesions of the pitching arm in adolescents. *JAMA* 1972; 220:264.

CHAPTER 16

Radiologic Aspects of Orthopedic Diseases

Dean F. Tamisiea, M.D.

Contained within this chapter are a radiologist's viewpoints and suggestions regarding the interpretation of bone roentgenograms that it is hoped will serve as a useful and practical guide for the busy family practitioner. Principles concerning roentgenographic positioning, anatomy, and pathology will be presented by utilizing a regional anatomic approach.

Additionally, the musculoskeletal applications of specialized radiologic modalities will be discussed. This will include comments on nuclear medicine procedures, diagnostic ultrasound, arthrography, xerography, angiography, and standard radiographic tomography. Importantly, the newer imaging technologies of computed tomography (CT) and magnetic resonance imaging (MRI) as they pertain to the evaluation of orthopedic problems will be detailed.

GENERAL CONSIDERATIONS OF ROENTGENOGRAPHIC BONE ANATOMY

Before beginning a detailed discussion of regional roentgenographic anatomy and pathology, a consideration of pertinent radiologic bone anatomy is important. A bone can be evaluated according to its various components (Fig 16–1).

Epiphysis

The primary growth center of a bone is termed the *epiphysis*. It contributes to the growth in length of the bone. It, as well as the following components, can be affected and changed in appearance by congenital, metabolic, nutritional, traumatic, and other disease processes.

Physis

The radiolucent band between the epiphysis and metaphysis constitutes the physis or epiphyseal cartilage plate. It is formed in part by the zone of provisional calcification.

Metaphysis

The metaphysis is characteristically splayed or funnel shaped. It is a favorite site for the development of benign as well as malignant lesions.

Diaphysis

The longer tubular segment of bone forms the diaphysis. The constituent parts include the central medullary cavity and spongiosa and the dense cortex lined internally by the endosteum and covered externally by periosteum.

Apophysis

There are several apophyses found throughout the skeletal system, the best example being the greater trochanter of the proximal portion of the femur. They do not contribute to bone growth but are considered accessory ossification centers.

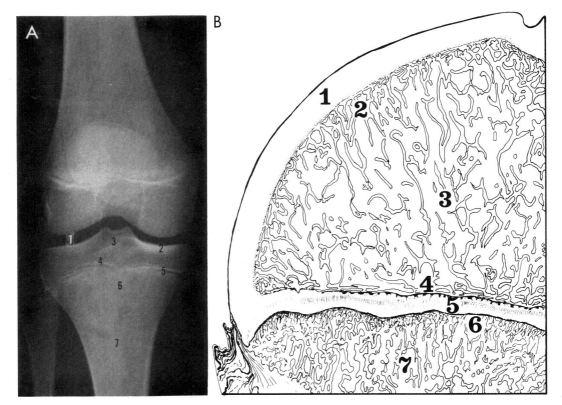

FIG 16–1.
Anatomy of a bone. **A,** radiologic terms: *(1)* articular cartilage does not show in the film; *(2)* white outline of the subarticular margin of the epiphysis; *(3)* epiphysis; *(4)* increased density of the terminal plate, inner bone margin of the epiphysis; *(5)* epiphyseal line, strip of lesser density, epiphyseal plate, diaphyseal-epiphyseal gap (roentgenographically, these terms exclude the recently calcified cartilage, which appears as part of the metaphysis); *(6)* metaphysis, including both calcified cartilage and newly formed bone, *(7)* diaphysis or shaft. **B,** histologic terms: *(1)* articular cartilage; *(2)* compact bone of subarticular margin; *(3)* epiphysis, spongy bone; *(4)* terminal plate; *(5)* physis, epiphyseal disc, growth cartilage (histologically, these terms include the calcified cartilage); *(6)* metaphysis, including only newly formed bone of primary ossification; *(7)* spongy bone of diaphysis. (From Pyle SI, Hoerr NL: *Radiographic Atlas of Skeletal Development of the Knee.* Springfield, Ill, Charles C Thomas Publishers, 1955. Used by permission.)

They tend to appear later than the epiphyses in normal bone development and form protrusions to which ligaments and tendons attach.

Epiphyses and apophyses occasionally fail to unite to the parent bone, and this results in unfused ossicles or accessory bones that are often misinterpreted as fractures. Most of these will be discussed under regional anatomic variations. When confronted with such problems as accessory bones, *An Atlas of Normal Roentgen Variants That May Simulate Disease* (Keats, 1988) and *Borderlands of the Normal and Early Patho-*

logic in Skeletal Roentgenology (Kohler and Zimmer, 1968) are excellent reference sources.

In addition to the status of nonfusion, epiphyseal and apophyseal centers can be divided before they unite and cause further confusion with fractures. Sesamoid bones, as seen in the hands and feet, can also be divided.

Bone Vessels

There is only indirect evidence of the presence of blood vessels on roentgenograms, and they are the nutrient canals and foramina. They enter the medullary cavity by way of foramina, most often near the midshaft of a long bone, and result in radiolucent channels. When viewed on the roentgenogram, one can be confused with a fracture.

Prominent nutrient canals frequently are seen in the diaphyses of the femur and tibia. Y-shaped nutrient canals occur in the midportion of the iliac bones of the pelvis and in the subspinous region of the scapulae.

ANALYTIC APPROACH TO BONE CHANGES

General Considerations

Rather than going into a great deal of confusing anatomic and pathologic detail, some basic fundamentals and principles related to bone roentgenograms will be discussed. The first and foremost rule is that every roentgenogram is abnormal until it is proved, after thorough examination, that everything is, indeed, normal. It may not work all of the time, but it encourages as complete a search of the film as possible. This results in two important objectives. First, it eliminates the method of instantaneous pattern recognition. Second, it prods the physician to search for even the slightest, most subtle change in bone roentgenographic patterns.

It is important to avoid tunnel vision; one should look at the "whole thing" from the corners of the film to the center. Evaluate separately the soft tissues, joints, bone density, architecture, and trabecular patterns. Scrutinize the medullary cavity and spongiosa as well as the cortex, periosteum, and endosteum.

In other words, attempt an analytic approach by evaluating each specific feature of bone. Visualize each detail separately. An obvious fracture catches one's attention, and the tendency is to forget the remainder of the picture, possibly missing an associated but unsuspected dislocation or even an early destructive tumor.

Taking two views of a bone at right angles is an important law in radiology. Never make a diagnostic interpretation on the basis of one view. The physician should not hesitate to obtain additional projections of the suspicious area if he is convinced that something is wrong. Comparative films of the opposite side are also often helpful, especially in younger patients whose growth centers cause more than enough confusion. And if the roentgenograms remain normal to the eye but clinical suspicion persists, have the patient return in 7 to 10 days for repeated films since it is not uncommon for a stress fracture, radial head fracture, or early osteomyelitis to have delayed appearances roentgenographically.

Once a bone lesion is discovered on an x-ray film, the physician is in the challenging position of forming a differential diagnosis. At first, the spectrum of possibilities might be quite broad, but by correlating historical, physical, and laboratory findings with the roentgenographic discovery, the spectrum can be narrowed to a few diseases and will, in most instances, lead to the correct diagnosis.

To permit the most accurate diagnosis, the differential list should be based on certain, specific bone responses that are most characteristic of the disease process. There are various distinctive visible reactions that bone may have to singular disease entities, such as the pattern of bone destruction or production, the type of periosteal reaction, and soft tissue involvement, if any.

Unfortunately, there are more diseases affecting bone than there are responses that bone can create. Consequently, there are more roentgenographic similarities than differences among the various bony lesions. For example, the periosteal reaction usually associated with Ewing's sarcoma, characteristically described as "onion skin," quite often occurs with osteomyelitis.

Conversely, there are specific disease processes that produce more than one kind of predictable bone reaction. Such is the case with osteomyelitis, whose periosteal response can appear benign but can also mimic malignant changes.

Any office or clinic that performs diagnostic x-ray film studies should have appropriate references available for proper positioning of the patient. Several technical books may be found to assist the nurse or technician when examining the various skeletal regions. A two-volume set by Merril, *Atlas of Roentgenographic Positions* and *Standard Radiologic Procedures,* is highly recommended.

Specific Parameters

There are certain specific parameters of bone that need careful attention. In the process of evaluating these, employing a systematic approach can lead to a logical conclusion. Among the criteria to be analyzed are an increase or decrease in bone density, alterations in osseous texture (trabecular pattern), periosteal reactions, and the conditions of the cortex, endosteum, and medullary spongiosa.

If any changes of these are observed, then the abnormality should be studied in terms of its size and configuration and the sharpness of its margins (transition zone); the specific bone involved and the position of the lesion within that bone (epiphysis, metaphysis, or diaphysis) should be noted. For example, leukemia, metastatic neuroblastoma, a benign simple cyst, and Brodie's abscess have a predilection for the metaphysis, whereas a chondroblastoma typically involves the epiphysis.

This is a simple, general outline with many more particulars coming into play. But by developing this type of approach, the many clues offered will help to determine the nature of the pathologic process and place the lesion into a certain category (for example, benign, malignant, infectious, traumatic, or metabolic). In Table 16–1 some of the specific characteristics of different bone lesions have been listed.

Many noteworthy textbooks are available that

TABLE 16–1.
General Characteristics of Different Bone Lesions

Characteristics of benign bone lesions
  Sclerotic margins (narrow transition zone)
  Homogeneous periosteal reaction
  Expansion of an intact cortex
Characteristics of solitary malignant bone lesions
  Permeative or moth-eaten destruction (wide transition zone)
  Irregular, sometimes spiculated periosteal reaction
  Preferential metaphyseal location
  Extraosseous extension with soft-tissue mass and occasional fluffy calcifications
Characteristics of metastatic lesions
  Absence of periosteal reaction
  Moth-eaten destruction of medulla and cortex
  Preferential diaphyseal location
  Pathologic fractures
  Multiple bone involvement
Characteristics of infection
  Often irregular periosteal reaction, no spiculation
  Bone destruction variable
  Diaphyseal involvement, often involving long segments
  Destruction of adjacent cartilage, crossing joints (majority of malignant neoplasms lack this ability)
  Sequestration and involucrum formation

cover this topic in greater detail (Edeiken and Hodes, 1989; Greenfield, 1975). However, there are two parameters that require more expanded discussion: types of bone destruction and periosteal reaction.

Patterns of Bone Destruction

Three roentgenographic patterns of bone destruction have been described according to Lodwick: geographic, moth-eaten, and permeative:

1. Geographic bone destruction is distinguished by single or multiple sharply marginated, relatively large, punched-out holes. Multiple myeloma and histiocytosis X (eosinophilic granuloma, Letterer-Siwe disease, and Hand-Schüller-Christian disease) tend to fit this pattern.

2. Moth-eaten bone destruction involves a lesion containing multiple, coalescing holes of moderate size that suggests a somewhat aggres-

sive process. Osteomyelitis and less pathogenic tumors may exhibit this form of destruction.

3. Permeative bone destruction is seen when the bony alterations are characterized by multiple, tiny holes that become smaller and fewer in number near the periphery of the lesion; as a result there is a wide transition zone from abnormal to normal bone. This will be seen in very aggressive tumors and poorly localized infections.

It is of interest that no matter what type of osseous resorption is taking place, as much as 50% of the bone must be destroyed before becoming evident roentgenographically. Radionuclide bone scans constitute a much more sensitive examination for determining the presence of bone replacement by the tumor or infection. In one recent comparative study, the accuracy of isotope imaging with technetium ^{99m}Tc phosphate complexes for skeletal lesion detection was 98%, as compared with 28% for standard roentgenography (Siberstein et al., 1973). Because of this fact, the use of skeletal roentgenographic surveys has declined in favor of nuclear scans. Nevertheless, although the sensitivity of scanning is high, its specificity is low, and therefore roentgenographic studies of the abnormal isotope areas are mandatory.

Types of Periosteal Reactions

When the outer periosteal membrane of bone is irritated, its constituent osteoblastic cells react by producing new bone. This new bone can take on either a solid or an interrupted appearance, and the specific form can assist in identifying the inciting cause (Table 16–2).

Solid periosteal reactions are usually indicative of a benign process. The new bone is consistently uniform in density. As seen in Table 16–2, the thickness and marginal characteristics vary according to the precipitating factor.

The interrupted forms of periosteal reactions are more commonly found in malignant disease, although benign lesions are occasionally responsible. The classic spiculated or sunburst pattern of osteogenic sarcoma and the lamellated or onion-skin periosteal reaction of Ewing's sarcoma come under this heading (see Table 16–2).

Of the various types of periosteal reactions, Codman's triangle is of special interest. This form is produced by a lifting up of the periosteum, which causes a break in its continuity and forms an angle. Thought to be pathognomonic of malignancy at one time, it is now known to develop in benign diseases as well. The sign can be induced by underlying infiltrating tumor cells, pus, or hemorrhage.

TABLE 16–2.

Roentgenographic Types of Periosteal Reactions*

Types	Examples
Solid periosteal reaction	
Thin	Eosinophilic granuloma, osteoid osteoma
Thin undulating	Hypertrophic pulmonary osteoarthropathy
Dense undulating	Vascular
Dense elliptical (with destruction)	Osteoid osteoma
Cloaking	Long-standing malignancy
	Chronic infection
Interrupted periosteal reaction	
Perpendicular (spiculated or sunburst)	Osteosarcoma, Ewing's sarcoma, infection
Lamellated (onion skin)	Osteosarcoma, Ewing's sarcoma, infection
Amorphous	Malignant tumors
Codman's triangle	Malignant tumors, infection, hemorrhage

*From Edeiken J, Hodes PJH: *Roentgen Diagnosis of Diseases of Bone.* Baltimore, Williams & Wilkins, 1967. Used by permission.

One other interesting periosteal condition is hypertrophic pulmonary osteoarthropathy. The uniform, thin, but solid undulating new bone, often associated with bone pain, is a relatively infrequent roentgenographic finding in individuals suffering from benign and malignant thoracic tumors, chronic obstructive pulmonary disease, and chronic lung infections. The exact mechanism is uncertain, but it may be related to decreased arterial oxygen tension.

REGIONAL ANATOMIC AND PATHOLOGIC ROENTGENOGRAPHY

Cervical Spine

Roentgenographic Examination
The standard roentgenographic views of the cervical spine include anteroposterior, lateral, and both posterior oblique views as well as an open-mouth anteroposterior projection of the odontoid process and the first two cervical vertebral segments (Fig 16–2). The majority of cervical spine studies are performed for the evaluation of trauma. In the more severely injured individual, the most important views are a cross-table horizontal beam lateral image and an anteroposterior supine film. By keeping patient movement to a minimum, potentially fatal spinal cord injury is prevented.

On the lateral exposure, C7 and occasionally C6 will often be excluded, especially in heavy, short-necked individuals. In such instances it becomes necessary to depress the shoulders by gentle but firm downward traction of the arms.

If the cervicothoracic junction still has not been adequately visualized and severe injury to the neck has been excluded, a so-called swimmer's view may be obtained. The patient lies in a prone-oblique position with the higher tube-side arm above the head and the lower table-side arm beside his body. The x-ray tube is angled 15 to 20 degrees toward the feet.

There are occasions when other special projections can be of assistance. Flexion and extension lateral views will often reveal minor degrees of subluxations resulting from damage to ligaments.

Dr. Don Weir of St. Louis University developed the "pillar view" for better evaluation of the lateral articulating masses, the superior and inferior articulating facets, and their intervening joints. Moreover, this view brings into focus the anterior and posterior margins of the lamina (Fig 16–3). The film is produced with the patient supine. Each side is done separately. The head is turned very slightly to one side, with the x-ray tube angled toward the feet 35 to 45 degrees and centered over the middle to lower vertebrae. The opposite side is then examined in a similar manner.

Roentgenographic Anatomy
In order to properly evaluate the cervical spine, a thorough understanding of its roentgenographic anatomy is an absolute prerequisite. Each component of the individual vertebrae should be appraised separately on all views.

Odontoid View. Of the seven cervical vertebrae, the first two are anatomically distinct. The odontoid represents a superior extension of the body of C2 and is actually the vestigial body of C1.

On the anteroposterior open-mouth film, the odontoid should be analyzed in terms of its position between the two lateral articulating masses of C1 (see Fig 16–2,D). The spaces between the lateral edges of the odontoid and the medial borders of the C1 articulating masses should be equal. However, minor degrees of rotation can produce spurious inequality of these interval distances. How can one determine this? The alignment of the densities of the spinous processes of C1 and C2 can be seen. If the C2 spinous process is to one side or the other, then rotation is present.

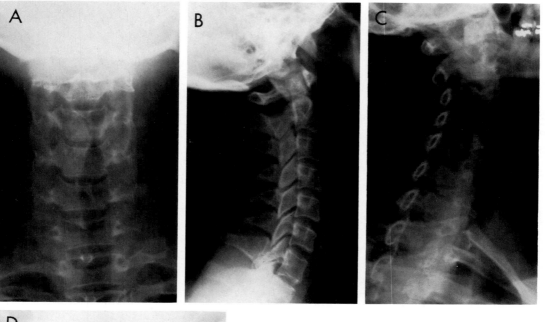

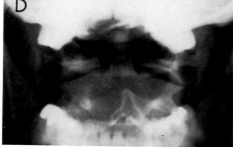

FIG 16–2.
Normal roentgenographic study of the cervical spine. **A,** anteroposterior view. **B,** lateral view. **C,** right oblique view. **D,** odontoid view.

Also on viewing the odontoid film, the transverse processes and lateral borders of the articulating masses of C1 and C2 should not be overlooked. The horizontal joints between the atlantoaxial articulating masses should be symmetric (see Fig 16–2,D).

Confusing artifacts superimposing on the odontoid can be misleading and can result in misinterpretation of fractures of this structure. The inferior margin of the posterior arch of C1 can overlie the base of the odontoid and create a "Mach" effect, a radiolucent line produced by overlap of the edges of two bones. In a similar fashion, the space between the two incisor teeth

may lay over the odontoid and yield an artifactual vertical cleft (Fig 16–4).

It is not unusual for the odontoid process to be completely obscured by the base of the occipital bone if the head is held too far in extension. In such circumstances, have the view repeated with the patient's head slightly more flexed.

Anteroposterior View. The straight anteroposterior film of the cervical spine demonstrates several specific structures. The vertical alignment of the spinous processes as well as the lateral margins of the articulating masses should be followed. The uncinate processes are the small tri-

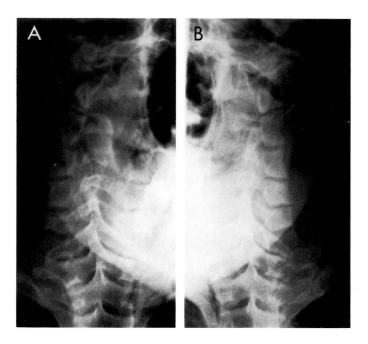

FIG 16–3.
Pillar views of the cervical spine. Right **(A)** and left **(B)** projections.

angular projections arising from the posterolateral margins of the vertebral bodies that by their apposition form the uncovertebral joints (also termed joints of Luschka). These establish the anterior boundaries of the intervertebral foramina. As synovial joints, they can be involved by degenerative osteoarthritis and produce the spurs that encroach on and narrow the foramina so as to result in impingement of the cervical nerve roots. In addition, being lined with synovium, they are subject to the alteration of rheumatoid arthritis and rheumatoid spondylitis. The foramina, however, are best evaluated on the oblique films.

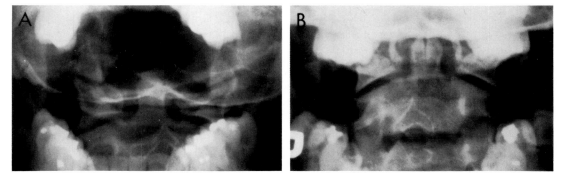

FIG 16–4.
Artifacts over the odontoid process simulating fractures. **A,** anterior arch of C1. **B,** cleft of the incisor teeth.

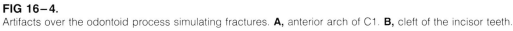

Lateral View.   Several important points must be remembered when viewing the lateral projection of the cervical spine (see Fig 16–2,B). Alignments of the anterior and posterior borders of the vertebral bodies, alignment of the lateral articulating masses, and alignment of the spinolaminar line are studied. The latter is formed by the anterior margins of the spinous processes, which also describe the posterior surface of the spinal canal. The superior extension of this line is in direct alignment with the posterior margin of the foramen magnum.

The distance between a line drawn through the posterior borders of the vertebral bodies and the spinolaminar line will provide the anteroposterior width of the spinal canal. This should measure no less than 13 mm from C3 through C7, being normally wider above C3. Any measurement less than this suggests the possibility of spinal stenosis.

The clivus at the base of the skull, which is a dense line continuous with the dorsum sella, is a helpful indicator for confirming normal craniovertebral alignment and should be included, at least in part, on all lateral studies of the cervical spine. A line drawn along its margin will pass through the posterior third of the odontoid.

The superior and inferior articulating facets will ordinarily be well visualized on the lateral film. The posterior borders of the lateral articulating masses should form a straight line (see Fig 16–2,B). If there is a slight offset, a facetal dislocation must be considered, although slight rotation can give a similar appearance. The view should be repeated if there is any confusion, and if the problem persists, tomography should be considered.

Measurement of the space between the anterior border of the odontoid and the posterior margin of the anterior arch of C1 is mandatory. This is an indicator of a possible transverse ligament tear and should measure no more than 5 mm in children and 3 mm in adults in neutral, flexion, and extension positions.

Finally, evaluation of the lateral cervical spine film is incomplete without an analysis of the prevertebral soft tissues. There are minor differences in the measurement from physician to physician and from patient to patient, but the width of the soft tissues at the level of the inferior margin of the C3 body should not exceed 5 to 7 mm. Any increase in this measurement indicates swelling from hemorrhage or infection.

Oblique Views.   The intervertebral foramina and surrounding elements, including the pedicles and uncinate processes, are the most important components demonstrated on the oblique views. The foramina on the right side are visualized on the left posterior oblique projection and those on the left on the right posterior oblique film (see Fig 16–2,C).

Trauma

Recognition of an abnormal cervical spine should be a relatively simple task once normal roentgenographic anatomy has been mastered. The primary objective, after a traumatic lesion has been identified, will be the establishment of whether or not the condition is stable. The stability of a fracture is best determined by grouping the type of injury according to the mechanisms of trauma, which are outlined in Table 16–3.

TABLE 16–3.

Classification of Cervical Spine Injuries According to the Mechanisms of Injury*

Flexion
  Subluxation
  Bilateral interfacetal dislocation
  Simple wedge fracture
  Flexion teardrop fractures
  Clay-shoveler's fracture
Flexion-rotation
  Unilateral interfacetal dislocation
Vertical compression
  Bursting fractures
    Jefferson's C1
    Bursting fractures, other levels
Extension
  Posterior neural arch fracture
  Extension teardrop fracture
  "Hangman's" fracture

*From Harris JH Jr: *Semin Roentgenol* 1978; 13:53–68. Used by permission.

From this classification, a statement of the instability of the injury can be made (Table 16–4).

Flexion Injuries.   There are a variety of flexion injuries, which are described below.

Subluxation.   The roentgenographic findings in this stable lesion may be minimal, often requiring flexion and extension lateral views for confirmation. The body and posterior elements remain intact, that is, show no fracture. However, there is major soft-tissue involvement. The interspinous and posterior longitudinal ligaments as well as the interfacetal joint capsules are disrupted at the affected level. This allows the involved vertebral body to rotate anteriorly about its anterior and inferior corner, along with upward and forward displacement of its inferior articular facet on the lower adjacent vertebra's superior articular facet. The interspinous distance widens, and the inferior intervertebral disc space narrows anteriorly and widens posteriorly. These alterations are accentuated on the flexion film

TABLE 16–4.

Classification of Cervical Spine Injuries Based on Stability*

Stable
  Subluxation
  Simple wedge fracture
  Unilateral interfacetal dislocation
  Bursting fracture, except Jefferson's fracture of C1
  Clay-shoveler's fracture
Unstable
  Bilateral interfacetal dislocation
  Flexion teardrop fracture
  Jefferson's bursting fracture of C1
  Hangman's fracture
  Extension teardrop fracture, unstable in extension but
    stable in flexion

*From Harris JH Jr: *Semin Roentgenol* 1978; 13:53–68. Used by permission.

(Fig 16–5). In young children under 8 years of age, with the head held in flexion, the second cervical vertebra will normally be displaced anteriorly over C3. This malalignment must not be mistaken for subluxation.

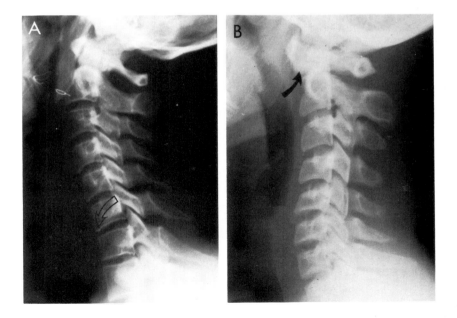

FIG 16–5.
Subluxation injuries of the cervical spine. **A,** mild subluxation of C6 and C7. **B,** atlantoaxial subluxation. Note the increased width of space between the odontoid and the anterior arch of C1 in **B.**

Bilateral Interfacetal Dislocation. A more severe form of subluxation, bilateral interfacetal dislocation represents a true unstable situation. The inferior articular facets of the involved vertebra not only move up and forward but also over the superior articular facet of the distal vertebra and come to rest within the intervertebral foramina. Oblique projections will be necessary to establish the diagnosis, but these have to be done with extreme caution. The changes on the x-ray film are related to a force sufficient to rupture all of the surrounding supporting ligaments at the level of the displaced vertebra. Occasionally, there will be an associated avulsion fracture.

Compression Fractures. Forceful flexion of the neck can result in an uncomplicated, simple wedge-shaped compression fracture of one and sometimes two or three vertebral bodies. Because they are stable, extension and flexion films are permissible.

Flexion Teardrop Fracture. Considered the most dangerous and unstable of all cervical spine injuries, flexion teardrop fractures are diagnosed on the cross-table lateral film only, with no indications or justification for acquiring further studies. The name of the lesion is derived from the fact that there is a fracture through the inferior and anterior corner of the body, but the major component is comminution of the body. The posterior fragments become displaced backward into the spinal cord, with consequential acute and severe neurologic deficits. The posterior neural arch is also frequently fractured.

Clay-Shoveler's Fracture. The name of this lesion is derived from the injury acquired by people in occupations in which heavy lifting is required. This injury consists of a fracture through the spinous process of either C6 or C7. There is no significant ligamentous damage, and therefore a stable condition exists. Since C7 is sometimes difficult to project on the lateral film, the fracture can be missed. A clue might be apparent on the frontal film, where an extraspinous

process fragment is sometimes evident as the result of inferior displacement. An unfused apophysis of a spinous process must not be misinterpreted as a fracture (Fig 16–6).

Flexion-Rotation Injuries. When the cervical spine is subjected to a rotational force in addition to flexion, a unilateral interfacetal dislocation may be observed (Fig 16–7). An inferior articular facet of one body is displaced over the adjacent superior articular facet of the next inferior vertebra on one side only. The dislocated facet is more or less locked in place, but due to associated ligament damage the lesion may be unstable; therefore, flexion and extension views are contraindicated. Oblique projections are most productive in identifying the displaced facet, but it may be suggested on the lateral film when the margins of the facets of a single vertebra do not superimpose on one another as the result of rotation. Additionally, a line drawn through the posterior borders of the bodies is offset at the level of the suspected injury.

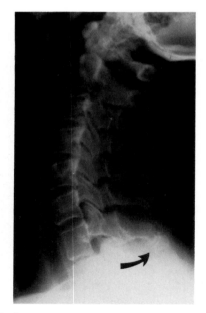

FIG 16–6.
An unfused apophysis of the spinous process of C7 simulates a fracture *(arrow)*.

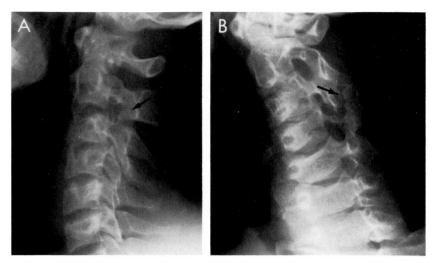

FIG 16–7.
Unilateral interfacetal dislocation. **A,** lateral view. **B,** oblique view.

Extension Injuries.   Various extension injuries are described as follows:

Posterior Neural Arch Fractures.   The neural arch of one vertebra may be compressed between the posterior elements of the two adjoining vertebrae during maximal forced extension. A unilateral or bilateral fracture may be sustained. If bilateral, the fragment can be displaced posteriorly, yet there will be no encroachment on the neural canal; thus the situation is a stable one (Fig 16–8).

Extension Teardrop Fracture.   Similar to the flexion variety, an extension teardrop fracture demonstrates a triangular-shaped fragment at the anterior-inferior margin of the body, most often involving C2, although other levels are affected. The injury, however, is not quite as severe because there is no posterior involvement. When the neck is held in flexion, there is stability of the spine since the posterior ligament complex is intact. However, instability occurs during extension since the minor fragment remains attached to the anterior longitudinal ligament but not to the parent body.

Hangman's Fracture-Dislocation of C2.   This lesion consists of vertical disruption of both pedicles of C2 and is created by flexion forces against the extended vertebrae. The body of C2 is thrust forward over C3, with concomitant rupture of both the anterior and the posterior longitudinal ligaments giving rise to an unstable injury (Fig 16–9).

Vertical Compression Fractures.   A considerable force directed through the vertical axis of

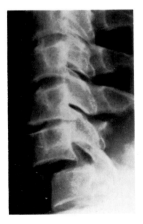

FIG 16–8.
Posterior neural arch fracture.

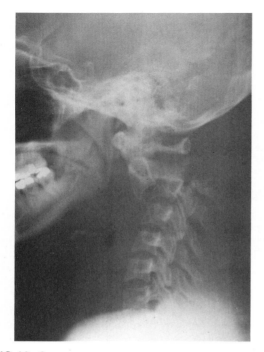

FIG 16–9.
Hangman's fracture-dislocation of the second cervical vertebra.

Although vertebra plana is not usually related to trauma, it might be mistaken for a compression fracture. This very rare condition, in most instances related to eosinophilic granuloma (histiocytosis X), has the appearance of a pancake with extreme, uniform flattening of the body but with preservation of the posterior elements. Some other possible causes for this unusual finding are metastasis, multiple myeloma, osteochondritis of the primary ossification center of the body (Calvé's disease) and postradiation osteitis.

Thoracic and Lumbar Spine

Roentgenographic Examination

The thoracic spine is ordinarily examined by means of anteroposterior and lateral films. However, due to the superimposition of the shoulders, the upper three to four vertebrae will be omitted from the lateral view, and if clinical symptoms point to this region, an oblique swimmer's projection should be obtained.

It is generally agreed that the above films will offer optimum information about the anatomy of the thoracic vertebrae. However, either or both oblique views of no more than 10 to 20 degrees can be obtained and provide a different aspect of a questionable or subtle change in the vertebral bodies or articulating facets.

Routine roentgenographic examination of the lumbar spine must be composed of anteroposterior, lateral, and both oblique projections as well as a cone-down lateral film of the lumbosacral joint.

Roentgenographic Anatomy
Anteroposterior View. On the anteroposterior study, the 12 thoracic and 5 lumbar bodies will show a slight increase in size from top to bottom. The height, width, and alignment of the bodies and their cortical margins, trabecular architecture, and density need to be scrutinized carefully.

Subsequently, the round-to-oval pedicles need to be evaluated separately. They overlie the superolateral corner of each body and, like them, be-

the spine (such as a large object falling on top of the head or a diving injury) can produce the so-called bursting fractures of the cervical vertebrae. The least common type is the Jefferson fracture of C1. The anterior and posterior aspects of the ring are fractured on both sides, with bilateral lateral displacement of the fragments. This unstable injury can be apparent on the open-mouth anteroposterior film but more reliably is distinguished on the lateral roentgenogram where the fractures are seen to extend through the posterior arches.

Vertical compression or bursting fractures more frequently involve the middle and lower cervical vertebral segments. The longitudinally oriented pressures cause the intervertebral discs to impact against the end plates of the bodies. Ordinarily there is no instability because the posterior elements remain intact. When viewed on the anteroposterior film, a vertical fracture line is identified within the involved body.

come progressively large inferiorly. The density and sclerotic cortical margins should be noted for any alterations because they are involved in a number of pathologic processes.

The interpedicular distance, a line drawn between the inner boundaries of a vertebral body's pedicles, is an important observation throughout the spine. It affords an indirect evaluation of the size of the neural canal.

The transverse processes in the thoracic spine become smaller from superior to inferior, are oriented posterolaterally, and are located behind the intervertebral foramina. The normal articulations of the ribs should not be overlooked. In the lumbar spine the transverse processes are more laterally oriented and are much larger, the processes of the third vertebra usually being the largest.

On the anteroposterior projection, the spinous processes provide another guide for the evaluation of alignment. Rarely, they may be absent because of aplasia or due to malignant or infectious destruction.

Additionally, on the anteroposterior view, the paravertebral soft tissues should be studied. An increase in the width of the soft tissues will alert the clinician to a possible fracture, neoplasm, or infection in the spine, the result of hematoma, infiltrating tumor cells, or bacterial extension, respectively. The psoas margins in the paralumbar region are fairly sensitive indicators to similar changes when they become obliterated. This abnormal change can also reflect lymphadenopathy or urinary lesions such as a perirenal abscess. In fact, when viewing the lumbar spine, the clinician should always attempt to delineate the psoas and renal margins as well as search for urinary tract calculi as causes of back pain.

Lateral View. One of the goals for studying lateral views of the thoracolumbar spine is to ensure normal alignment of the anterior and posterior borders of the vertebral bodies. Furthermore, the cortical outlines and the internal structure of the bodies must be mentally recorded. Any narrowing of the intervertebral disc spaces

can be established. In the thoracic spine, the intervertebral foramina can be seen on end but require oblique views for their proper visualization in the lumbar area.

The inferiorly directed spinous processes, as seen on the lateral film, may require a "hot" light to be adequately seen but should not be neglected for reasons mentioned previously.

Oblique Views. Important anatomic features are introduced on the oblique views of the lumbar spine. These details have been covered more extensively in Chapter 7. On the left posterior oblique film (left side down against the film), the left half of the posterior neural arch elements, including the intervertebral foramina, are identified, whereas the right half of these components are viewed on the opposite projection. In the cervical spine, the reverse condition exists.

Developmental Variations and Congenital Abnormalities

Confusing anatomic variations are seen in the developing and mature spine. In infancy the vertebral bodies are egg shaped on lateral view. The upper and lower anterior corners are beveled until the apophyseal vertebral rings appear about each end plate. They fuse with the body by the 15th year, but occasionally they remain ununited and, except for the presence of a complete sclerotic border, often are confused with a corner fracture (Fig 16–10).

On the anteroposterior film, a vertical radiolucent cleft is seen superimposing on the vertebral bodies (Fig 16–11). This represents the normal uncalcified portion of the posterior neural arch and spinous process and is not to be confused with spina bifida. At approximately 3 to 5 years of age, these will ossify and fuse. When they do fail to fuse completely, the cleft persists as a spina bifida occulta. This can occur anywhere in the spine, but is most common at L5. These are of no clinical importance.

True spina bifida is the result of a very wide defect in the posterior neural arch, usually involving multiple vertebrae and commonly found

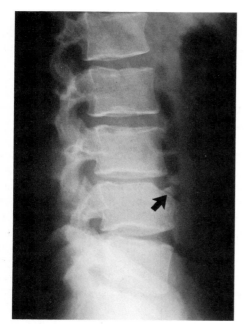

FIG 16–10.
An unfused ring apophysis of a lumbar vertebra as seen here can be confused with a fracture.

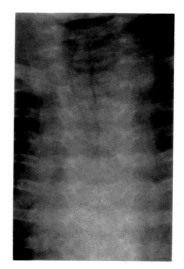

FIG 16–11.
Normal thoracic spine of an infant. Note the vertical cleft of the neural arch.

in the lumbar region. The widened spinal neural canal is evidenced by an increased interpedicular distance. These may be associated with a meningocele that produces a prominent posterior soft-tissue density on the roentgenogram.

This wide gap of the dorsal arch and increased interpedicular width should also bring to mind the possibility of diastematomyelia, a condition in which the cord is divided by an intraspinal cartilaginous, fibrous, or bony spur. This has a predilection for the thoracolumbar junction. Syringomyelia can produce a similar appearance in the cervical spine where there is cystic dilation of the cord. The same type of appearance can also be seen with intraspinal tumors such as lipomas or dermoids.

Vascular channels may give rise to confusing appearances. Blood vessels perforate the anterior cortical borders of each body and form a radiolucent line termed the clefts of Hahn. A similar vascular defect that becomes more apparent in adulthood may exist along the posterior margin of the body.

Hypoplasia of the vertebrae, fusion or block vertebrae, and hemivertebrae constitute a few of the other spinal anomalies that may be encountered (Fig 16–12).

Trauma

The focus of attention will now be shifted to some of the traumatic lesions involving the thoracolumbar spine. The majority of injuries will disturb the muscular and ligamentous structures surrounding the spine. Just as in the cervical spine, the only visible roentgenographic findings may be scoliosis and/or straightening of the normal curvatures, which indicates muscle spasms.

When a fracture is present, the usual appearance is that of a wedge-shaped compression deformity, the result of hyperflexion forces. Avulsion-type corner fractures of the anterosuperior body result from extension forces. They appear as a very sharp, nonsclerotic fragment as opposed to an unfused apophysis.

Quite frequently, the dilemma of determining the age of a fracture presents itself. In long-standing compression fractures, degenerative changes with hypertrophic spurs arise along the articular margins, and there may be an unpre-

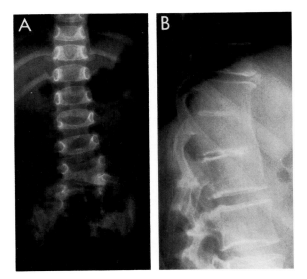

FIG 16–12.
Anomalies of the spine. **A,** hemivertebra of the lumbar spine. **B,** fusion or block vertebrae.

dictable degree of eburnation. Yet at times, these changes are absent, and the determination of age may be difficult if not impossible. Radioisotopic bone scans that utilize technetium 99m phosphate compounds then become a valuable aid. Within 2 to 5 days of the injury, a recent collapse will show an increased uptake of the isotope, whereas older lesions will show no activity. However, the abnormal uptake may remain detectable for 18 to 24 months or longer, depending in part on the extent of the fracture and its location.

Wedge-shaped deformities of the vertebral bodies necessitate differentiation from other causative processes such as Scheuermann's disease. This represents a form of osteochondritis or aseptic necrosis that involves the end-plate ring apophyses and is seen in adolescents. Described as juvenile kyphosis, it predominates in the thoracic region. Schmorl's nodes commonly accompany this spinal affliction. These are rounded-to-oval protrusions of the anterior margins of the end plates and develop from focal intrabody herniation of the nucleus pulposus.

Biconcave deformities of the bodies, or so-called fish vertebrae, have a predisposition for the thoracic and lumbar location. They represent a chronic progressive form of compression characteristically seen in postmenopausal patients with osteoporosis. Vertebral body compression fractures with a history of minimal or no trauma should alert the physician to the possibility of a metastatic or primary malignant process.

Another important traumatic lesion, particularly of the lumbar spine, that can be easily ignored is the transverse process fracture (Fig 16–13). The importance of its recognition rests with the fact of frequently related renal injury. It is important not to mistakenly call the unfused apophysis of the transverse process a fracture.

A seldom-seen injury to the lumbar vertebrae is the Chance fracture (Fig 16–14). An extreme flexion force, often related to seat belt injuries, causes a fracture through the spinous process, across the neural arch or lamina, and into the posterosuperior aspect of the vertebral body. An isolated fracture of the spinous process is uncommon in the thoracic and lumbar regions.

One more pitfall to watch for in the assessment of spinal trauma is the unfused ossification center of the articular facets, which can resemble a fracture (Fig 16–15). In evaluating the poste-

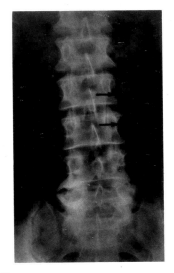

FIG 16–13.
Transverse process fractures of the lumbar spine. Note the lucent fracture lines *(arrows)* at the bases of the processes of L3 and L4 on the left. Incidentally, the patient demonstrates lumbarization of the S1 segment.

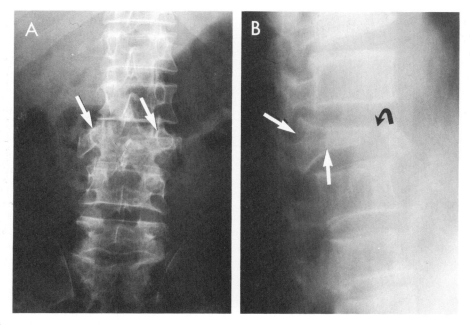

FIG 16–14.
Chance fracture of the lumbar spine that extends through the body into the posterior neural elements and can be seen in individuals wearing seat belts. **A,** anteroposterior view demonstrating lateral displacement of the pedicles *(arrows).* **B,** lateral view showing a fracture extending through the body *(curved arrow)* and involvement of the neural arch *(straight arrows).*

rior elements, it is important to keep in mind the entities of spondylolysis and spondylolisthesis (see Chapter 7).

Tumors

Except for metastatic neoplasms to the spine, tumors—both benign and primary malignant lesions—are very infrequent. The vertebrae are the most commonly affected portion of the skeleton for metastasis and account for approximately 40% of all secondary tumors of bone. A few of the common and not-so-common tumors will be disussed.

Hemangioma. Hemangiomas of the vertebral body may be the most common benign tumor, although few have been documented pathologically. Typically, their appearance is that of increased vertical trabeculations producing a somewhat striated pattern (Fig 16–16). They should not be confused with Paget's disease or

osteoblastic metastasis, whose descriptions are forthcoming.

Aneurysmal Bone Cyst. Of the benign tumors of the spine, aneurysmal bone cysts are possibly the next most frequent after hemangiomas. Of course, they are more commonly found in the extremities, especially the distal portion of the femur. In the spine they tend to involve the posterior elements as well as the body. Possessing a thin shell of peripheral bone, they are expansile and cystic in nature. Roentgenographically, a malignant appearance can be seen with a predominant cystic pattern. Unlike other tumors, benign and malignant alike, aneurysmal bone cysts have the unique capability of crossing over the cartilaginous disc space to involve adjacent vertebrae. A malignant chordoma also has this potential.

Osteoid Osteoma. A benign tumor that can produce significant and disabling pain is the os-

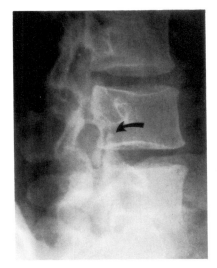

FIG 16–15.
Unfused apophysis of the superior articular facet of L5 *(arrow).*

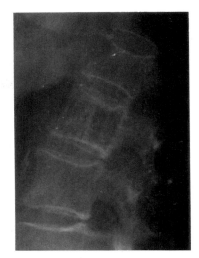

FIG 16–16.
Hemangioma of a vertebral body.

teoid osteoma. Most frequently found in the extremities, this tumor can involve the spine on rare occasions and must be considered in the differential diagnosis of back pain. It is one of many causes of scoliosis. The lesion is almost always limited to the neural arch, a position that often prevents its detection on conventional roentgenographs. Tomography and isotopic bone scanning may be required for its recognition. It is composed of a small radiolucent nidus sometimes containing calcifications. A very dense reactive sclerosis surrounds the central nidus and often obscures it.

Osteoblastoma.   An osteoblastoma is a benign lesion that classically involves the spine, primarily the dorsal elements. Because of its varied histologic appearances, it has been described as a giant osteoid osteoma, and certain cases may even mimic osteogenic sarcoma.

A wide variety of primary malignant tumors may involve the spine, only a few of which will be mentioned. Such tumors may be seen anywhere in the spine but have a preference for the sacrococcygeal region.

Multiple Myeloma.   The most common primary malignant tumor of bone is multiple myeloma. The classic picture of "punched-out" lesions, particularly evident in the skull, is characteristic but not that frequent. The usual presentation is diffuse demineralization. Multiple vertebral compression deformities form in a progressive nature.

Sarcoma.   Osteosarcoma, fibrosarcoma, and chondrosarcoma involve the spine only rarely and usually in the sacrum. These tumors may arise in an area of previous irradiation, Paget's disease, or fibrous dysplasia.

Round-Cell Tumors.   Ewing's sarcoma and reticulum cell sarcoma are rarely encountered in the vertebral column. They have more of a predilection for the appendicular skeleton but must be included in the differential diagnosis of destructive lesions.

Hodgkin's Lymphoma.   Hodgkin's disease can occasionally be seen within the bony spine and may present as an osteolytic or osteoblastic alteration or a combination of the two. More commonly, however, para-aortic lymph node involvement with lymphoma will produce erosive changes of the vertebral cortical margins.

In the same way and as an interesting sidelight, an aortic aneurysm can cause pressure destruction of the vertebra. A massively enlarged heart such as that in mitral stenosis can produce extrinsic changes of the thoracic spine. It is of interest that elderly individuals who ordinarily demonstrate degenerative spurs of the thoracic spine will only show them to any extent on the right side; apparently, the pulsating aorta prevents their formation on the left.

Chordoma and Sacrococcygeal Teratoma.

There are two primary malignant tumors of the spine that are classified as developmental. A chordoma is an invasive lesion arising from remnants of the primitive notochord and therefore can presumably occur anywhere along the vertebral column, although there are no reported cases of its occurrence in the thoracic region. The sacrum is the most popular site and accounts for approximately 50% of cases. An intracranial chordoma located along the clivus represents about 30% of cases, and the remaining 20% originate in the cervical and lumbar areas. Roentgenographically, the tumor presents as an expansile, lytic process with moderate soft-tissue extension. As noted previously, it may cross the disc space cartilage, an uncommon occurrence of any tumor but typical of infections. In one third of the tumors, calcifications are observed.

The second type of developmental primary malignant tumor is a sacrococcygeal teratoma. Sixty percent of these lesions, however, are benign but exhibit some degree of localized infiltration. They are found in infants within the pelvis around the parasacral region. Malformation of the spine can be an associated finding. They appear, roentgenographically, as variable-sized soft-tissue masses, often with calcifications or ossifications within them. The rectosigmoid colon is extrinsically displaced forward. Destructive changes will be present to some extent within the sacrococcygeal bony structure.

Infection

For obvious reasons, infections involving the spine have decreased in frequency over the years. Nevertheless, this must be considered in the differential diagnosis of a painful back and abnormal roentgenographic findings.

Acute bacterial infections or pyogenic spondylitis can involve either the disc space, the vertebral body, or both. The former condition, termed pyogenic discitis, is more common in the younger population, apparently on the basis of a healthy vascularization of the cartilage and, therefore, easy access by blood-borne bacteria. This results in a closed-space infection that can secondarily extend into the bodies.

On the other hand, infection of the vertebral body, particularly its anterior two thirds, is more commonly identified in the adult. Originating in the substance of the body, the infection may then secondarily involve the interspace by extension.

An important principle in pathophysiology should be re-emphasized at this point. Cartilage serves as no barrier to the extension of infection and thereby is vulnerable to destruction. Conversely, the disc cartilage is very resistant to malignant cellular infiltration so tumors tend to remain confined to the body.

In both pyogenic discitis and vertebral osteomyelitis, the earliest roentgenographic findings may be joint space narrowing. Depending on the aggressiveness of the offending bacteria and the time of institution of therapy, the surrounding bone will show varying degrees of demineralization brought on by hyperemia. The end plates will then demonstrate progressive loss of continuity with irregular destruction and focal areas of subchondral reactive sclerosis. Extension into the posterior third of the body, then into the dorsal appendages as well as into the adjoining vertebrae, may occur. The body may eventually collapse. Some degree of surrounding soft-tissue swelling is invariably present and detectable on roentgenograms.

Tuberculosis of the spine, or Pott's disease, is an extreme rarity among the abnormal spine

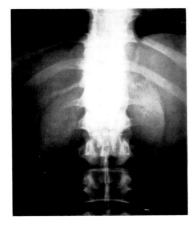

FIG 16–17.
Pott's disease of the spine. The chronic tuberculous process has resulted in calcified paravertebral psoas abscesses.

not always the situation. An occasionally prominent feature is a large paravertebral soft-tissue mass that constitutes the abscess. In later phases, there may be extensive calcification within this mass. The bony structures will show a decrease in density, and there will be narrowing of one or more of the disc spaces. The margins of the end plates will manifest irregular destruction, and a mottled sclerotic and lytic appearance will extend into the bodies, which display varying degrees of compression (Fig 16–17).

Paget's disease

One of the distinctive roentgenographic characteristics of spinal Paget's disease is that the disorder involves the entire vertebra—the body and all of the posterior elements, including the transverse and spinous processes (Fig 16–18). Generally, there is an increase in density produced by a thickened trabeculae. A picture frame appearance can be imparted to the body, the result of a dense peripheral margin of thickened cortex. Furthermore, there is an actual increase in volume of the entire vertebra. This finding, along with total vertebral involvement, distinguishes Paget's disease from an osteoblastic metastasis.

studies of today. The vertebral column remains the most common skeletal site for this chronic infection. The midthoracic and thoracolumbar junctions constitute the most prevalent sites of involvement.

Because of its insidious and chronic nature, the spinal lesions are usually advanced when first examined roentgenographically, although this is

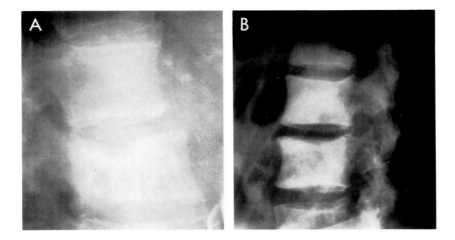

FIG 16–18.
Spinal Paget's disease and osteoblastic metastasis. **A,** Paget's disease demonstrates increased trabeculations, a bone-within-bone appearance, and increased volume including the pedicles. **B,** osteoblastic metastasis.

The Shoulder

Roentgenographic Examination

In the majority of cases, a complete and optimal roentgenographic study of the shoulder girdle need only include upright—standing or sitting—anteroposterior views with the humerus in internal and external rotation. These two projections will usually permit adequate evaluation of the bony structures constituting the shoulder.

On these roentgenograms the complete clavicle should be visualized as well as the entirety of the scapula and at least the proximal third of the humerus. Special attention should be given to the alignments of the glenohumeral, acromioclavicular, coracoclavicular, and sternoclavicular joints. The tuberosities of the humeral head and its articular surface should be specifically scrutinized. The acromium and coracoid processes, in addition to the borders and flat surfaces of the scapula, require attention.

The standard examination, of course, may require modification because there are certain situations when special views must be obtained for better delineation of specific structures. In an acutely injured shoulder in which immobilization of the shoulder is required, the humerus will ordinarily be held in internal rotation. In order to obtain roentgenograms of the humerus in external rotation without moving the arm, the patient can be positioned by rotating him 40 degrees posteriorly with the affected side toward the film. Because of pain, this requires that the patient be sitting or standing.

Upright exposures are also beneficial in demonstrating fat-fluid levels. This occurs when a fracture has extended into the joint through the articular cortex; this most often happens with fractures of the greater tuberosity. Such information is useful since articular cartilage damage is certain, and the patient should be informed that degenerative osteoarthritis in time is a possibility.

When there is suspicion of a fracture involving the shaft of the humerus below the neck, in addition to an anteroposterior view, a transthoracic lateral projection is necessary for evaluation of alignment (Fig 16–19). The glenohumeral relationship can also be accessed with proper exposure, but because of superimposed ribs, fractures above the neck are difficult to see. Instead, a trans-scapular study will be more helpful (Fig 16–20). This view is obtained by having the patient face the film at an angle of 45 degrees with the affected side toward the film holder. The resultant picture forms a Y where the acromium, coracoid, and scapular body intersect. The humeral head will be superimposed on the Y. This is useful not only for fractures but also for posterior dislocations. This trans-scapular examination is always utilized when studying the scapula in addition to the routine anteroposterior roentgenogram.

Posterior shoulder dislocations are notorious for their ability to avoid detection on the standard anteroposterior views, and the tangential projection is an excellent means for detecting the abnormality. This is performed by angling the x-ray tube approximately 30 degrees so that the central ray passes tangentially across the glenoid

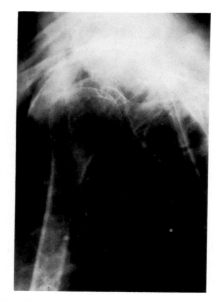

FIG 16–19.
Transthoracic view of the shoulder.

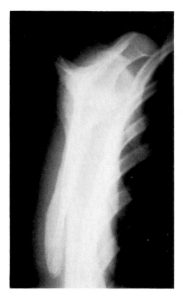

FIG 16–20.
Trans-scapular view of the shoulder.

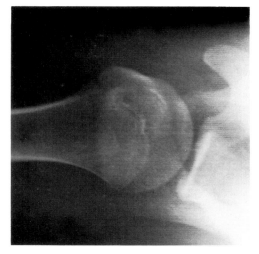

FIG 16–21.
Axillary view of the shoulder. Note the glenohumeral relationship, the hooklike coracoid process, and the acromium behind the head of the humerus.

articular surface. In this manner the glenohumeral relationship is much better defined than on the conventional straight anteroposterior view.

The axillary film also provides another perspective of the shoulder anatomy (Fig 16–21). The acromium, coracoid, glenohumeral joint, and humeral head are viewed in a different plane. By holding the film against the top of the shoulder, the picture is produced by abducting the arm and centering the x-ray tube through the axilla. The study requires a special "grid" cassette for the film. It is helpful in determining the presence of a humeral head displacement, but it is not recommended when a dislocation has just been reduced since the required abduction may reluxate the joint.

The clavicle itself requires two projections in the anteroposterior plane in order to evaluate it properly. One film should be made perpendicular to the plane of the body, while the other exposure is made with a 15- to 20-degree cephalad angulation.

The acromioclavicular joints are best inspected with an anteroposterior film and tilting

the x-ray tube 15 degrees toward the head. Comparative films are necessary to determine the presence of a separation, and this should be performed with and without weight bearing.

A more difficult area to examine roentgenographically is the sternoclavicular joint. Due to bony superimposition, tomography may be required, but since this is not universally available, both oblique and lateral views may suffice. However, if these attempts are unsuccessful, the patient can be positioned prone. The x-ray tube is then centered through the sternoclavicular joints and angled toward the head at a 35-degree tilt.

Roentgenographic Anatomy and Developmental Variations

Needless to say, a considerable degree of confusion can be created by the ossification centers of the shoulder. The proximal humeral epiphysis does not become visible, as a rule, until the fourth to eighth month of life. There are two and occasionally three separate centers. By the 20th year, the proximal epiphysis fuses to the shaft of the humerus.

Before complete closure of the epiphyseal suture, the lucent line has a peculiar angulated appearance (Fig 16–22). Overlap of the suture line occurs no matter what projection is employed and consequently produces an image simulating a fracture.

A deceptive appearance of the proximal humeral shaft is the deltoid tuberosity, which, incidentally, receives the tendinous attachment of the deltoid muscle. The thickened cortex in this area may bring to mind the periosteal reaction of infection or tumor.

On a congenital basis, there may be a complete absence of the clavicle or at least partial underdevelopment of its lateral end. This represents hereditary cleidocranial dysplasia, a disease that also affects the skull, pelvis, hips, and other skeletal regions.

The outer end of the clavicle appears less dense than the middle and sternal aspects, the result of a lesser thickness of overlying soft tissue. Soft tissues are also responsible for a discrete line density paralleling the superior border of the clavicle that measures no more than 4 mm in width and is described as the "accompanying shadow." This shadow may be thickened in cases of subtle fractures.

The rhomboid fossa is a familiar anatomic variation of the clavicle and is found along the inferior border at its medial aspect as a notch-like depression. This represents the location of the insertion of the costoclavicular (rhomboid) ligament, which secures the first rib to the clavicle. Its irregular appearance has been misinterpreted as a destructive process.

Trauma

Of all the joints in the body, the shoulder is the most frequent site of dislocations. Over 97% are anterior in type and can be described as subglenoid or subcoracoid, depending on the location of the humeral head. Invariably this form of dislocation can be visualized by a single anteroposterior roentgenogram (Fig 16–23).

Whenever a dislocation occurs, it is not unusual to have an associated fracture; this should be searched for on the film. With an anterior dislocation, a fracture of the greater tuberosity may exist; the lesser tuberosity is vulnerable in posterior dislocations. The lower glenoid margin is also susceptible in either type of dislocation. An infraction of the articular cartilage without a visible fracture is also possible in dislocations and may require arthrography to demonstrate.

Not infrequently with intra-articular extension of a fracture in the absence of true dislocation, an intact joint capsule may become progressively distended with blood, and if enough blood accu-

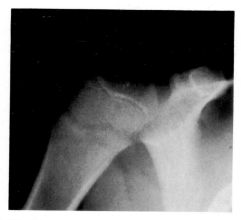

FIG 16–22.
Normal proximal humeral epiphysis in a child.

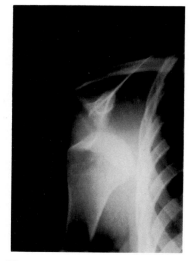

FIG 16–23.
Anterior dislocation of the shoulder, subglenoid in type.

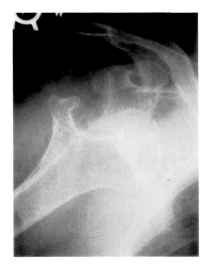

FIG 16–24.
Hill-Sachs deformity in chronic recurring anterior shoulder dislocation.

mulates, there will be inferior displacement of the humeral head away from the glenoid. This condition is termed pseudosubluxation, or "hanging shoulder."

With chronic recurring anterior dislocations, a defect becomes apparent along the superolateral aspect of the humeral head. This cortical infraction, present because of impaction against the anteroinferior rim of the glenoid, is commonly re-

ferred to as Hill-Sachs deformity. This abnormality is usually best demonstrated on an internally rotated anteroposterior view (Fig 16–24).

The less frequent posterior dislocation is much more difficult to visualize roentgenographically. The problem arises because the humeral head on the standard anteroposterior projections shows no apparent separation from the glenoid fossa when in fact it is separated. The posterolateral orientation of the glenoid articular surface accounts for this to some extent. Ordinarily, in the normal shoulder the head of the humerus overlaps about three fourths of the glenoid fossa. When it becomes posteriorly dislocated due to lateral displacement of the head, this overlap is less, but the change may be very subtle. This perplexing situation can usually be solved by employing the 30-degree tangential view, the axillary projection, or the trans-scapular film (Fig 16–25).

A very rare form of dislocation of the shoulder joint is luxatio erecta, a condition where the humeral head is located under the glenoid rim and the humeral shaft is directed above the head in fixed abduction (Fig 16–26). A lateral fall on an elevated arm will produce such an abnormality. The acromium process of the scapula acts as a fulcrum pushing the head of the humerus down and out of the glenohumeral joint. The dynamics

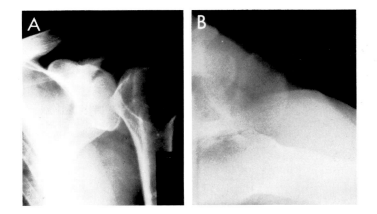

FIG 16–25.
Posterior shoulder dislocation. **A,** anteroposterior view showing some discrepancy in the glenohumeral joint. **B,** axillary view demonstrating posterior displacement of humeral head from the glenoid fossa (see Fig 16–21 for a normal axillary film).

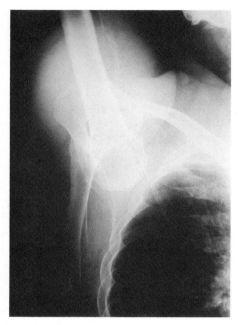

FIG 16–26.
Luxatio erecta of the shoulder. Note the superior orientation of the humeral shaft and the head of the bone locked under the glenoid.

of the applied forces can result in a fracture of the acromium, the lower lip of the glenoid, or the greater tuberosity of the humerus. Oftentimes, there is an associated tear of the rotator cuff.

Fractures involving the proximal portion of the humerus are classified according to involvement of the head, either tuberosity, or the surgical or anatomic neck. Additionally, a fracture-displacement of the yet unfused epiphysis may occur.

For descriptive purposes, anatomists describe the surgical neck as that portion of the humerus just inferior to the tuberosities where there is a normal narrowing. The constriction or shallow groove at the articular margin of the head of the humerus is referred to as the anatomic neck.

Fractures of the proximal portion of the humerus must be evaluated by at least two views at right angles to one another. An anteroposterior view alone with a transthoracic lateral projection will fulfill this criteria, but obliquely directed x-ray films may be necessary to best demonstrate displacement and/or angular deformity.

Transverse subcapital fractures of the surgical neck along with avulsions of the greater tuberosity are the most commonly encountered injuries to the shoulder. A fracture-displacement of the ununited epiphysis creates a more difficult diagnostic challenge. The normal epiphyseal line itself, as already alluded to, makes interpretation troublesome. The normal epiphysis has a uniform width and dense margins, whereas a fracture will demonstrate varying thickness with a sharp, nonsclerotic edge. Often there is impaction or distraction of the fragments causing some degree of overlapping, which makes the diagnosis somewhat simpler. Of course, if the presence of an abnormality is uncertain or indeterminate, an accurate comparison with the opposite uninjured shoulder should be performed.

The infraglenoid area of the scapula is the most common location of fractures of this bone. The normal lucent nutrient canal in this region with its dense margins should not offer much concern. Instead of a discrete fracture line, only a zone of increased density will offer any clue to the injury. The clinician should also search for underlying rib fractures.

A complete fracture of the clavicle in most circumstances will exhibit overriding of the fragments when they involve its midportion. Due to the forces applied by the pectoralis minor muscle as well as the weight of the arm, the lateral fragment is displaced inferiorly in most cases. An incomplete or nondisplaced fracture may be so subtle as to avoid detection initially, but the two standard views, including straight anteroposterior and cranially angulated projections, will in most instances reveal the fracture.

Tumor

The proximal aspect of the humerus is a relatively common location for a benign solitary cyst, which may appear as either simple or multiloculated (Fig 16–27). Such cysts are found within the metaphysis and exhibit destruction of the

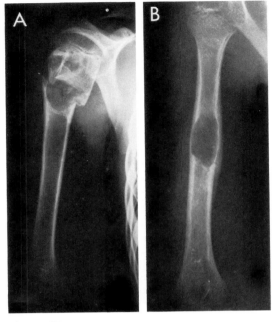

FIG 16–27.
Benign cysts of the humerus. **A,** a multiloculated cyst in the metaphysis shows a fresh pathologic fracture. **B,** a simple solitary cyst in the midshaft demonstrates a healing fracture.

medullary spongiosa with more or less expansion of the bone. Thinning of the cortex can attain paper thickness, and pathologic fractures are a very common event, even in the absence of significant trauma. When initially discovered, the cysts extend to the epiphyseal line but do not involve the growth center itself. When followed serially until fusion of the epiphysis, the cyst appears to "migrate" toward the middle of the shaft as growth of the bone ends progresses.

Primary malignant tumors of the shoulder are a rarity and are often of the sarcomatous variety. Osteogenic sarcoma as well as the round-cell tumors, Ewing's sarcoma, and reticulum cell sarcoma have already been described.

Secondary metastatic disease is much more prevalent than primary lesions, particularly disease of the proximal aspect of the humerus. As with cysts, pathologic fractures frequently accompany these malignant changes.

Arthritis

The roentgenographic alterations of osteoarthritis of the shoulder are similar to those seen in the knee and will be described under that heading. The process, however, more often has a post-traumatic relationship.

Rheumatoid arthritis of the shoulder, as in other joints, will demonstrate articular erosions without much bone production or osteophyte formation as is seen in osteoarthritis. However, unique to this area, erosions of the lateral ends of the clavicles may be present. This pathologic change, nevertheless, is not specific for rheumatoid arthritis and may be seen in hyperparathyroidism and other less common diseases.

Calcific Tendinitis

Calcific tendinitis represents a disease entity that is particularly prone to develop in the shoulder. The majority of roentgenographic examinations performed for this disease are negative for abnormal changes. The radiographic diagnosis is made by the identification of calcifications involving the tendinous insertions of the rotator cuff muscles into the head of the humerus. This most commonly affects the supraspinatus tendon as it crosses over the superior articular surface of the humeral head and inserts into the greater tuberosity. Pathogenically, the presence of calcium infers organization of a focal hematoma resulting from tearing of some of the tendon's fibers. The subacromial bursa overlies and is in contact with the supraspinatus tendon and, due to this close relationship, may become secondarily inflamed. In fact, rupture of the puttylike calcifications into the bursa heralds the onset of subacromial bursitis. The density of the calcium can be seen to extend along the lateral aspect of the humeral head as it finds its way into the subdeltoid extension of the subacromial bursa.

The Elbow

Roentgenographic Examination

Standard examination of the elbow includes a straight anteroposterior film with the forearm fully extended and supinated as well as a true lateral view with the joint flexed 90 degrees and the forearm supinated. Not uncommonly, particularly with trauma, the patient is unable or unwilling to extend or flex the elbow. To delineate the distal humeral articulating surface when the elbow is held in flexion, the anteroposterior view can be obtained by orienting the central beam of the x-ray tube perpendicular to the distal humeral shaft. In the same way, the proximal radial and ulnar details and relationships can be observed by pointing the tube perpendicular to their shafts. Medial and lateral oblique exposures may become necessary to better analyze the radial head and shaft, the humeral condyles, or the coronoid process of the ulna.

Roentgenographic Anatomy

Before considering specific elbow lesions, pertinent roentgenographic anatomy of the elbow must be considered. Evaluating the different bony landmarks and their relationships can prove extremely useful.

In children a great deal of confusion arises because of the ossification sequence of the growth centers. The capitellum, trochlea, and the medial and lateral epicondyles compose the centers of the distal portion of the humerus. In addition, the elbow contains the olecranon apophysis and the radial head epiphysis (Fig 16–28).

The first of the distal humeral epiphyses to appear is the capitellum, which develops by the age of 2 years. At about 6 years of age the medial epicondylar center becomes visible. Next to become evident is the trochlea at 10 years of age, and finally, the lateral epicondyle appears near the 12th year of life.

The radial head epiphysis calcifies at about the same time as the medial epicondyle, in the vicinity of the sixth year. Before the age of 10 years, the olecranon ossification center is not visible.

The ossification centers normally fuse between the ages of 14 and 16 years, although union of the medial epicondyle may not occur until the 18th year.

Following their union, the medial and lateral epicondyles form the flared segment of the distal third of the humerus. Between the condyles on both the ventral and dorsal surfaces are indentations identified as the coronoid and olecranon fossae, respectively, as they relate to the anatomic segments of the ulna. This area may be very thin and appear as a zone of rounded rarefaction on the anteroposterior film. In fact, an actual open-

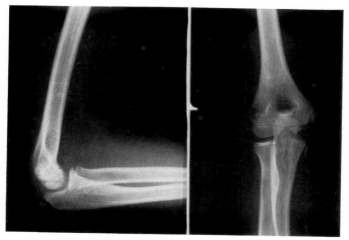

FIG 16–28.
Normal elbow of a 9-year-old child. *Left,* lateral view; *Right,* anteroposterior view.

ing, termed the supratrochlear foramen, is occasionally present.

Contained within these recesses are the fat pads, fairly sensitive indicators of the presence of a distended joint capsule. In the normal elbow, providing a true lateral flexion film is obtained, the posterior fat pad is not visible. The anterior fat pad forms a slim triangular lucency adjacent to the anterior humeral cortex. With the presence of joint fluid, such as blood resulting from an intra-articular fracture, one or both of these fat pads will be elevated. The so-called fat-pad sign is not specific and may be seen in conditions other than trauma, such as pyarthrosis or rheumatoid arthritis. In cases of injury, a positive fat-pad sign should be searched for from the beginning and, if found, should initiate further investigation for an occult fracture, particularly of the radial head (Fig 16–29). Oblique views may be required, and if necessary, a repeat examination may be done in 7 to 10 days, at which time a fracture should be apparent. On occasion, no fracture will be found, and the distended joint may be on the basis of a cartilage infraction or capsular tear. In adults an intra-articular fracture may be present in the absence of fat-pad eleva-

tion, but in children it is a more reliable indicator, being found in approximately 90% of elbow fractures (Rogers, 1978).

Two other helpful relationships will be of assistance when evaluating normal elbow anatomy. The first is the anterior humeral line. On the lateral film, a line is drawn along the anterior margin of the humeral shaft and extended through the joint. If the capitellum is divided into equal thirds, this line normally passes through the middle third. It is a simple and useful index in analyzing the normal 140-degree angle that the articular structures form with the shaft of the humerus. This easy maneuver often will alert the physician to a subtle transcondylar fracture in children: the line will be seen to extend through or anterior to the anterior third division of the capitellum (Fig 16–30).

The second practical indicator is the radiocapitellar line, denoted by a line drawn through the longitudinal axis of the radius. This line will always pass through the capitellum, no matter what projection is being viewed. When the radial head is dislocated, this relationship no longer exists. Whenever there is a fracture of the ulnar shaft, this procedure should be utilized since the

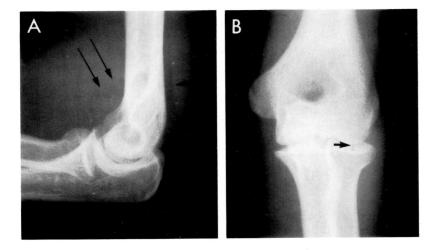

FIG 16–29.
Radial head fracture with a positive fat-pad sign. **A,** lateral view showing elevation of both anterior and posterior fat pads *(arrows).* **B,** a fracture line through the radial head *(arrow)* is well delineated on the anteroposterior projection.

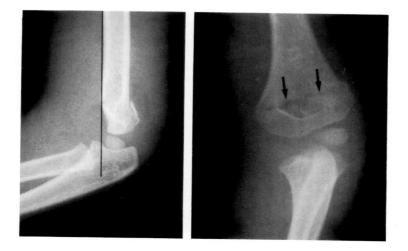

FIG 16–30.
Transcondylar fracture of the humerus. *Left,* lateral view revealing anterior and posterior fat-pad elevation. An obvious fracture is identified, but note how the anterior humeral line extends anterior to the capitellum. *Right,* Anteroposterior view clearly outlining the fracture *(arrows).*

radial head is often dislocated in what constitutes a Monteggia fracture.

Trauma

Sixty percent of all elbow fractures in children are of the supracondylar type. The lateral epicondyle is involved about 15% of the time, and the medial epicondyle accounts for 10% of all fractures. The radial and olecranon ossification centers are infrequently traumatized.

In adults the radial head or neck mark the most common elbow area for fractures. Unlike the pediatric age group, adults seldom suffer fractures of the distal third of the humerus.

A supracondylar fracture should more aptly be called a transcondylar fracture because it extends across the condyles and is seen through the coronoid and olecranon fossae (see Fig 16–30). The anterior humeral line will indicate posterior displacement of the distal fragment when the fracture is complete, which is seen in 75% of cases. The remainder, however, are incomplete, and visualizing the fracture line may be impossible. Almost always the posterior fat pad will be elevated.

When the lateral epicondylar epiphysis is traumatized, it usually contains a fragment of metaphyseal bone. Because it serves for the attachment of forearm extensor tendons, the fragment becomes displaced posteriorly and inferiorly.

Little Leaguer's elbow, discussed in Chapter 5, describes an injury in which the medial epicondyle is separated. Ordinarily the avulsed center is best identified on the anteroposterior film, often lying adjacent to the capitellum. In rare instances the fragment may become displaced into the medial joint space, where it can simulate the trochlear ossification center before its actual appearance.

The coronoid process is frequently avulsed in posterior dislocations of the elbow and is impacted against the trochlea. Whenever an elbow dislocation occurs, the radius and ulna are displaced lateral and posterior to the humerus in almost all instances. In children, when the radius and ulna are medial to the humerus, there is not a dislocation but rather a fracture through the entire distal humeral epiphysis. This is extremely important to recognize since treatment of the two are entirely different.

The Wrist and Hand

Roentgenographic Examination

Routine roentgenographic study of the wrist consists of posteroanterior, oblique, and lateral projections. The oblique film is achieved by orienting the wrist at a 45-degree angle to the plane of the film with the ulnar side down.

There are several special wrist views that are necessary for the evaluation of specific anatomic features. One of the more frequently employed studies is that for the carpal navicular bone. A fracture of this bone may easily escape detection. When clinical symptoms point to a navicular injury yet the routine study appears normal, this view becomes mandatory. The palm is placed against the film holder with the thumb and index finger spread apart. The tube is angled 45 degrees toward the elbow. This results in an elongated appearance of the navicular, but the distortion is minimal, and it is projected free of superimposition from the other carpal bones (Fig 16–31). The midportion of the navicular, where the majority of fractures occur, is clearly outlined.

Roentgenographic examination of the phalanges and metacarpals is performed with posteroanterior and oblique films. When the fingers are evaluated, the individual digits should also be examined with true lateral views.

Roentgenographic Anatomy, Developmental Variations, and Pathology of the Individual Bones

In this section on the hand and wrist, anatomy, variations, and abnormalities (especially those of the individual carpal bones) will be considered together.

The carpus is composed of a proximal and distal row of four bones each. In order to remember their names, the infamous mnemonic of ". . . Tilly's pants . . ." still applies, but a picture is sometimes more than words can describe (Fig 16–32).

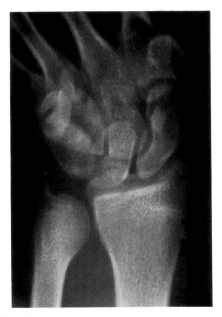

FIG 16–31.
Angulated navicular view. An incidental finding is a dense bone island within the body of the carpal navicular bone.

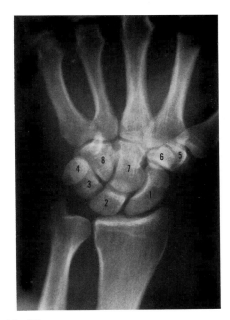

FIG 16–32.
Normal carpal bones: *1*, navicular; *2*, lunate; *3*, triquetrum; *4*, pisiform; *5*, greater multangular (trapezium); *6*, lesser multangular (trapezoid); *7*, capitate; *8*, hamate.

The proximal row is concave in alignment toward the hand, whereas the distal row is more or less convex in the same direction as seen on the anteroposterior film. The navicular, lunate, triquetral, and pisiform bones constitute the proximal column; the distal row is made up by the greater multangular (trapezium), lesser multangular (trapezoid), capitate, and hamate bones. For proper interpretation, each bone should be identified and scrutinized separately.

Throughout the skeleton, constitutional disease such as congenital hypothyroidism (cretinism) and other endocrine and metabolic diseases affect and alter the time of appearance and growth rate of ossification centers, but the wrist and hand provide one of the most sensitive indicators of growth retardation of bone age. A handbook for the normal growth and development of the hand and wrist is found in most radiology departments (Greulich and Pyle, 1959).

There are a few, infrequently described congenital abnormalities affecting the carpus. Agenesis or hypoplasia of one or more of the bones may be found. Fusion anomalies or synostoses are also occasionally seen.

Anatomic variations occur with such frequency that some of the more common ones will be described to permit differentiation from pathologic conditions.

Accessory bones do appear about the carpal bones but are very infrequent. They are mentioned merely to make one aware of their existence, and they need to be recalled when considering the possibility of an avulsion fragment.

Small, well-defined, round-to-oval areas of increased density are often identified in any of the carpal bones, metacarpals, and phalanges. They represent clinically insignificant bone islands (see Fig 16–31).

Tiny, rounded lucencies with well-delineated sclerotic margins coincide with vascular channels, but cystlike areas are also frequently encountered within or along the cortical borders of any of the hand or wrist bones, especially the carpal bones. These may be the result of medullary fibrosis or hemorrhagic cysts. When related to the articular cortex, these cysts are the result of synovial herniation in osteoarthritis when the other classic signs of this disease are present. Erosive cysts at the justa-articular margins are diagnostic of rheumatoid arthritis.

In the forthcoming discussion, all of the individual wrist and hand bones will be considered separately.

Navicular.   The navicular bone becomes visible somewhat late, usually by the fifth to sixth year. This bone may be entirely absent (agenesis), or it may become assimilated (fused) with the radial epiphysis. A small hypoplastic navicular may result in a malformed radial-carpal joint. Quite often a tubercle arises from the distal and lateral corner of the bone. A partial division of the navicular resulting from incomplete fusion of two ossification centers can simulate a fracture. This condition will require follow-up studies to determine healing, but the same may be found in the contralateral wrist.

Serial examinations of a fractured carpal navicular bone at about 3- to 4-week intervals are imperative in view of the possible complications. These include malunion, nonunion, and aseptic necrosis. The latter presents as a progressively increasing sclerosis of the proximal fragment as a result of vascular interruption to this segment.

Transverse fractures of the navicular most often involve the midportion, but any segment can be involved, including avulsions of the lateral tubercle. Dislocations of the navicular will be discussed in the following section with the lunate bone.

Lunate.   In the vicinity of the fourth to fifth year of life, the lunate bone becomes visible by ossification. Like the navicular, it may develop from two separate centers; if these centers fail to fuse, complete or partial fracturelike lines result.

One of the most notable pathologic changes affecting the carpal lunate is Kienböck's aseptic necrosis. This form of osteochondritis has been described in more detail in Chapter 6.

The carpal lunate is infrequently fractured but

is involved in one of the more important traumatic lesions of the wrist—dislocations. Three important types of wrist dislocations have been described. The first is a transnavicular perilunate dislocation (Fig 16–33). In this condition, there is a fracture at the midnavicular. The proximal pole fragment and the lunate maintain their normal relationship with the radial articulation, but the distal pole segment of the navicular bone and the remaining carpal bones become displaced posteriorly.

In a perilunate dislocation, the navicular is intact, and it along with the carpus becomes dorsally dislocated. The lunate remains in normal position.

The third type of carpal displacement is a pure lunate dislocation (Fig 16–34). The articular relationship between the lunate and the capitate is disrupted. The lunate rotates anteriorly, which is best appreciated on the lateral view. On the anteroposterior film, the lunate takes on a somewhat triangular appearance, which should alert the clinician to this abnormality.

Triquetrum. The triquetrum, or triangular bone, appearing between the second to third year, probably is the second most frequently fractured bone of the carpus. This usually consists of a posterior chip fracture, identified on the lateral roentgenogram, and is usually of no clinical importance.

Pisiform. The last and smallest bone of the carpus to ossify is the pisiform, usually in the ninth or tenth year of life. Because it often develops from multiple centers, its early appearance has often been misinterpreted as a fracture or aseptic necrosis. Traumatic lesions of the pisiform are almost nonexistent, although fractures and dislocations have been reported in the literature.

Greater Multangular. Progressing on to the distal row, the first bone to be considered is the greater multangular, or trapezium. Appearing at approximately the fifth year, this carpal bone should be observed for its concave articulation with the base of the first metacarpal bone. A fu-

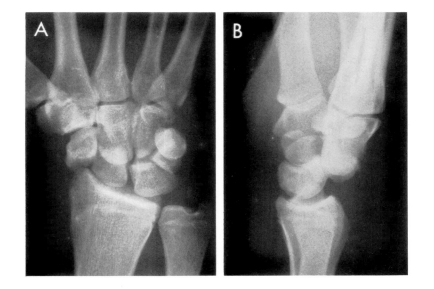

FIG 16–33.
Transnavicular perilunate dislocation. **A,** posteroanterior view. Note the obvious displaced fracture of the navicular and the overlap of the proximal pole fragment and the capitate, which should alert one to the presence of more than just a simple fracture. **B,** lateral view showing typical posterior displacement, particularly of the capitate, with the lunate maintaining its normal position.

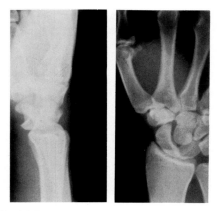

FIG 16–34.
Pure lunate dislocation. The lateral view *(left)* reveals the semilunar articular margin of the lunate faces forward. On the frontal view *(right)* note the abnormal relation of the lunate to the navicular, capitate, and triquetrum.

sion between the two is not infrequent. In addition, it exhibits a tendency for fusion with the navicular. This bone, along with the lesser multangular, is somewhat difficult to evaluate because of the superimposition of the two.

Degenerative osteoarthritic alterations are very common at the greater multangular joint at the first metacarpal bone. Joint narrowing, subarticular sclerosis, and spurring are characteristic findings of this process.

Lesser Multangular.   The lesser multangular, or trapezoid, makes its appearance sometime after the navicular is visualized. It is rarely involved in pathologic processes, including trauma. Synostosis between it and the adjoining capitate has been observed.

Capitate.   The first carpal bone to ossify and the largest of the eight is the capitate. Cystlike lesions seem to predominate in the capitate bone. Its position appears to protect it from trauma.

Hamate.   Finally, the last carpal bone to be visualized is the hamate. To the inexperienced observer the uncinate process or hamulus, the bony protuberance of the hamate extending toward

the palm, will appear as a lucent lesion with a sclerotic border when seen en face in the antero-posterior projection. Because avulsion fractures of this hooklike process may happen, it is helpful to obtain an oblique view of the wrist with the posterior surface of the small finger resting against the film. This will project the hamulus free of overlapping bones.

Distal Radius and Ulna.   When analyzing the wrist roentgenogram, the distal radius and ulna can hardly escape attention. We are all aware of what constitutes a Colles' fracture and its reverse, a Smith fracture, but subtle impaction fractures of the distal third of the radius may evade detection. A helpful rule to follow is to measure the anterior angle of the tilt of the distal articular margin of the radius, which normally measures 15 degrees on the lateral view. The only indication of a fracture may be straightening or reversal of this tilt.

A transverse fracture of the radial styloid may be an isolated finding and constitutes the so-called chauffeur's fracture. A styloid fracture of the ulna usually accompanies another fracture, but it may be an isolated finding.

Dislocations of either or both the distal radius and ulna must not be overlooked, and this is easily accomplished if a true lateral roentgenogram is not performed. The displacement is invariably posterior.

Metacarpals and Phalanges.   When describing the individual fingers, the term "ray" is employed. Each of the five rays is composed of a metacarpal and its three associated phalanges (proximal, middle, and distal).

A number of congenital abnormalities exist at birth. Included are fusion of two or more of the digital rays, a condition referred to as syndactyly. Duplicative anomalies, or polydactyly, can involve any of the rays. Arachnodactyly of the fingers occurs in the generalized skeletal disorder of Marfan's syndrome; here the digits are elongated and very thin.

When assessing the metacarpal bones, there

are several important anatomic features to be considered (Fig 16–35). The epiphysis of the first metacarpal bone (the thumb) is located proximally, whereas the growth center occupies the distal aspect of the remaining four metacarpals. This property is consequential in terms of an examination made for assessing the presence of fractures in the growing patient. But, as is usual, there is always some variation to confuse the issue. On occasion the clinician may see what appear to be epiphyses involving the distal first metacarpal or the proximal second metacarpal; these are appropriately termed *pseudoepiphyses.*

Sesamoid bones about the hand and wrist deserve mention because of their frequency and occasional mistaken identity as fractures. They typically overlap the heads of the metacarpal bones. A fracture of a sesamoid is very rare, being more commonly found in the foot.

The appearance of the phalanges, particularly the terminal ones, is extremely variable, and the variants, for all practical purposes, should be

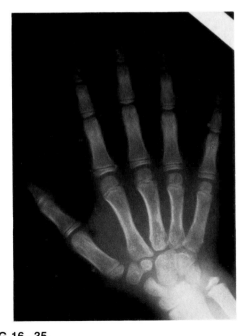

FIG 16–35.
Normal hand bones of a 9-year-old child. Note the position of the epiphyses of the metacarpal bones.

considered normal. The ungual tuberosity or tuft of the distal phalanx can have many shapes and sizes, yet a number of disease processes may alter them considerably. Deformity and erosive changes of the tufts are seen in scleroderma, sarcoidosis, psoriasis, and leprosy.

Cystlike or erosive changes in the tufts can be ascribed to glomus tumors, which produce pressure erosion of bone and are accompanied by severe pain. Enchondromas can involve any of the phalanges and are prone to pathologic fracture.

Of all of the fractures involving the fingers, those of the tuft are probably the most common and may be avulsion types or comminuted. When analyzing the injured finger, the importance of obtaining a true lateral view, in addition to anteroposterior and oblique projections, cannot be stressed too much (Fig 16–36). This becomes particularly apparent in cases of volar plate injuries. A fragment of bone is avulsed from the palmar aspect at the base of the middle phalanx and involves the proximal interphalangeal joint. The result of hyperextension forces, the fragment may be obscured on all but the lateral film.

Degenerative osteoarthritis is a relatively common disorder of the terminal interphalangeal joints of the elderly. The deformity is characterized by joint space narrowing, irregularity of the articular margins, subarticular sclerosis, and hypertrophic spurs. Clinically, palpable Heberden's nodes are a distinctive, characteristic finding of this disease.

Rheumatoid arthritis produces distinctive transformations in the joints of the hand and wrist. The earlier roentgenographic finding may be periarticular soft-tissue swelling. Later demineralization about the joint with slight widening of the joint space will be noted—the result of inflammatory hyperemia with intra-articular fluid and synovial thickening. This progresses to juxta-articular cortical erosions, which are related to synovial hypertrophy and panus formation. Eventually the joint space becomes narrowed, and classic ulnar subluxations occur. Unlike degenerative osteoarthritis, there is no reactive spur production in rheumatoid arthritis.

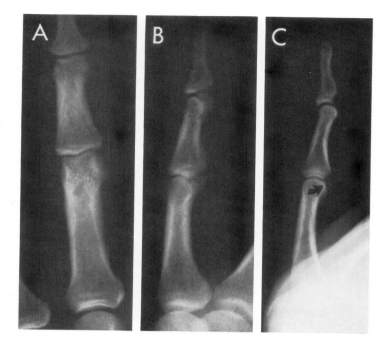

FIG 16–36.
Volar plate fracture of the finger. **A,** posteroanterior view. **B,** oblique view. **C,** lateral view. Note that the fragment is identified only on the lateral film *(arrow).*

Hyperparathyroidism produces a pathognomatic change in the hands. Typically, there is subperiosteal resorption along the radial aspect of the middle phalanges.

The Pelvis and Hips

Roentgenographic Examination

The anteroposterior view is the only standard projection required for roentgenographic examination of the pelvis. This film should include the entirety of the body pelvis, from iliac crests to the ischial tuberosities, which inherently encompasses the sacrococcyx and sacroiliac joint. Furthermore, both hips will be imaged on the film, and this should include the femur to the subtrochanteric region (below the lesser trochanter) whenever possible.

There are special projections that will aid the analyses of certain pelvic segments and clarify suspected regions. Films performed in the an-

teroposterior direction with the x-ray tube angled 30 degrees toward the head (cephalad) and 30 degrees toward the feet (caudad) are practical under certain circumstances. These will give a different perspective of the sacroiliac joints, sacrococcyx, the iliac wings, and the anterior pelvic arch (the ischiopubic rami). Nondisplaced fractures of the rami may go undetected initially on the straight anteroposterior exposure but can be clearly delineated on these angled projections.

The anteroposterior views may suffice for complete preliminary pelvic assessment in cases of trauma. Minimal motion of the patient is the best policy to prevent possible compromise to already injured soft tissues, for example, blood vessels and urinary bladder. However, oblique films can be helpful adjuncts on follow-up studies. The supine patient is first rotated 45 degrees with the right hip down against the film (right posterior oblique) and then to the left 45 degrees (left posterior oblique). Because of the outward orientation of the sacroiliac joints, oblique films allow the viewer to look straight down the joints without confusing overlap of the free edges. Moreover, the ischiopubic rami and the margins of the obturator foramen will be visualized in a different manner. The posterior margin of the acetabulum can also lend itself to more direct inspection. Acetabular fractures, a topic that will be disussed later, require not only oblique roentgenograms but also lateral films for proper evaluation.

When the focus of attention is the hip, it is useful to include both sides on a single film for comparative reasons. The straight anteroposterior roentgenogram of the pelvis and hips is an appropriate examination, but it is a must to view the hip from the lateral aspect when at all possible. This can be achieved in one of two ways: (1) a frog-leg position with the femur maximally rotated externally or (2) a horizontally directed roentgenogram with the tube placed along the inner aspect of the thigh and directed through the hip to a grid film placed alongside the hip. This latter method is generally the desired technique in cases of fracture, because the patient usually will not tolerate rotation of the leg and hip and little or no motion of the injured part is preferred.

Roentgenographic Anatomy and Developmental Variations

The pelvis is formed by two innominate bones, each consisting of an ilium, an ischium, and the pubis, which are distinct entities in youth but fuse to form a singular solid structure in the adult. The sacrum serves as a posterior bridge between the two by way of the essentially non-mobile sacroiliac joints.

The epiphyses and apophyses of the pelvis and hips ordinarily do not unite until the second decade of life. The apophyses of the iliac crest normally make their appearance by the 12th to 15th year and fuse by 21 to 25 years of age. They are separated from the body of the ilium by no more than 2 to 3 mm, often have an irregular rippled appearance, and may show segmentation into two or more parts.

Small centers of ossification arise from the anterior inferior iliac spines by the 13th year and fuse 2 to 3 years later. Athletes are prone to avulsion of these centers, and this should be looked for when there is localized pain in a sports-related injury. Oblique films are most useful in such situations, and a view of the opposite side is almost always needed to make the diagnosis.

Cheerleader's "splits" can create a similar avulsion of the ischial tuberosity apophysis on one or both sides (Fig 16–37). The time of appearance and fusion of these ossification centers parallels those of the iliac crest.

Until the eighth year of life, a radiolucent cartilage separates the ischium and pubis along the inferior ramus (Fig 16–38). This area of normal development is frequently misjudged as a fracture. During the process of union, this region appears more dense and expanded so as to give the

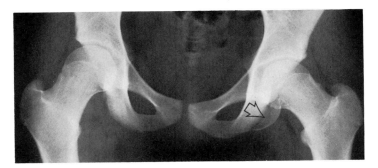

FIG 16–37.
Avulsion fracture *(arrow)* of the ischial tuberosity on the left side.

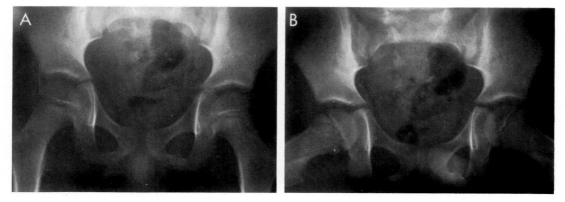

FIG 16–38.
Normal pelvis and hips of a 10-year-old child. **A,** anteroposterior view with the hips in the neutral position. **B,** anteroposterior view with the hips in the froglike lateral position. Note the triradiate cartilage and the bulbous appearance of the ischiopubic synchondroses of the inferior rami.

impression of callus formation or tumor. The bilateral appearances are often asymmetric.

The triradiate cartilage forms a Y-shaped configuration at the acetabulum and constitutes the junctures of the pubis, ischium, and ilium (see Fig 16–38). This will become completely filled in with bone at about the time of puberty. There have been many occasions when this, too, has been called a pelvic fracture.

In evaluating the symphysis pubis, it is more important for the inferior margins to align, whereas the superior borders are frequently and normally offset. Ordinarily, the width of the symphysis pubis joint measures no more than 8 mm in adults and 10 mm in children. Widening of the joint is characteristic of late pregnancy.

The posterior margin of the acetabulum, somewhat obscured by the femoral head and requiring an oblique view to see adequately, may arise from a separate ossification center and easily simulate a fracture because of its linear appearance. This variation is often a bilateral finding. A variable-sized ununited center, the os acetabuli, may persist throughout life and is located along the superolateral margin of the acetabulum (Fig 16–39).

Proceeding now to the anatomy of the hip, the developmental features are of utmost impor-

tance. The femoral capital epiphysis appears during the first year. Synostosis of the head with the femoral neck is completed by the 18th year, but a cartilaginous fissure may persist. A central indentation along the articular margin of the femoral head corresponds to the fovea centralis, where the ligamentum teres is embedded.

The greater trochanter apophysis becomes visible by the fifth year and unites at the same time as the femoral capital epiphysis, namely, 18 years. The line of fusion may also persist for a long time and result in confusion.

In addition to the bones themselves, there are certain soft-tissue densities about the hips and pelvis that demand attention. The shadows of the obturator internus, the iliopsoas, and gluteus medius muscles are ordinarily outlined by radiolucent adipose tissue. Because of their close approximation to the joint capsule, blood or pus that will distend the joint will be reflected on the roentgenogram by displacement of these fat stripes.

Trauma

A rather significant degree of correlation exists between the presence of an extracapsular subtrochanteric hip fracture and a pathologic process. In other words, do not take for granted that such

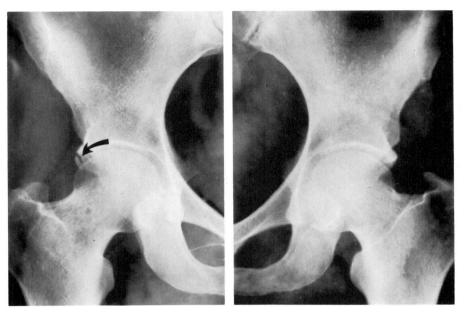

FIG 16–39.
Os acetabuli. The right side demonstrates this normal variant *(arrow)*. None is seen on the left.

a fracture is related purely to trauma since this is a favorable site for metastasis.

Hip dislocations have been discussed in Chapter 9. From a radiologist's point of view, it is useful to comment on some of the roentgenographic changes seen in this type of injury. First of all, hip dislocations are classified as anterior, posterior, and central. In the most common posterior form of dislocation, the injury may not always be readily apparent on the anteroposterior film. There may be a slight difference in the size of the femoral heads as a result of slight rotation of the displaced hip. Shenton's line may be askew. This is a continuous, smooth line formed along the sweep of the inner margin of the femoral neck, and it normally follows the inferior boundary of the arched contour of the superior ischiopubic ramus. Any disruption of this line would indicate a dislocation. The posterior lip of the acetabulum may be fractured, but as previously noted, a persistent unfused apophysis is sometimes located here.

When an anterior dislocation is present, the femoral head may lie medial and below the acetabulum, sometimes superimposed on the obturator foramen. However, the head infrequently may overlie the acetabular roof and simulate a posterior dislocation. This will require a horizontal groin lateral roentgenogram for differentiation.

When either a posterior or an anterior dislocation has been reduced, postreduction roentgenograms should be inspected for associated fractures. Also, the width of the hip joint space requires measurement. A difference of more than 2 mm should make one suspect the possibility of interposed tissue, such as a portion of the torn capsule, which will necessitate surgical removal. Short of surgical exploration, the diagnosis may need tomography or even hip arthrography with radiopaque material.

A central dislocation of the hip is always associated with an acetabular fracture; hence, the condition is termed a central fracture-dislocation (Fig 16–40). A central acetabular fracture, however, may exist without a dislocated hip. There

FIG 16–40.
Central fracture dislocation of the hip.

verse type extends from the anterior acetabular margin backward through the ischial spine, whereas the oblique form is directed more superiorly to the greater sacrosciatic notch. Both actually divide the innominate bone into superior and inferior segments.

The second variety of acetabular fracture, as discussed previously, involves the posterior rim. This most often is produced by a posteriorly dislocated hip.

Two other categories of acetabular fractures are depicted in the schematic drawing of Figure 16–41: anterior (iliopubic) and posterior (ilioischial) column fractures. Oblique films will be required for their proper interpretation.

In addition to acetabular fractures, the remainder of the pelvis can be fractured in various ways. It is best to classify these as either stable or unstable.

Stable fractures can be categorized into avulsions, ischiopubic rami fractures, iliac wing fractures, and fractures of the sacrococcyx. Avulsions of the anterior superior and inferior iliac spines

are four basic types of acetabular fractures, but the central form constitutes the most common.

As seen in Figure 16–41, a central acetabular fracture may be transverse or oblique. The trans-

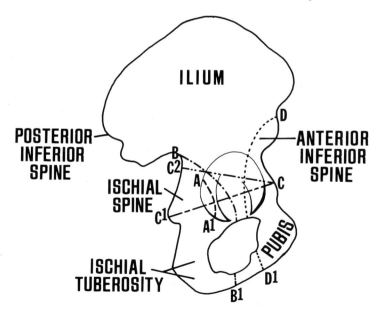

FIG 16–41.
Types of acetabular fractures. This drawing of a lateral view of the pelvis describes the basic fractures that can involve the acetabulum: A-A^1 = posterior rim fracture; B-B^1 = posterior column fracture (ilioischial); C-C^1 = central transverse fracture; C-C^2 = central oblique fracture; D-D^1 = anterior column fracture (iliopubic). (From Thaggard A, Harle TS, Carlson V: *Semin Roentgenol 1978;* 13:117–133. Used by permission.)

as well as the ischial tuberosities have already been discussed.

The most frequent pelvic fractures are those involving the ischiopubic rami. Occasionally, these may be stress-type infractions. Their visualization may call for cephalic and caudal tilt films.

A fracture of the iliac wing often results from a direct lateral blow to the pelvis. These are best depicted with an oblique roentgenogram.

Anteroposterior and lateral exposures of the sacrococcyx are required for the assessment of fractures, but it is often useful to include an anteroposterior cephalic (upward) tilt projection. Overlying intestinal content can obscure a fracture in this area, and linear tomography may be required.

A variety of fractures and/or dislocations result in unstable conditions of the pelvis. Among the more common types that might be encountered is the straddle fracture (Fig 16–42,A). This situation exists when there are vertical fractures involving the superior and inferior ischiopubic rami on both sides. Less frequently, the fractures are unilateral but with separation of the symphysis pubis. Approximately 30% of such injuries will have associated urethral or bladder trauma.

More serious forms of unstable fractures are classified as double vertical fracture-dislocations (see Fig 16–42). There are three such types, and all have in common a double component involving the pelvic ring, anterior and posterior to the acetabulum.

When there are unilateral vertical fractures of the ischiopubic rami or a dislocation of the symphysis pubis in combination with a fracture about the ipsilateral sacroiliac joint or a dislocation of that joint, the condition is termed Malgaigne's fracture (Fig 16–42,B and C). The hemipelvis on the involved side may become displaced up or down and create a true unstable situation.

A "sprung pelvis" is another form of an unstable double vertical injury. Here, there is separation of one or both sacroiliac joints and a disjunction of the symphysis pubis (Fig 16–42,D). Careful inspection of the sacroiliac joints should be made in any patient with displacement of the pubis.

The third type of double vertical pelvic injury is the so-called bucket-handle fracture (Fig 16–42,E). There will be fractures through the upper and lower rami of the anterior pelvic ring. The opposite or contralateral sacroiliac joint will be separated or will demonstrate a juxta-articular fracture.

CT has revolutionized the radiologist's ability to evaluate fractures of the pelvis. The transverse images provide greater anatomic detail, which allows one to distinguish important relationships and significant fragment displacements not readily apparent on the standard x-ray films. Furthermore, alterations in the soft tissues can be better determined, such as the development of associated hematoma formation. Totally unsuspected fractures that are not apparent on routine films often are visualized by CT. Furthermore, the sacroiliac joints are much better depicted (Fig 16–43).

Tumor

Our attention is now directed to neoplastic disease of the pelvis. Primary tumors are seldom seen and usually present no diagnostic dilemmas. Most of these are similar to those described in the discussion of the spine.

On the other hand, metastatic disease is quite common in the pelvis and constitutes approximately 12% of all bone metastatic sites. Difficulty in distinguishing minimal involvement may be related to confusing overlying intestinal gas and fecal material. Here is where the sensitivity of nuclear bone scanning will help to solve these difficult situations.

Not infrequently a pelvic roentgenogram will be seen that shows a marked increase in density. The majority of these cases will represent either diffuse osteoblastic metastasis or Paget's disease. The differentiation, as already observed, can often be made utilizing basic characteristics of each (Fig 16–44). Notably, Paget's disease will disclose increased volume of bone and a greatly thickened trabecular pattern. Moreover, it may be confined to one side of the pelvis, a less likely

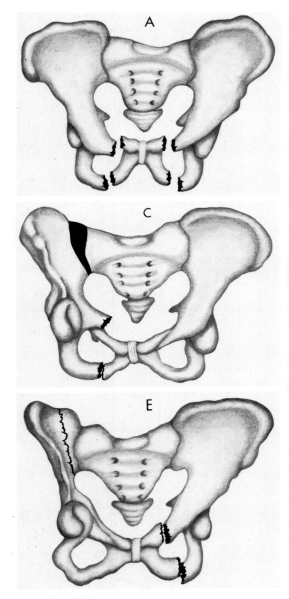

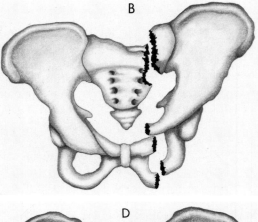

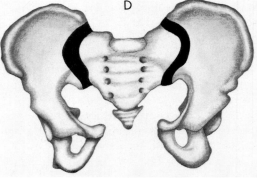

FIG 16–42.
Types of unstable pelvic fractures. **A,** straddle fracture. **B,** Malgaigne's fracture with an ipsilateral double vertical fracture. **C,** Malgaigne's fracture with dislocation of the sacroiliac joint. **D,** sprung pelvis. **E,** bucket-handle fracture. (From Dunn AW, Morris HD: *Bone Joint Surg* 1968; 50:1639–1648. Used by permission.)

occurrence in metastasis. In a small percentage of individuals (fewer than 1%), Paget's disease may transform to osteogenic sarcoma.

Infection
Infections involving the hips and pelvis, such as acute pyogenic arthritis and tuberculous osteomyelitis, are extremely rare today. Secondary seeding of infection, either directly from pelvis

inflammation or through the blood stream, can take place and result in either an infected joint or osteomyelitis.

Sacroiliac Joints

A discussion concerning diseases affecting the sacroiliac joints should prove beneficial. There are a number of conditions that can alter the

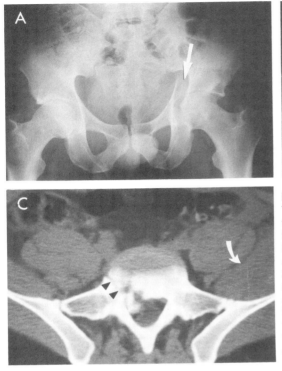

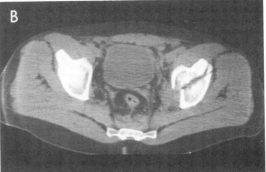

FIG 16–43.
These CT images of the pelvis dramatically disclose the extent of fractures not apparent on a routine x-ray film. Note also the unsuspected displaced fragment at S1 that extends into the central neural canal. Additionally, a fracture of the right transverse process of L5 was documented on the CT films that was not appreciated on the standard x-ray films (not shown). **A,** routine pelvic x-ray film showing an obvious fracture of the left hemipelvis *(arrow).* **B,** comminuted fracture of the acetabulum. **C,** unsuspected fracture of S1 *(arrowheads).* Note the large hematoma *(curved arrow).*

joints in characteristic roentgen patterns and distributions.

A frontal projection of the pelvis usually does not afford an adequate view of the sacroiliac joints, and it becomes necessary to perform a 45-degree oblique x-ray film due to their posterolateral oblique orientation. However, the addition of an anteroposterior film with the tube angled 20 to 35 degrees toward the head can project the joints' articular surfaces to better advantage.

Anatomically, the sacroiliac joints in part are true synovial joints with restricted mobility. The joint spaces themselves occupy only the lower half to two thirds of the joints—the upper por-

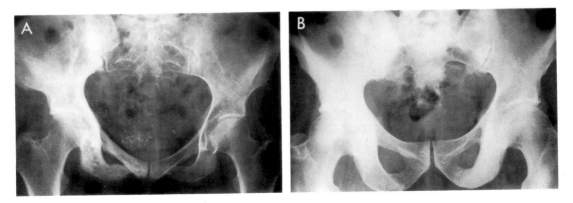

FIG 16–44.
Increased bone density in the pelvis. **A,** Paget's disease. **B,** osteoblastic metastasis.

tion being formed by interosseous ligaments. In adults, the spaces normally measure 2 to 5 mm in width.

In older individuals, the joints quite often reveal the changes of degenerative arthritis. This most often is bilateral and symmetric in distribution. The joint spaces narrow, and a thin line of sclerosis forms along the iliac aspect. Osteophytes or spurs commonly accompany the process, particularly along the anterior aspect. These can be focal and sclerotic and may be confused with an osteoblastic metastasis when seen on the frontal film. The spurs can extend inferiorly from the joints as well.

Excluding infection, a variety of inflammatory diseases may produce sacroiliitis. Listed among these are rheumatoid arthritis, rheumatoid spondylitis, psoriasis, Reiter's syndrome, and inflammatory intestinal disorders such as ulcerative colitis, regional enteritis (Crohn's disease), and Whipple's disease. Although there may be subtle differences among these, differentiation is often impossible and requires correlation with clinical and laboratory findings.

Because they are lined with synovium, the sacroiliac joints, like other synovial joints, may be involved with rheumatoid arthritis, but only in advanced cases. The alterations may involve only one side, but both are usually included and almost always in an asymmetric fashion. Demineralization about the joints is seen along with distinctive subarticular erosions that eventuate in narrowing of the spaces. Spurring and ankylosis (fusion) are not features of rheumatoid arthritis in the sacroiliac joints.

On the other hand, ankylosing spondylitis (Strümpell-Marie disease) is often bilaterally symmetric. The roentgenographic changes are distinctly different from those of rheumatoid arthritis. However, the sacroiliac joint alterations of rheumatoid arthritis and the other noninfectious inflammatory lesions can be very similar and preclude a differentiation in some cases. The fundamental findings of ankylosing spondylitis involve the ilium initially and consist of irregular deossification, articular erosions, indistinct subchondral

line density, and spotty sclerosis. Subsequent reactive new bone formation often bridges the joint space and can eventuate in actual ossification and obliteration of the joints. Another distinguishing peculiarity of rheumatoid spondylitis as it pertains to the pelvis is a fine-to-coarse spiculated or "whiskering" appearance that may develop along the inferior margins of the ischial tuberosities.

The distribution and pattern of involvement caused by the sacroiliitis of intestinal diseases may be similar to that of rheumatoid spondylitis. But psoriasis and Reiter's syndrome more often are unilateral or show asymmetry of each side and lack any bony bridging. The separation of these entities might be facilitated by moving up to the lumbar spine, where the classic changes of rheumatoid spondylitis, the "bamboo spine," may be identified. The bony bridges or syndesmophytes between the vertebral bodies (as seen in ankylosing spondylitis and bowel disease spondylitis) are smooth, uniform, thin, and symmetric. Those found in psoriasis and rheumatoid arthritis present as irregular, asymmetric, and thick outgrowths.

Gouty arthritis involving the sacroiliac joints occurs in long-standing and severe cases in a minority of individuals with this affliction. One or both joints may exhibit involvement. The most striking features are those seen in other skeletal regions: irregular, often large, subarticular erosions and related sclerosis.

The Knee

Roentgenographic Examination

The basic minimum examination of the knee consists of supine anteroposterior and flexed lateral views. The latter film should be obtained with the knee bent at least 45 degrees, although this may be impossible in an acutely injured, fluid-filled joint or in a severely osteoarthritic knee.

Certain situations will call for other views. Internal and external oblique films may help visualize otherwise nonvisible subtle fractures of the tibial plateaus or femoral condyles. These features, as well as the intercondylar space and the tibial spine (intercondylar crest), can also be evaluated with a tunnel film. The "sunrise" or tangential projection affords another perspective of the patella and the femoropatellar joint. A fat-blood level may be detected on an across-the-table horizontal beam roentgenogram and indicate an intra-articular fracture in which marrow fat and blood have been extruded into the joint.

Stress films, including valgus and varus manual forces, can bring out ligamentous injuries or laxity. Standing anteroposterior weight-bearing studies give information related to subtle joint space narrowing in degenerative osteoarthritis. Occasionally, tomography will elucidate abnormalities not identifiable on standard films. With the advent of better fluoroscopic equipment, intra-articular changes of the invisible cartilaginous menisci, articular cartilage, and ligaments can be successfully evaluated by means of double air-contrast arthrography.

Roentgenographic Anatomy and Developmental Variations

The distal femoral epiphysis normally appears in the ninth month of gestation and therefore is utilized in determining fetal maturity. At birth it measures approximately 5 mm. The distal femoral epiphysis normally fuses at 20 years of age. As in other areas of the skeleton, the epiphyseal line may persist as a faint track.

The intercondylar fossa, best evaluated on the tunnel film, forms a smooth arch. It serves primarily as a compartment for the proximal origins of the anterior and posterior cruciate ligaments.

The joint space, divided into medial and lateral compartments, normally measures 3 to 5 mm in height. It represents the thickness of the articular cartilages of the femur and tibia as well as the medial and lateral semilunar cartilages.

The proximal tibial epiphysis becomes visible by ossification in the last 2 months of fetal life. Like the femoral epiphysis, it fuses to the shaft by the 20th year. Between the ages of 7 and 15 years, the tongue-shaped anterior and inferior extension of the epiphysis is visible and forms the anterior tibial tuberosity or spine (Fig 16–45,A). The tuberosity is an extremely variable structure that develops in an irregular fashion and often has a fragmented appearance. This should not be confused with a fracture or Osgood-Schlatter disease. Its features on the antero-posterior view can be particularly bewildering (Fig 16–45,B). On the frontal view, a radiolucent cleft often appears over the proximal tibial shaft.

The articular surfaces of the proximal third of the tibia present a varied number of appearances, and this is especially true of the intercondylar eminence of the tibial spine. There are two major crests, lateral and medial. Occasionally, the clinician may identify an anteromedial tubercle to which the anterior cruciate ligament attaches. A similar but less frequently found posterolateral tubercle marks the insertion of the posterior cruciate ligament. The "tunnel" view of the knee usually demonstrates this anatomy to the best advantage. Small avulsion fragments arising from the crests and presenting as loose intra-articular bodies will be best projected on this x-ray film view.

The patella is considered a large sesamoid bone embedded in the quadriceps tendon. It should always be examined with a tangential film in addition to the lateral and frontal roentgenograms. On the anteroposterior projection, the details of the patella may become completely lost in the shadow of the distal portion of the femur, and hence pathologic changes may be overlooked, thereby requiring tangential, lateral, and sometimes oblique views.

Ossification of the patella is irregular in nature and arises from multiple foci. In the young it may be divided into several segments. It often has a granular appearance with irregular borders. Before complete fusion of the patellar ossification centers, there can be confusion with fractures, or its irregular outline may suggest osteochondritis (Fig 16–46).

One of the more difficult problems associated with roentgenographic appraisal of the patella is the commonly observed anomaly of patella par-

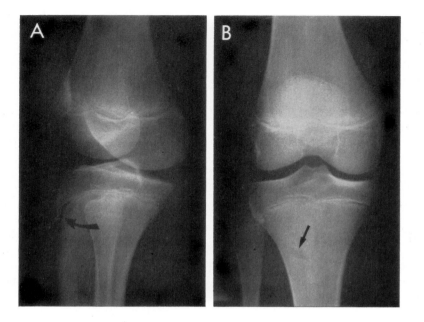

FIG 16–45.
Normal appearance of the anterior tibial tuberosity in a 12-year-old. **A,** lateral view. **B,** anteroposterior view. Note the radiolucent line *(arrow)* superimposing the tibial metaphysis.

tita. This condition is usually bilateral but must be differentiated from fractures. A bipartite status is the most prevalent form, but multipartite patellae also exist, and as many as six different segments have been reported. In the usual instance, or bipartite state, a radiolucent line separates a smaller segment that almost always occupies the upper-outer quadrant, although many other rare variations are found. There have been cases described for patellar partition into anterior and posterior portions.

A somewhat distracting osseous shadow, the fabella, is seen in 10% to 20% of knees along the posterior aspect (Fig 16–47). A small sesamoid bone of varying size and shape, it lies within the lateral head of the gastrocnemius muscle and is best seen on the lateral view. Many times it overlies the border of the lateral femoral condyle and appears as an avulsion fragment on the anteroposterior film. The bone is most often a bilateral finding and is seen more often in males. It must be differentiated from a fracture, loose joint body, foreign body, and phlebolith.

The soft tissues about the knee deserve partic-

ular attention and must not be overlooked on the knee roentgenogram. The fundamental observation in the presence of joint effusions is an anterior displacement of the patella and an elongated oval area of increased density above the patella that represents fluid in the suprapatellar bursa. A small amount of fluid may not produce these changes.

Not uncommon, short slivers of ossification immediately above and below the patella and usually attached to it represent the tendons of the quadriceps muscle and the patellar ligament, respectively. They can be misleading shadows to the unwary and probably represent the end result of tendinitis, much like that seen in the rotator cuff tendons of the shoulder.

Usually on the basis of degenerative processes, the menisci may become calcified. These must be differentiated from calcifications occurring in the articular cartilage, a process seen in degenerative osteoarthritis but also in pseudogout (chondrocalcinosis), a rare disorder in which calcium pyrophosphate is deposited in the cartilage.

It is not too surprising to visualize a radiolu-

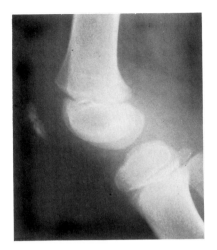

FIG 16–46.
Normal appearance of the patella in an 8-year-old. Note the irregular, fragmented, and sclerotic character simulating osteochondritis.

cent slit within the knee joint and, usually more frequently, within the hip and shoulder joints of children. This phenomenon is linked to a vacuum effect and is caused by pulling on the extremity or by producing forced adduction or abduction. It is important that this not be interpreted as abnormal. Nevertheless, in the elderly population it is a pathologic observation and may be seen in severe arthritis with degeneration of the cartilage. The finding is a potential perception in a vertebral spine with advanced degenerative disc disease.

Trauma

The majority of roentgenograms done for trauma to the knee will be normal. At times a joint effusion will be demonstrated, but fractures are infrequent. Fractures can involve one or both femoral condyles, the tibial tuberosity, or the proximal third of the fibula as well as the patella. As many views as are necessary should be utilized to evaluate these injuries.

Femorotibial dislocations are rare, can be anterior or posterior, and are often associated with a fracture. The major concerns in such situations are tearing of the collateral and cruciate ligaments and, more acutely important, severing of the popliteal artery, which will require angiography for proper assessment.

Tumor

Of the many benign tumors involving the knee region, osteochondroma is probably one of the more frequent, with the exception of benign cortical defects. The latter are peripherally located, round-to-oval radiolucencies that often measure no more than 2 cm. They have a sharply defined

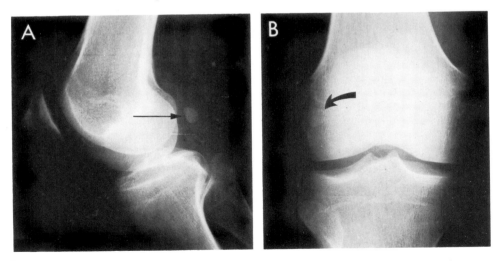

FIG 16–47.
The fabella (arrows). **A,** lateral view. **B,** anteroposterior view.

sclerotic margin and are common in the metaphyseal areas of the distal portion of the femur and the proximal and distal thirds of the tibia. They are asymptomatic and discovered incidentally on roentgenograms performed for other reasons. With advancing age they tend to disappear.

The osteochondroma is seen as a bony protuberance of variable size, contiguous with the femoral or tibial metaphyseal or diaphyseal bone marrow and extending away from the joint in the direction of the tendons and muscles (Fig 16–48). Osteochondromas have an invisible cap of cartilage. Solitary osteochondromas are less frequently demonstrated about other joints of the body. When these exotoses are multiple, they constitute a hereditary bone dysplasia designated as diaphyseal aclasis.

Aneurysmal bone cysts are found in the neural arches of the vertebrae, in the ends of long bones, and most frequently in the distal third of the femur. They become very expansive but are confined by a thin layer of cortical bone and contain many septa of bone.

A giant-cell tumor characteristically involves the distal portion of the femur. It is considered a benign vascular lesion, but occasionally it transforms into a locally invasive malignant process. There is a gradual eccentric expansion of a thinned cortex, but not to the same extent as an aneurysmal bone cyst. A "soap-bubble" appearance is quite characteristic. The lesion involves the closed epiphysis and metaphysis and extends to the subarticular cortex but not into the joint.

Although not ordinarily considered under the topic of tumors, bone infarcts, frequently located in the distal third of the femur, can create confusing roentgenographic changes. They occur in caisson disease, pancreatitis, and various vascular disorders. Any segment of bone, epiphysis, metaphysis, or diaphysis can be involved, but the alterations are confined to the medullary cavity. They appear as irregular sclerotic longitudinal streaks, occasionally with fine cystic patterns resembling a corkscrew (Fig 16–49).

The knee has the dubious distinction of being the most common site for the development of osteosarcoma. The metaphysis of the distal portion of the femur accounts for approximately 75% of all osteogenic sarcomas. This primary bone malignancy tends to occur during puberty, with boys being more commonly affected than girls. The roentgenographic changes take many forms, either being purely osteolytic or showing a mixed destructive and osteosclerotic pattern (Fig 16–50). Extensive soft-tissue involvement is the rule. Periosteal reaction can be exuberant, eventually forming the typical spiculated "sunburst" appearance, although this is not always present.

Under the heading of round-cell tumors, Ewing's sarcoma is manifested as a solitary lesion arising in the diaphysis and metaphysis of long bones, particularly the femur; however, it has been observed with relative frequency in the humerus and ulna as well as the pelvis. Originating in the bone marrow, it produces a characteristic

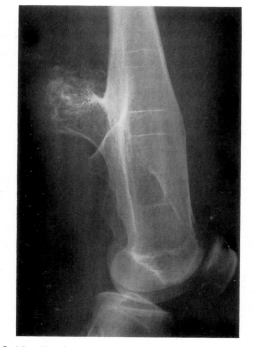

FIG 16–48.
Osteochondroma of the knee.

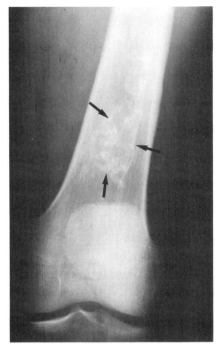

FIG 16–49.
Bone infarct of the distal third of the femur *(arrows)*.

layered periosteal thickening resembling an "onion skin." A variable patchy dissolution without significant expansion is imparted to the osseous architecture. Unfortunately, the symptoms of fever and pain and the sarcoma's roentgenographic manifestations can resemble those of osteomyelitis in the child and adolescent, and indeed the distinction may be extremely difficult to make.

Arthritis

Osteoarthritis is a familiar affliction of the knee (Fig 16–51). Degenerative wear and tear produce the changes with progressing age, but secondary post-traumatic arthrosis is also a leading offender. Minimal joint space narrowing will be one of the earliest roentgenographic changes reflecting wearing and thinning of the articular cartilage. Standing weight-bearing films might be required to demonstrate this finding. The decreased height of the joint space may be accompanied by increasing sclerosis of the subarticular

region of the tibia, quite often the medial condyle. The femoropatellar joint will undergo similar alterations of narrowing and associated sclerosis of the articular surface of the patella. Eventually the process leads to bony spurs arising from the articular margins of the femur, tibia, and patella. These osteophytes may become significantly large so that function is impaired.

Subchondral cysts, which are not always evident, are a unique feature of osteoarthritis, even in joints other than the knee. They are well-defined round-to-oval lucencies, one or more in number, and measure anywhere from a few millimeters to 3 to 4 cm. One proposed theory for their evolution states that, because they are lined with synovium, they represent protrusions of the membrane through a defect in the articular cartilage. A small channel forms a direct communication between the cysts and the joint space, and this has been proved on pathologic dissections. A change in the intra-articular fluid and pressure dynamics of the disorganized joint is thought to be the mechanism for their formation.

The actual size of the intercondylar fossa, as seen on the tunnel view, may enlarge somewhat in osteoarthritis. This feature, however, is more pronounced in rheumatoid arthritis and the arthrosis of hemophilia with repeated intra-articular hemorrhages.

Osteochondritis

There are several disease entities classified as osteochondritis or aseptic necrosis involving the knee. The abnormalities of osteochondritis dissecans have already been described (Chapter 10). Osgood-Schlatter disease is another form involving the anterior tibial tubercle. As mentioned previously, there is a significant variation in the roentgenographic appearance of the normal tuberosity, and the diagnosis is primarily a clinical one. Even though there may be sclerosis and/or fragmentation, this does not necessarily constitute Osgood-Schlatter disease. The only roentgenographic abnormality, almost universally present in the acute phase, is overlying soft-tissue swelling. The principal purpose for obtaining the

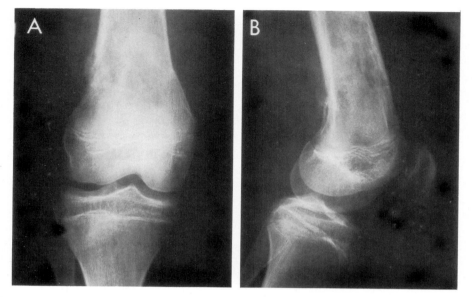

FIG 16–50.
Osteosarcoma of the knee. **A,** anteroposterior view; **B,** lateral view. Note the mottled bone destruction with interrupted periosteal reaction and soft-tissue extension.

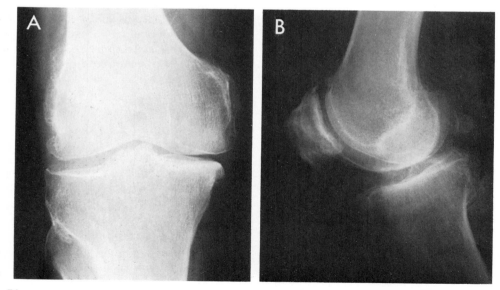

FIG 16–51.
Osteoarthritis of the knee. **A,** anteroposterior view; **B,** lateral view.

films is to exclude some other lesion, such as tumor or infection.

One other type of osteochondritis that might be encountered in the knee is Blount's disease, or tibia vara. For some unknown reason, possibly stress, a localized growth disturbance occurs along the medial-posterior aspect of the tibial metaphysis. The changes may appear between the ages of 1 through 12 years and culminate in outward bowing of one or both legs.

Roentgenographically, the medial tibial metaphysis is widened and forms a broad spur that extends both medially and posteriorly. The medial surface of the tibial epiphysis becomes flattened and produces a slope of concavity where this growth center is normally convex.

Without correction, the fully developed knee may exhibit a persistent downward slope of the medial tibial articular surface. The medial femoral condyle hypertrophies to compensate for the tibial deformity.

The Ankle and Foot

Roentgenographic Examination

Three views are mandatory for proper evaluation of the ankle, and three projections are necessary for the foot examination. As elsewhere in the skeleton, modified and special films can clarify suspicious areas.

For the ankle, the three films include anteroposterior, lateral, and oblique projections (Fig 16–52). The oblique study, or mortise view, is obtained by rotating the foot internally 10 to 15 degrees. Even though the calcaneus, tarsal bones, and bases of the metatarsal bones are not considered anatomically a part of the ankle, they should be included since associated or isolated injuries to these structures may be found when symptoms point only to the ankle. A good example of this is a fracture of the base of the fifth metatarsal bone.

An external oblique view might be requested when there is still a question of an abnormality in the absence of findings on the three standard x-ray films. A subtle fracture of either malleoli may be brought out in this way.

In the presence of soft-tissue swelling following trauma but without an associated fracture, ligamentous damage must be considered. Stress anteroposterior filming utilizing manual abduction and adduction of the heel may be indicated. Widening of the ankle mortise strongly suggests a tear in either or both the medial deltoid ligament

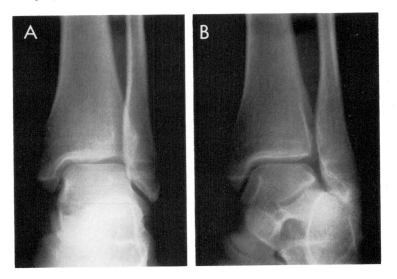

FIG 16–52.
Normal ankle films. **A,** anteroposterior view; **B,** oblique (mortise) view (see Fig 16–53 for lateral view details).

or lateral collateral ligaments. Because of pain, maneuvering the ankle for stress views may require local anesthesia.

The standard roentgenographic study of the foot should include anteroposterior, internally rotated oblique, and lateral projections. Because of superimposition, the metatarsal and phalangeal bones cannot be evaluated to any extent on the lateral film, but the talus, calcaneus, and tarsal bones are relatively clearly outlined. Additionally, the talocalcaneal, talonavicular, and calcaneocuboid joints are well depicted. On the anteroposterior film, the cuboid and lateral cuneiform bones are superimposed, and the bases of the metatarsals tend to be obscured by overlap. These bones are projected into profile with internal oblique films. An externally rotated oblique view will delineate the first metatarsal and medial cuneiform bones.

The toes should be examined with anteroposterior and internal and external oblique films. An individual toe that causes concern requires a lateral view. This may be performed by having the patient hold the toe in extension with a pencil while the other toes are held in flexion, a maneuver that also is utilized for finger roentgenograms.

The heel is best demonstrated with lateral and axial (tangential) films. However, as will be pointed out later, oblique exposures sometimes aid in the study of this bone.

Roentgenographic Anatomy, Variants, and Pathology

Ankle. The ankle mortise is formed by the distal third of the fibula (lateral malleolus), styloid process of the tibia (medial malleolus), the horizontal articular plate of the tibia (plafond), and the dome-shaped articular surface of the talus (tenon) (see Fig 16–52).

On the lateral view, the width of the joint space between the tibia and talus narrows from anterior to posterior in the normal subject. Because of this, most ankle dislocations are anterior, except where there is a disruptive fracture of the mortise.

As has been mentioned previously with other growth centers, a linear sclerotic zone of bone condensation or a lucent line of incomplete union may persist in the distal portion of the tibia where the epiphyseal line existed. Additionally, just as in the distal thirds of the radius or femur, a variable number of regular transverse bands of increased bone density may be observed in the tibial metaphysis. These so-called growth lines are normal; they tend to disappear with age and should not be confused with a pathologic process such as the lines of lead poisoning.

Not infrequently, the tip of the medial or the lateral malleoli arises from separate ossification centers that fail to fuse. The resultant os subtibiale and os subfibulare can be variable in size, but like all accessory bones, they have a well-defined thin cortical margin throughout their circumference. This will differentiate them from recent fractures.

Because of the high frequency of accessory bones in the ankle and foot, comparative views are recommended since the findings are usually but not always bilateral. If the distinction between fracture and an accessory ossicle is difficult, the clinician should consider one of several textbooks dealing with normal variants (Birkner, 1978; Keats, 1984; Kohler and Zimmer, 1968).

One of the best-known accessory skeletal elements of the ankle in addition to the os subtibiale and os subfibiale is the os trigonum (Fig 16–53). Situated behind the talus near the posterior aspect of the talocalcaneal joint, it is best viewed on the lateral roentgenogram. Its shape and size are variable, and it may measure a centimeter or more. Despite its frequency, it still is commonly misinterpreted as a fracture.

Rarely, the os trigonum may be mimicked by a fracture of the posterior tubercle of the talus. This may occur when the posterior talar process becomes wedged between the posterior articular rim of the tibia and the calcaneus with severe forced plantar flexion.

On the anteroposterior projection of the ankle, the Achilles tendon is seen as a thick band of slightly increased density behind the tibia. The resultant shadow at times can create a bewilder-

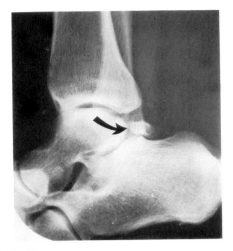

FIG 16–53.
Os trigonum *(arrow).*

ing roentgenogram. On the mortise film, the clinician may see a horizontal V-shaped lucency through the medial margin of the talus. This corresponds to the inner margin of the talocalcaneal joint.

Overlap of the cortical margins of the fibula and tibia occurs in most views of the ankle, except a correctly positioned mortise film. This results in an apparent radiolucent defect termed a "Mach" effect and often leads to fracture misinterpretation.

On the lateral view of the ankle, distension of the joint capsule with blood can be discerned in either or both the anterior or posterior soft-tissue compartments. Such a finding is often indicative of a fracture of the distal portion of the tibia or talus but not the lateral malleolus since the synovial membrane of the capsule invests only the talus and tibia but not the distal third of the fibula.

Benign cortical defects are a relatively frequent finding in the distal portion of the tibia in children and are just as common in the femur and tibia about the knee. Their characteristics have been described under the section of the knee. They are easily distinguishable on roentgenograms from more serious lesions.

The distal third of the tibia is a favorite site for

the development of Brodie's abscess. This lesion results from a sharply localized pyogenic infection of low virulence. This isolated form of osteomyelitis, seen primarily in children, quite often involves the metaphysis. Its intramedullary location is usually eccentric. It is seen on roentgenograms as a central irregular lucency surrounded by a thick capsule of sclerotic bone.

Foot. Overlap of the individual bony elements of the foot tends to make evaluation of the roentgenographic anatomy somewhat difficult. Anatomically, the bones of the foot include the phalanges, metatarsals, cuboid, the three cuneiforms, navicular, and the calcaneus, as well as the talus, although the latter is also considered a component of the ankle.

Of the tarsal bones, the talus is second only to the calcaneus as the most frequent bone to be fractured. The majority of these injuries are chip and avulsion types. They may occur along the anteroposterior surface of the neck, and therefore a lateral film is required. Such fractures have also been described along the medial, lateral, and posterior processes. A fragment of the posterior eminence may simulate the os trigonum. Less commonly, the talus is fractured through the neck.

The talus is more susceptible to dislocation than the other tarsal bones because it is the only bone in the lower extremity not having direct muscle attachments. Furthermore, due to its tenuous vascular supply, post-traumatic aseptic necrosis of the talus may eventually take place.

The calcaneus anatomically consists of a body and a large posterior tuberosity. The sustentaculum tali forms a platform of bone along the inner superior surface of the body that provides support to the anterior portion of the talus. The posterior facet, behind the sustentaculum tali, is that portion of the talocalcaneal (subtalar) joint that slopes downward, as seen on the lateral reentgenogram, and into which the lateral triangular process of the talus projects (Fig 16–54).

The apophysis of the posterior calcaneal tuberosity appears early in life and fuses in or

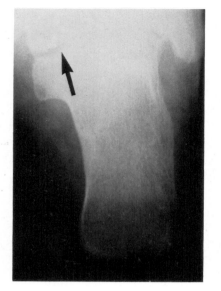

FIG 16–54.
Axial view of the os calcis. Note the sustentaculum tali (arrow).

about the 17th year. The margins of the apophysis and the posterior tuberosity can look quite irregular and ragged. The apophysis itself may exhibit fragmentation and varying degrees of sclerosis (Fig 16–55). Sever's disease, a form of osteochondritis or aseptic necrosis (discussed in a

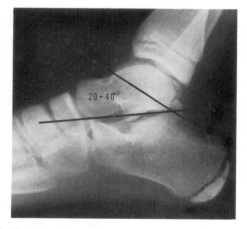

FIG 16–55.
This lateral film of an ankle demonstrates Boehler's angle. Normal measurement is 20 to 40 degrees.

previous section), has been ascribed to this ossification center, but much like Osgood-Schlatter's disease of the knee, the diagnosis is principally clinical since the normal x-ray film appearance is extremely inconstant. Once fused, the area may show multiple irregular striations and some irregularity of the margins. It is of interest that in rheumatoid spondylitis the posterior surface of the tuberosity may display typical "whiskering" or fraying of its margins much like that seen in the ischial tuberosities of the pelvis.

In order to properly evaluate the heel, especially in cases of trauma, in addition to the lateral film a tangential (axial) projection (Fig 16–54) as well as both oblique views are required. To obtain the axial exposure, the patient is seated on the table with his heel against the film. A towel or long piece of gauze is placed around the ball and toes of the foot, and the individual is instructed to flex the foot by pulling on the cloth. The tube is angled 40 degrees toward the head and centered over the heel. Multiple axial films from angles of 20 to 40 degrees may be necessary to properly demonstrate the location and extent of a fracture.

Fractures of the os calcis are often the result of a fall from a height feet first; crushing injuries with compression and comminution are produced. In 10% of such cases, the fractures are bilateral, and in a similar percentage there will be an associated injury of the lumbar or thoracic spine due to the vertical compression forces dispersed into the back.

The lateral convex and medial concave surfaces of the calcaneus should be well delineated on the axial view. If the film is accurately exposed, the sustentaculum tali along the medial aspect will also be identified.

When viewing the os calcis on the lateral examination, it is mandatory that Boehler's angle be measured. This is formed by the intersection of (1) a line drawn from the dome of the os calcis at the talocalcaneal joint to the anterior process of this same bone and (2) a line extending from the posterior tubercle to the dome of the calcaneus (see Fig 16–55). Normally this measures 20 to 40 degrees. With compression fractures, this angle will be reduced. Subtle compression fractures may be overlooked without measuring this angle.

Stress fractures of the os calcis do not become manifested immediately after injury, similar to other bones of the body. It may take 10 or more days before a line of sclerotic endosteal new bone is detected that parallels the posterior border of the heel.

Exostoses or spurs are a common finding in the heel. They can arise from the posterior or inferior margin of the tuberosity. The posterior bony outgrowths extend in the direction of the Achilles tendon. Inferior or plantar spurs grow toward the sole of the foot within the plantar fascia. These excrescences may lead to local irritation and subsequent pain.

A somewhat rounded-to-triangular area of lucency that is relatively well circumscribed will occasionally be observed in the body of the calcaneus on the lateral roentgenogram (Fig 16–56). This finding can create interpretive difficulties since it simulates a cyst. This has been proved anatomically to represent a normal area of thinned, deficient trabeculae. This is usually an incidental finding and can be very disturbing when seen.

When considering the tarsal navicular bone roentgenographically, there are several lesions that deserve discussion because of their relatively common occurrence. Traumatic injuries to the

tarsal navicular are uncommon. Avulsion fractures along the dorsal surface may be found near the talonavicular joint and require differentiation from an os supranaviculare. The medial tuberosity that serves for the insertion of the posterior tibial tendon may be subjected to forces resulting in fracture. Importantly, such a fracture may be associated with a fracture of the cuboid bone, often with dorsal subluxation of the navicular. An accessory bone, the os tibiale externum, located behind the tuberosity is more frequent than tuberosity fractures and may be confused with one (Fig 16–57).

Of all of the tarsal bones, the cuboid initially has the most striking features due to its multifragmented appearance. After a short interval, the fragments become united into one solid structure.

Rarely encountered, cuboid anomalies are synostoses to the calcaneus, talus, navicular, or metatarsals. Accessory bones closely related to the cuboid are the relatively common os peroneum and less frequent os vesalianum. Their distinction from avulsion fractures is not always simple.

It is a rare occasion for the cuboid to exhibit an isolated fracture. Ordinarily, there are associ-

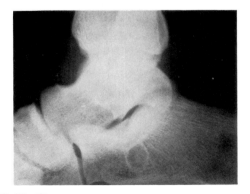

FIG 16–56.
Normal lucency within the os calcis simulates a cyst.

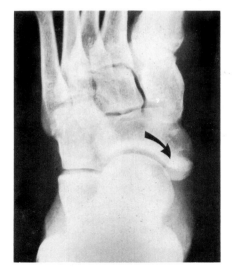

FIG 16–57.
Os tibiale externum (arrow).

ated tarsal injuries, usually the tuberosity of the navicular or anterior process of the calcaneus.

The three cuneiform bones are anatomically labeled and numbered as follows: (1) medial or internal, (2) middle, and (3) lateral or external. Like the navicular and cuboid bones, the internal cuneiform may demonstrate multicentric ossification. A not-so-infrequent finding is division of the first cuneiform into dorsal and plantar segments representing a true bipartite condition. Isolated fractures of any of the three cuneiforms are definitely an uncommon situation.

With the correct roentgenographic projection on the internal oblique film, the joint space between the first and second cuneiform bones can appear quite wide and might lead the clinician to a false impression of a separation. The middle and external cuneiforms often elude appropriate inspection due to their inconspicuous positions within the framework of the bony arch.

In the growing foot, the epiphyseal centers of the metatarsal bones are essentially similar in location to those of the hand. They appear in the third year and normally fuse about 15 years of age. Each of the metatarsals contains one epiphysis, but the fifth metatarsal also possesses an apophysis at its proximal end. The epiphyses of the second through fifth metatarsals are distal, whereas that of the great toe is proximal. On rare instances, the clinician may encounter pseudoepiphyses at the bases of the lateral four metatarsals, particularly the third and also the head or distal aspect of the first metatarsal. Occasionally, a cleft divides the epiphysis of the great toe metatarsal bone and should not be misconstrued as a fracture.

Several interpretive challenges are presented by the appearance of the base of the fifth metatarsal bone. The longitudinally oriented shell-like apophysis can be roentgenographically dissimilar in the feet of the same individual and vary in size and shape. Furthermore, it may persist unfused throughout life, but this is an uncommon event. Ordinarily the distinction between the apophysis and a fracture is relatively simple since the growth line is oriented to the axis of the shaft, whereas a fracture is transverse in almost all in-

stances (Fig 16–58). An accessory bone, the os vesalianum, alluded to previously, is located near the junction of the proximal metatarsal tuberosity and the cuboid. This fact should be remembered when evaluating trauma to this area.

A moderate degree of overlap of the bases of the metatarsal bones is noted to a greater or lesser degree on all views, but more so on anteroposterior projections. With the "Mach" effect in mind, this can and has led to the diagnosis of many erroneous fractures. The internal oblique film tends to reduce this problem to some extent.

When viewing the foot, the tarsometatarsal joints form a somewhat curvilinear line convex toward the toes. This is disrupted only by the recessed base of the second metatarsal bone, which results from a relatively short middle cuneiform. The base of this metatarsal is therefore wedged between the first and third cuneiform bones. Furthermore, the medial margins of the base of the second metatarsal and the middle cuneiform are always in line (Fig 16–59).

In the proximal space between the bases of the first and second metatarsal bones may be found the os intermetatarseum. It is located

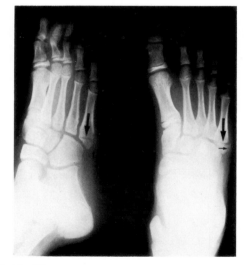

FIG 16–58.
Transverse fracture *(large arrows)* through the base of the fifth metatarsal bone. Note the normal shell-like apophysis *(small arrow)* that will increase in size before fusion.

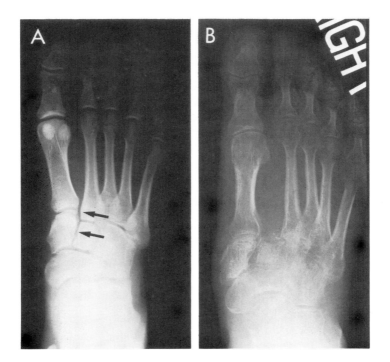

FIG 16–59.
A, normal alignment of the second metatarsal and middle cuneiform bones *(arrows)*. **B,** lateral dislocation of the three middle metatarsal bones.

along the dorsal surface and, like most accessory ossicles, can assume variable sizes and shapes. Radiopacities in the form of arteriosclerotic vascular plaques can also be seen in this same interdigital space. Both of these can simulte avulsion fractures.

There is one traumatic lesion involving the metatarsal area that deserves special attention but, fortunately, is infrequent. The Lisfranc fracture-dislocation involves the tarsometatarsal junction and consists essentially of dorsal displacement of the metatarsal bases. Two basic forms exist: homolateral and divergent. In the homolateral type, the lateral four metatarsals are dislocated posteriorly and laterally, often with associated fractures at the bases. The divergent type exists when the first metatarsal is displaced medially and the others are dislocated laterally. The disfigurations may be subtle, and the normal straight alignment of the second metatarsal and middle cuneiform bones should be utilized (see Fig 16–59).

SPECIALIZED RADIOLOGIC STUDIES OF THE MUSCULOSKELETAL SYSTEM

Nuclear Medicine Procedures

In a few of the previous sections, the use of radioactive isotopes in the evaluation of certain bone disorders has been touched upon. For some time now it has been known that phosphorus compounds will be metabolized in bone at a rapid rate and this assimilation can be readily detected by a scintillation camera when the substance is tagged by the radiotracer technetium

99m. Areas of very rapid bone turnover (such as those seen in healing fractures, aggressive tumors, and infections) can readily be detected by bone scanning.

There are occasions when fractures are extremely subtle or undetectable on standard roentgenograms, such as fractures that may be seen in the hip. Two to 5 days are required following the injury before scans demonstrate the fracture optimally. Abnormal increased activity may persist for up to 2 years or longer, depending on the severity of the injury. Nuclear scans can be particularly helpful in determining the age of compression deformities of the vertebral bodies.

Staging of tumors for therapeutic protocols has been greatly enhanced by the improved quality of bone scans over the past few years. Skeletal scintigrams are extremely sensitive to the presence of metastatic lesions, although their specificity is not as good as routine x-ray films. All patients with diagnoses of bronchogenic carcinoma, breast carcinoma, carcinoma of the prostate, and hypernephroma in addition to those who have a number of other tumors known to metastasize to the osseous system should have a baseline bone scan for staging purposes.

Benign tumors are less frequently evaluated by radionuclide bone scans. One exception, however, is the osteoid osteoma, a painful lesion that can affect the spine as well as the extremities and go undetected by the usual methods of examination. This tumor will take up the isotope intensely and reveal its location.

The presence and progress of osteomyelitis and its response to therapy can be adequately documented by bone scintigraphy. Gallium-133 can also be utilized due to its affinity to inflammatory and neoplastic processes, but it is seldom used in the study of bone infections. It can, however, quantitate soft-tissue involvement.

Reflex sympathetic dystrophy, described more extensively in a previous chapter, oftentimes can be followed by serial bone scans to determine whether it is quiescent, progressing, or improving.

Diagnostic Ultrasound

Exquisite image resolution and anatomic detail are possible with state-of-the-art, real-time diagnostic ultrasound systems. High-precision, small-parts transducers in the range of 7.5 to 10 mHz are now available that afford excellent structural delineation of the thyroid gland, testicles, and breast lesions, as well as vascular studies combined with Doppler flow measurements. Bone cannot be imaged with ultrasound; that along with its inability to be transmitted through air is a distinct disadvantage. However, soft-tissues provide an excellent medium for evaluation by sonography. The muscles of the extremities in particular can be examined easily and without discomfort to the patient.

Soft-tissue tumors, although uncommon, if unresectable can be followed by sequential sonographic studies, with their response to therapy recorded. Invasive characteristics such as osseous, neural, or vascular involvement cannot be depicted with ultrasound as well as with CT or MRI, however. Biopsies of such masses are easily performed under the guidance of ultrasound.

Sonography offers one of the best approaches to the detection of abscesses in the soft tissues. The location and extent can be adequately shown. Furthermore, ultrasonically guided needle aspiration of inflammatory masses for culture and sensitivity as well as drainage adds another dimension to the procedure.

Arthrography

Many joints in the body are accessible to needle entry and can be opacified for radiographic visualization by the introduction of iodinated contrast media, air, or both (double-contrast arthrography). Fluoroscopic spot films or overhead roentgenograms can then be obtained in multiple projections to delineate the intrinsic intra-articular anatomy.

The knee and shoulder are the most frequently examined joints, but the wrist, elbow, hip, and ankle as well as the temporomandibular joints may be studied by arthrography. The greater availability of the arthroscope and increased surgical expertise in its use have led to a decline in the number of knee studies, but the orthopedic surgeon occasionally will request the examination in difficult diagnostic cases.

Arthrographic procedures carry a low morbidity, are easily tolerated as an outpatient examination, and are quite simple to perform. Sterile technique is required in all cases along with local lidocaine (Xylocaine) anesthesia. Shoulder arthrography has its greatest application in the study of rotator cuff tears (Fig 16–60). It is also useful in the analysis of adhesive capsulitis (frozen shoulder), arthritis, synovitis, and capsular integrity, besides being helpful in the detection of loose bodies and abnormalities of the biceps tendon. The cartilaginous rim of the glenohum-

eral joint, the glenoid labrum, can be depicted and examined for tears and degeneration similar to examination of the knee menisci.

Adequately performed arthrography of the knee will define pathologic conditions of the medial and lateral meniscal cartilages, cruciate ligaments, collateral ligaments, articular cartilage, synovium (i.e., Baker's cyst), and joint capsule (Fig 16–61).

Xerography

The physical principles relating to x-ray xerography need not be detailed here other than to state that the resultant images are imprinted upon a special form of paper and that soft-tissue detail is much greater than that obtained with standard roentgenograms. However, by itself it offers no great advantage over x-ray films in the interpretation of bone. Of course, its largest application is in the field of mammography.

Xerography can provide information regarding the soft tissues that is not available on x-ray film images. It can be particularly helpful in detecting relatively nonopaque foreign bodies such as glass and wood. On occasion, the process will reveal anatomic data about primary soft-tissue tumors that are not visible otherwise, such as microcalcifications. Extension of tumors or inflammatory lesions of the muscles into bone may be best depicted by xerograms than by radiographs.

Infrequently subtle fractures will be identified or more apparent than on routine x-ray films. The fine periosteal reaction related to stress fractures may be detected more readily on xerograms.

Angiography

Angiography has a somewhat limited role in orthopedics. Its principal contribution is in the area of trauma when fractures of the extremities are infrequently complicated by vascular injury (Fig 16–62).

Less often, the evaluation of primary osseous or soft-tissue neoplasms can be aided by employ-

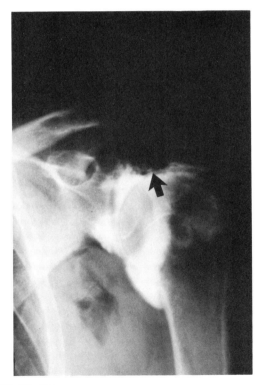

FIG 16–60.
An example of a double air-contrast arthrogram of the shoulder demonstrates a tear of the rotator cuff *(arrow)*.

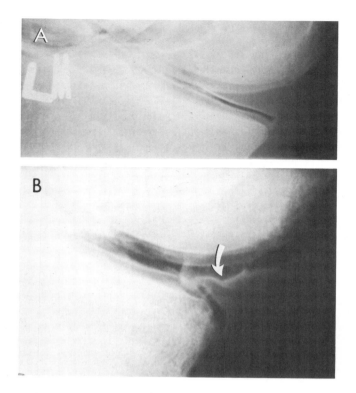

FIG 16–61.
These images demonstrate a normal-appearing medial meniscus **(A)** and a tear of the meniscus **(B)** *(arrow),* as seen on arthrography.

ing angiograms (Fig 16–63). Preoperative assessment of the degree of vascularity of the lesion in addition to its major blood supply can be invaluable to the surgeon's approach.

Standard Radiographic Tomography

There is a limited, potentially rewarding number of applications of standard x-ray tomography in the assessment of the skeleton. Simple linear tomography or more sophisticated pluridirectional tomographic systems can be indicated in certain instances of traumatic, neoplastic, or infectious processes involving the peripheral skeleton or the spine.

Subtle but clinically important fractures may be outside the limits of visibility on plain radiographs. But if symptoms should warrant, tomog-

raphy may be indicated to be certain of the presence or absence of pathology, such as in the case of a suspected carpal navicular fracture, a possible subcapital fracture of the hip, or a case in which a vascular groove needs to be differentiated from a true fracture (i.e., in the scapula). Questionable fractures involving the spine, particularly the odontoid or posterior neural arch elements, may require tomographic study.

The early changes of osteomyelitis or an osteogenic sarcoma may not be detected on plain films yet may be clearly delineated by the use of tomograms. Benign osteoid osteomas will give a characteristic appearance of a central lucent nidus surrounded by dense sclerosis, and this usually requires sectional filming in order to be seen.

Image detail is obviously improved over stan-

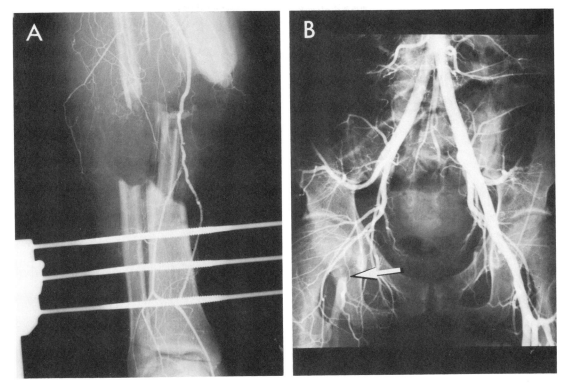

FIG 16–62.
Both of these angiograms are examples of the importance of angiography in cases of trauma in which arterial injury is suspected. **A,** a lower extremity study shows extensive vascular damage with complete disruption of the anterior and peroneal arteries and severe irregularity of the posterior tibial artery. **B,** this young man received blunt trauma to the pelvis. A routine x-ray film failed to reveal a fracture, but angiography demonstrates complete severance of the external iliac artery *(arrow)* with loss of all pulses to the extremity.

dard x-ray films by tomography. Although it is much less expensive than CT, it has some major practical disadvantages. It cannot define the intricate intrinsic bone detail, nor can it demonstrate the exquisite soft-tissue anatomy that CT scanning is capable of showing.

Computed Tomography

Detailed cross-sectional depiction of musculoskeletal anatomy and pathology has clearly established CT as a secondary diagnostic modality in the evaluation of bone, joint, and soft-tissue abnormalities. It is the imaging procedure that can clarify findings on conventional roentgenograms, standard tomography, and bone scans. The CT scan demonstrates greater sensitivity and specificity than do these other methods. Additionally, CT has a definite position in assessment of the spine, particularly the lumbar region, and this is most applicable in complex fractures and lesions affecting the spinal canal such as herniated discs.

The accuracy of CT depends on the presence of fat in the surrounding soft tissues to define individual muscles, vessels, and nerves. In cases in which there is a paucity of fat, CT has a limited role. Such is the case in the distal parts of extremities and in infants as well as in thin or emaciated patients.

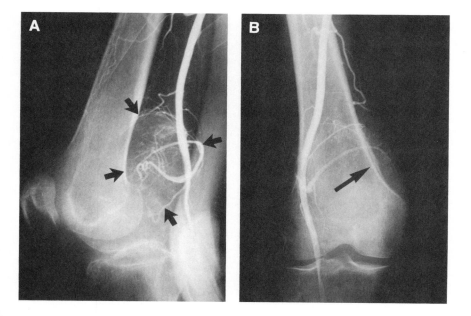

FIG 16–63.
An angiogram of a lower extremity in an elderly male with a large soft-tissue mass above the knee. The study delineates the neovascularity and mass displacement of the tumor (**A**, *arrows*) with secondary erosion of the adjacent bone (**B**, *arrows*). Pathologic findings disclosed this to be a fibrosarcoma.

In primary bone tumors, CT can accurately describe marrow and soft-tissue extent, including vascular and nerve involvement. Conventional roentgenograms cannot identify such details, which can influence the surgeon's approach or help in the selection of radiation ports.

Evaluation of metastatic bone disease is more appropriately performed by standard filming and radionuclide bone scanning. However, CT may be extremely helpful in areas of complex anatomy, such as in the spine or pelvic regions. Not infrequently, a person with known cancer demonstrates a single abnormal focus on a nuclear bone scan. It has been found that nearly 40% of these individuals eventually are proved to have bone metastasis. CT can be invaluable in the workup of these solitary bone scan abnormalities.

Distinguishing between benign and malignant soft-tissue tumors is easily accomplished by CT. Benign lesions are sharply demarcated and uniformly homogeneous and are confined to a single muscle or compartment. They may compress or displace vessels and nerves but, of course, do not invade them, which can be identified by CT. Conversely, malignant soft-tissue masses have no well-defined margins because of their infiltrative nature and naturally invade and distort adjacent nerves and vessels. Extension into adjoining bone is also well demonstrated by CT. Furthermore, malignant tumors often involve multiple muscle groups and compartments.

CT can be very useful in selected trauma cases, particularly those involving complex anatomic areas such as the spine, pelvis, hips, and shoulders. The cross-sectional image display of CT eliminates the overlapping structures and depicts the spatial relationship of fracture fragments to joints, muscles, nerves, and vessels. In addition, it can detect and define the extent of associated hemorrhage and hematoma formation (see Fig 16–43).

On occasion, infectious processes involving bone, joints, and soft tissues can be best demonstrated by CT. Osteomyelitis of long bones and infections of the spine and intervertebral discs, however, usually do not require CT, except when the diagnosis is in doubt with the more conventional means. Soft-tissue abscesses may at times be difficult to distinguish between tumor or hematoma. Early in the process, an abscess may have the same density as surrounding muscles, but it eventually undergoes central necrosis with liquefaction and acquires a low density center with an irregular peripheral high-density wall. The presence of air within an abscess suggests communication with the skin surface or air-forming bacteria.

Magnetic Resonance Imaging

Clinical indications for MRI are becoming well established. Applications of this newest diagnostic modality, particularly in the central nervous system, are well known and increasingly utilized. However, the development and usefulness of MRI in musculoskeletal disorders has become, to say the least, overwhelming. Recent developments in computer software and techniques have led to an increased usage of MRI in evaluation of the spine and extremities, and it has replaced CT in a number of areas.

MRI has multiplanar capabilities, that is, it can image in the sagittal, coronal, as well as the axial (transverse) planes in addition to oblique variations of these, thus providing more useful information than CT does, which is limited to the axial plane. Furthermore, unlike CT, it possesses greater contrast resolution and better delineates muscles, tendons, ligaments, fat, and fluids. Since it does not utilize ionizing radiation, MRI has no harmful effects and, indeed, is thought to be risk free for most patients. MRI contraindications include pregnancy (unknown teratogenic effects), those patients with pacemakers and electrostimulating devices, and individuals with intracranial ferromagnetic metal clips and metallic foreign bodies in close proximity to vital structures, which can be displaced by the strong magnetic force. Most prosthetic devices and surgical clips

today are nonferromagnetic and do not cause any significant problems to the patient or degrade the images.

In general physical terms, MRI employs a strong, uniform magnetic field into which the patient is placed. Specially designed surface conduction coils are placed near or around the region to be examined. Somewhat like a compass in the earth's magnetic field, the person's cellular hydrogen nuclei (protons) will align themselves appropriately. The polarized nuclei are in an elevated energy state, and via the coils a specified radio wave is transmitted through them and, as the result of a complex physical change, produces the release of energy that is tissue characteristic. This energy, in the form of radio waves, is then detected and amplified and the data collected by a computer, where it is processed into an image.

A number of disease entities affecting the spine and the soft tissues, bones, and joints of the extremities can be exquisitely demonstrated by MRI. These include musculoskeletal infections, bone and soft-tissue tumors, and various traumatic lesions. In addition, a long list of miscellaneous conditions are adequately evaluated such as congenital abnormalities, osteonecrosis, myopathies, arthritides, and bone marrow disorders. The discussions that follow will touch on a few of these and illustrate when MRI can be helpful in certain clinical situations.

MRI of the Spine

The vertebral bodies and their posterior neural arch components as well as the surrounding muscles can be *well demonstrated* with MRI. Additionally, the intervertebral discs are optimally visualized. MRI also depicts the contents of the central neural canal, including the cord, nerve roots, dura, and ligamentum flavum. The neural foramina and associated exiting nerve roots can be identified on sagittal and axial views. Figure 16–64 illustrates the normal midline sagittal appearance of the cervical, thoracic, and lumbosacral spine. Standard MRI protocol consists of 3- to 5-mm contiguous sagittal images from the neural

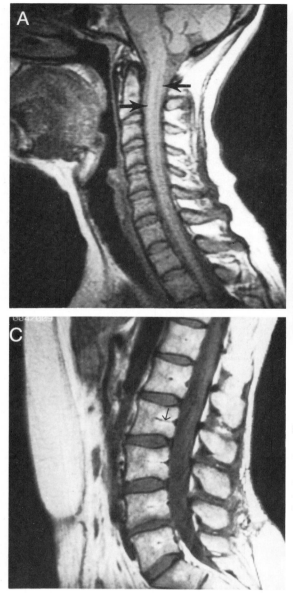

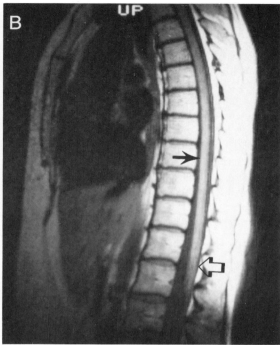

FIG 16-64.
Normal midline sagittal MRI of the entire spine. **A,**
cervical spine. **B,** thoracic spine. **C,** lumbar spine. Note
in detail the cord *(closed arrows)*, the conus medullaris
(open arrow), and the bones and intervertebral discs.
Also note the vascular channels in the posterior aspects
of the vertebral bodies *(vertical arrow)*.

foramina from one side to the other (Fig 16–65).
Selected axial images through the intervertebral
disc spaces are also performed (Fig 16–66). Occasionally coronal views are obtained that simulate x-ray contrast myelography.

Congenital Malformations. MRI of congenital
malformations of the spine in some instances

may be the only means of delineating the abnormality. Saggital cervical spine films clearly depict
the Arnald-Chiari malformation with herniation
of the cerebellar tonsils through the foramen
magnum. There may be an associated syringomyelia dissecting the cord, and this can be extremely well seen on MRI studies. MRI provides a
noninvasive way to evaluate meningoceles and

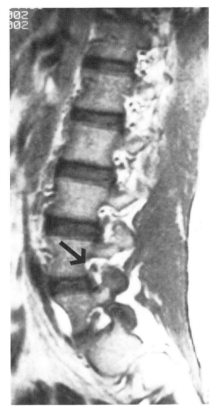

FIG 16–65.
Off-midline sagittal MRI of the lumbar spine demonstrates the neural foramina and their exiting nerve root *(arrow)*.

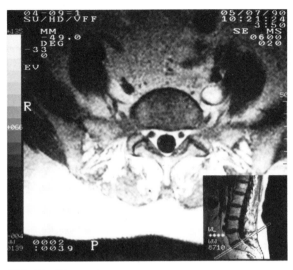

FIG 16–66.
Selected axial image of the L5, S1 disc space (see the sagittal inset with the *cursor*). Note the dural sac and two descending nerve roots *(black)* surrounded by the epidural fat *(white)*.

meningomyeloceles. With these entities, a tethered cord and associated lipoma are well appreciated below the conus medularis.

Spinal Trauma.   Because of increased examination times and the limitation in the use of life-support equipment that is affected by the magnet, acute trauma of the spine is best evaluated by plane x-ray films and CT rather than MRI. An MRI study of the cervical spine, for example, may take up to 30 minutes or more to perform, whereas a modified or limited CT examination can take as little as 10 minutes. However, delayed post-traumatic complications can be extremely well depicted by MRI. The site and extent of fractures and the displacement of fragments are probably best defined on CT but can be properly

accessed by magnetic imaging. The direct effect of displaced fragments on the cord and nerve roots may be determined by MRI. It also clearly identifies the integrity of the cord and the presence of intramedullary hemorrhage. Epidural and subdural hematomas around the cord are also visibly documented.

Disc Disease.   The role of MRI in the assessment of disc herniation, degenerative disc disease, and spondylitis with osteophyte formation as compared with CT and contrast myelography currently is undergoing considerable scrutiny in clinical practice. Most studies agree that the accuracy of the three modalities in these disease states are relatively equal in lumbar spine evaluations; however, the diagnostic sensitivity in the cervical and thoracic regions seems to favor MRI. CT at these spinal levels is very limited unless intrathecal contrast is used since the cord and dural sac are not well demonstrated. MRI shows these structures well. Contrast myelography is equally sensitive in detecting abnormalities, but the fact that MRI is essentially noninvasive favors its use.

The clinical diagnosis of a herniated intervertebral nucleus pulposus can be very dramatic but on occasion can be very subtle. After following a conservative clinical approach for a period of time without improvement of symptoms, the clinician may elect to evaluate the patient by some type of imaging procedure to diagnose and document the presence or absence of a herniated disc. Graphic visualization of a herniated disc can be an imaging challenge by any method. In the cervical region, bulging, protruding, and herniated discs lend themselves readily to MRI evaluation (Fig 16–67), although the distinction between bulging and herniation may at times be impossible. Lumbar spine disc herniation, however, continues to be accessed equally by CT or MRI (Fig 16–68). The choice of procedure will depend on availability, economic considerations, and to some extent, patient selection. An equivocal CT study may require MRI to best delineate the lesion, but less often the opposite is true.

One area of difficult clinical management is the postoperative spine. Contrast myelography or CT seldom can distinguish between postsurgical scar tissue and a recurrent herniated disc. With the introduction of an intravenously administered "contrast" agent, MRI is capable of making the distinction between the two. Gadolinium is a stable paramagnetic metal ion that is combined with diethylenetriamine pentaacetic acid (DTPA). When injected, the substance can enhance tissues with adequate vascularity by changing their magnetic field. Disc material, being essentially nonvascular, will not enhance, whereas scar tissue, which possesses a vascular supply, will.

Spondylitis. Early degeneration of the intervertebral disc material can be identified by MRI even before changes occur on x-ray films and CT; these changes include disc space narrowing and spur formation. A change in signal intensity (brightness) of the disc on the MRI sagittal images heralds the beginning of the pathologic process (Fig 16–69). As the disease progresses with disc space compression and production of osteophytes, MRI aids in defining the degree of spinal

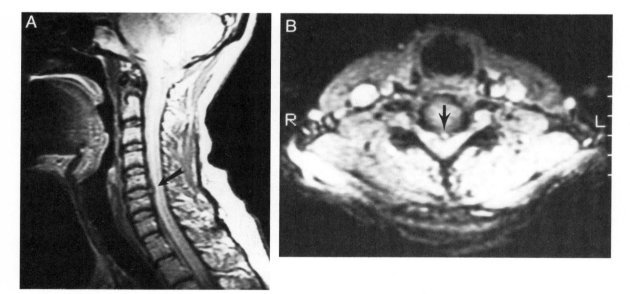

FIG 16–67.
Herniated disc of the cervical spine at the C5–6 level (arrows). **A,** sagittal, and **B,** axial views. Note on the lateral image an appearance simulating paste being squeezed from a tube. Also note deformity of the dural sac.

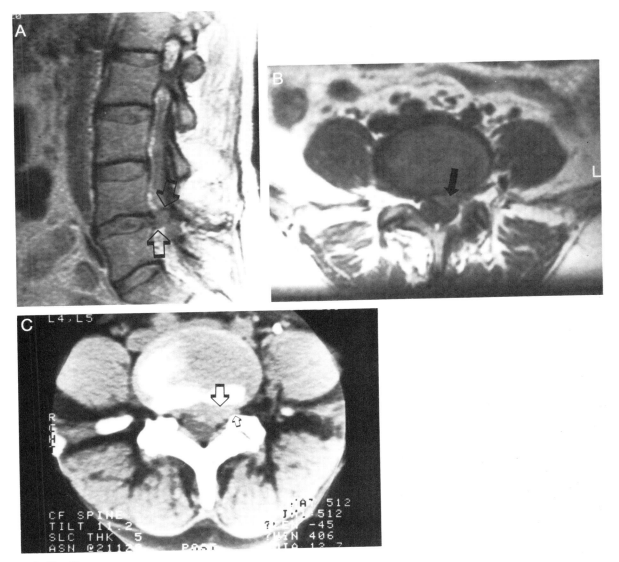

FIG 16–68.
Herniated disc of the lumbar spine at the L4–5 level *(arrows)*. **A,** sagittal, and **B,** axial MRI images. Note the deformity of the dural sac and the enchroachment on the left neural foramen. **C,** CT image of the same disc.

stenosis that can occur on the central neural canal and the neural foramina in both the axial and sagittal planes. The encroachment of degenerative spurs on the dural sac, their displacement of nerve roots, and their effect on the cord are all adequately assessed by MRI (Fig 16–70).

Infection. MRI of infectious processes in and about the spine can be very rewarding. Figure 16–71 demonstrates an unsuspected epidural abscess of the lumbar spine in an individual presenting with a relatively sudden onset of lower extremity neurologic symptoms including back

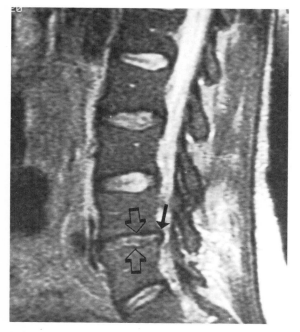

FIG 16–69.
Degenerative disc disease of the lumbar spine at the L4–5 level. Narrowing of the interspace is evident, and osteophyte formation is noted *(open arrows)*. Also note the decreased signal intensity (darkness), greatest at L4–5 but involving all discs; this indicates the decreased water content of the degenerating nucleus pulposus. Posterior osteophyte *(closed arrow)*.

pain, fever, and elevated white blood cell count. A lung infection was thought to be the source for this hematogenously introduced infection.

More common but still infrequent are spinal infections occurring after surgery to the spine. Osteomyelitis of the bony vertebrae with extension into the discs and eventual advancement into the epidural space can be easily pictured by MRI. The use of gadolinium can even further improve the ability to detect infections of the spine.

Tumor.   MRI has been found to be highly sensitive for the detection and characterization of tumors involving the spine. Gadolinium plays an important role in the evaluation of these lesions.

Secondary or metastatic neoplasms are the most commonly encountered tumors that involve the spine (Fig 16–72). These may be hematogenous, such as from lung or breast cancer; lymphatic, such as that from the prostate; or by direct extension from a contiguous lesion. Better definition of the margins of these tumors is afforded by the use of gadolinium, which distinguishes the tumor from surrounding edema and thereby better establishes radiation ports.

Primary spinal tumors are divided into intradural intramedullary and intradural extramedullary as well as extradural lesions. Intramedullary neoplasms may not be optimally visualized on unenhanced MRI due to extensive infiltration, associated edema, or intratumor necrosis or hemorrhage. Ependymomas and astrocytomas constitute the most common intramedullary tumors. A less common lesion is the hemangioblastoma. All three are best evaluated on MRI after gadolinium injection.

Intradural extramedullary tumors are commonly found to be meningiomas, neurofibromas or schwannomas (Fig 16–73). On conventional unenhanced MRI studies, these may be difficult or impossible to identify, especially if they are less than 5 mm. Larger lesions can displace the dural contents and are more easily detected by these indirect signs.

Metastases constitute the majority of extradural tumors and, as noted, are best evaluated by magnetic imaging. One area, however, where MRI has an obvious advantage over any other imaging procedure is in the presence of diffuse leptomeningeal spread of tumor. There is a marked increase in signal arising from the thickened leptomeninges following gadolinium administration.

Miscellaneous Spinal Lesions.   Demyelinating diseases, of which multiple sclerosis is the most common, are characteristically sensitive to magnetic imaging detection. Histopathologically, the lesions are multifocal destructive myelin zones of as yet unknown etiology that can involve the optic nerves, brain, and spinal cord. They present as areas of increased signal intensity (bright), are of

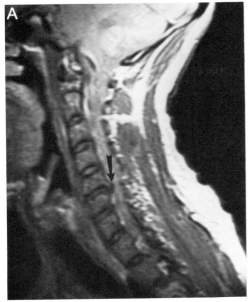
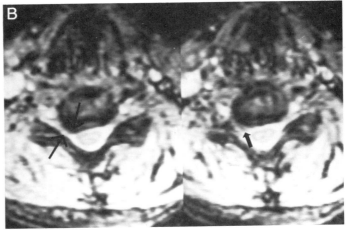

FIG 16–70.
Degenerative disc disease of the cervical spine at the C5–6 level. **A,** sagittal, and **B,** axial images. A large posterior spur *(arrows)* deforms the dural sac extending to the right and is creating stenosis of the neural foramen and subarticular recess.

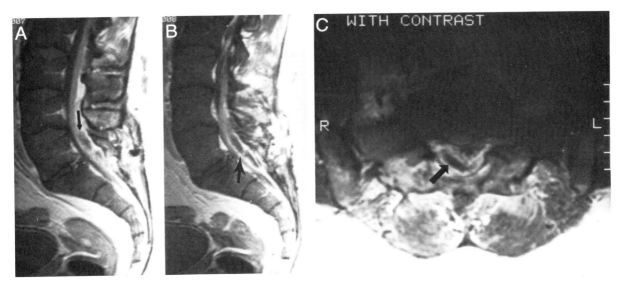

FIG 16–71.
A and **B,** sagittal lumbar spine images at two different planes, and **C,** axial image at the same L5, S1 level. An irregular dark (low signal intensity) area *(arrows)* signifies an epidural abscess.

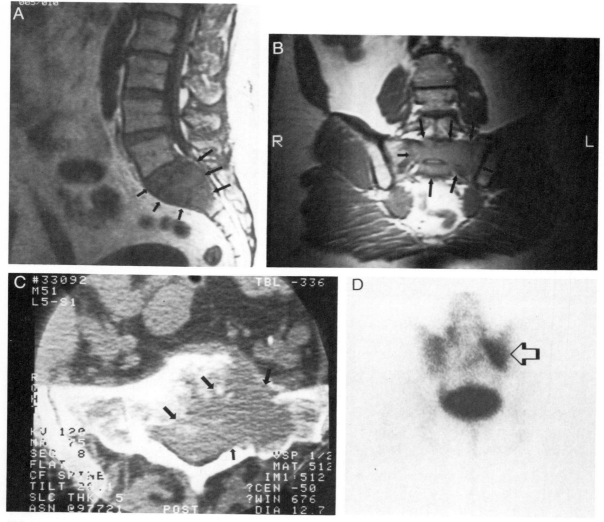

FIG 16–72.
Metastasis *(arrows)* to the sacrum from an occult lung cancer. **A,** sagittal, and **B,** coronal MRI. **C,** CT image. **D,** nuclear bone scan of the pelvis. All three modalities show sensitivity to the process, but MRI provides more anatomic information.

variable size and distribution, range from a few millimeters to several centimeters, and are scattered throughout the white matter. There appears to be a direct relationship between the number and size of these "plaques" and the severity of the symptoms. In addition, as the symptoms wax and wane, so does the appearance of the lesions seen on MRI.

Involvement of the spinal cord by multiple sclerosis is uncommon, but when discovered, the lesions tend to be elongated or linear rather than round or oval as seen in the brain, where they are typically periventricular in location. Lesions in the thoracic and lumbar cord are less frequently identified than in the cervical cord. Symptoms are variable and can range from weak-

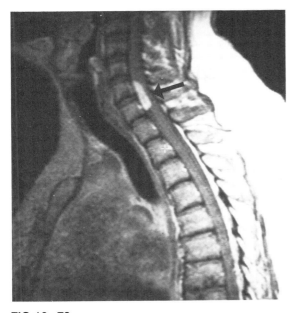

FIG 16–73.
Meningioma of the cervical spine *(arrow)* displays high signal intensity (bright).

ness and/or paraesthesias in one or more limbs, gait disturbances, or problems with micturition.

Although a rare event today, postradiation transverse myelitis is also susceptable to MRI detection. In addition to signal derangements in the

cord, radiation also causes changes within the marrow of the vertebrae that can be easily identified only by magnetic imaging.

Musculoskeletal MRI

Diagnostic orthopedic applications of MRI for disorders of the bones, joints, and soft tissues of the extremities are rapidly gaining acceptance. Although MRI will not totally replace the use of CT, nuclear imaging, or even conventional x-ray films in evaluation of the musculoskeletal system, there are certain areas and specific abnormalities that are best examined by the magnet.

Because of its excellent inherent contrast resolution, MRI can superbly delineate the separate soft-tissue components of the extremities (Fig 16–74). Muscles, tendons, ligaments, fat, cartilage, and fibrous tissue are all excellently displayed. Although the calcium of cortical and trabecular bone possesses no magnetic signal, it can be defined by the adjoining marrow and surrounding muscles and tendons. This property of magnetism, however, prevents MRI from defining cortical stress fractures. Tumoral calcifications and ossifications, as well as early cortical destruction and endosteal and periosteal reaction, which are adequately seen on CT, cannot be optimally identified by MRI, which gives it a distinct disad-

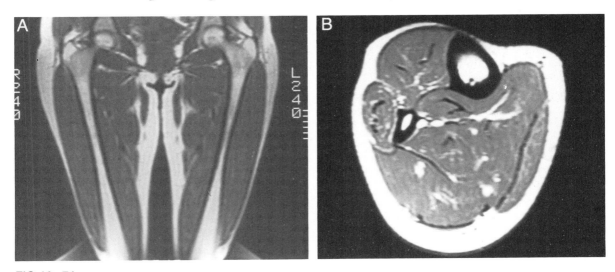

FIG 16–74.
A, coronal MRI of the femur and thigh. **B,** axial image of the tibia and fibula and associated soft-tissue detail.

vantage in such situations. Nevertheless, despite these limitations, MRI has become the diagnostic modality of choice for the evaluation of bone and soft-tissue trauma such as cartilage, ligament, tendon, or muscular damage.

Tumor. The surgical approach for the treatment of malignant bone and soft-tissue tumors today is a conservative one. The objective is limb salvage and restricting resections to a limited degree, thereby providing as much functional capabilities as possible. The multiplanar display of MRI and its excellent contrast resolution aid greatly in defining the size, location, and extent of a tumor. It can adequately assess marrow involvement, skip lesions, and invasion of adjoining muscles, compartments, blood vessels, and nerves (Fig 16–75). Of great importance is establishment of the integrity of adjacent joints and articular surfaces (Fig 16–76).

MRI cannot, unfortunately, differentiate between benign or malignant tissue characteristics. Certain types of tissues such as fat or the vessels of a hemangioma have distinctive appearances (Fig 16–77). Fluid-filled cystic lesions can be separated from solid masses with MRI, and this can aid in appropriate assessment such as needle aspiration or biopsy.

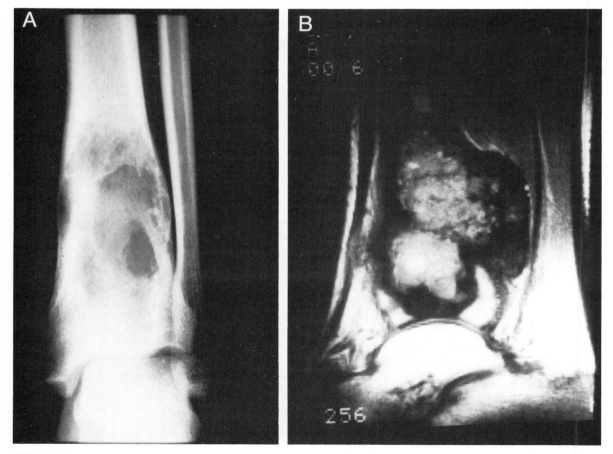

FIG 16–75.
Chondrosarcoma. **A,** anteroposterior roentgenogram of the distal third of the tibia. **B,** sagittal MRI of the same area.
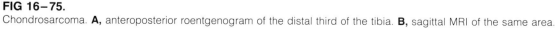

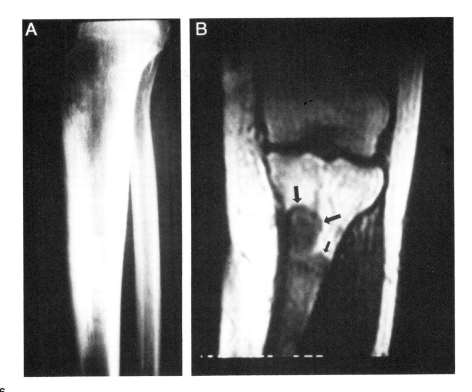

FIG 16–76.
Osteosarcoma. **A,** lateral roentgenogram of the proximal third of the tibia. **B,** coronal MRI of the same area. The medullary extent of the disease *(arrows)* is easily identified by MRI.

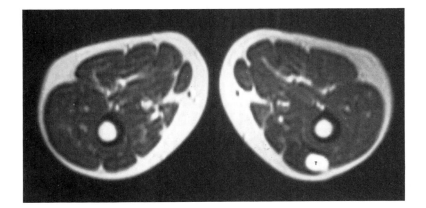

FIG 16–77.
Benign lipoma. Axial MRI of the thighs demonstrates a sharply marginated lesion *(T)* with high signal intensity.

Infection. The diagnosis and treatment of osteomyelitis, pyogenic arthritis, and soft-tissue infections of the extremities can be challenging. The earlier the detection and the better the process is delimited by imaging, the more precise will be medical and surgical approaches and the better will be the outcomes. Evaluation by standard x-ray films, conventional tomography, radionuclide bone scans, and CT all have a place, but each has its limitations and may delay appropriate therapy.

Bone infections may not become evident on x-ray films and tomography until up to 40% to 50% of the bone is destroyed, which may take up to 10 or 14 days following the onset. As has been previously discussed, nuclear bone scans are very sensitive but nonspecific and may not differentiate tumor from infection, nor can they adequately define the anatomic extent of the disease. Gallium 67– and indium 111–labeled leukocytes are radioisotopes that are more specific for infection than are technitium 99m–labeled phosphorus compounds, but again they provide poor resolution.

CT is helpful in determining cortical bone and periosteal findings but is less sensitive to marrow or surrounding soft-tissue changes. Also, because it is limited to transverse planes, the true upper and lower margins of the infection may be missed. Additionally, in cases of infections involving internal metallic fixation devices, the artifacts produced by CT prevent delineation of the abnormalities. The MRI artifacts produced by such devices are much less marked.

Hematogenous osteomyelitis, most often seen in children, commonly begins in the bone marrow of long bones in the lower extremities. On MRI studies, the intramedullary tissues will demonstrate signal changes of inflammation at an early stage. Furthermore, the anatomic extent of the process can be clearly demonstrated to include soft-tissue extension, joint involvement, and skip areas. If unresponsive to medical management, this can be valuable in planning surgical debridement.

MRI has been found to be of value in the evaluation of postsurgical bone, joint, and soft-tissue infections. Most metal fixation appliances today are nonferromagnetic and cause only minimal distracting image artifacts on MRI. This property is a significant problem with CT. Subtle bone changes immediately adjacent to metal implants, however, may be obscured by the minimal artifacts seen on MRI, and early infectious changes may be missed.

Trauma. The primary diagnostic modality for the study of skeletal injuries does not include magnetic imaging. These are reserved, of course, for standard roentgenologic procedures. However, an evaluation of soft-tissue injury, especially deep tissues, becomes more difficult with conventional tests. MRI, because of its multiplanar ability and its exquisite soft-tissue contrast and resolution, is gaining greater acceptance for elucidating extraosseous injuries.

Contusions of soft tissue that result in hemorrhage, edema, and inflammation as well as hematoma formation can be depicted by MRI. The location and size of the process and, importantly, the involvement of adjacent muscles, tendons, ligaments, blood vessels, and nerves are easily assessed. This can serve as a guide to excision and evacuation procedures when required.

As a result of severe muscle contraction or direct trauma, muscles, ligaments, and tendons can be torn or ruptured. Such findings, especially in the shoulder, knee, and ankle but also in other locations, will be directly visualized by magnetic scanning, something that up to now was difficult to do even with arthrography and might only be surmised clinically or by direct surgical exposure.

Evaluation of the knee joint is presently approached by direct visualization via arthroscopy, which has essentially supplanted arthrography. Orthopedic surgeons, however, are beginning to rely more frequently on the noninvasive accurate diagnostic images provided by MRI. The menisci, cruciate and collateral ligaments, the articular cartilage, the synovial capsule, and surrounding muscles are extremely well depicted on MRI scans (Fig 16–78). Recent studies have shown MRI to have an accuracy of 90% for meniscal tears and 95% for cruciate ligament tears (Fig 16–79). Magnetic imaging can define early degeneration of menisci and cartilage and even intrameniscal tears not visible by endoscopy. Loose intra-articular osteochondral bodies are easily detected by MRI.

The diagnostic capabilities of MRI in examin-

ing the shoulder have only recently been realized due to the development of better-designed, dedicated surface coils and updated computer software programs. Although arthrography is still being utilized and in some instances combined with CT, MRI appears to be taking the same direction as it did in knee evaluations and is becoming more frequently utilized. Coronal oblique, sagittal oblique, and axial planes of imag-

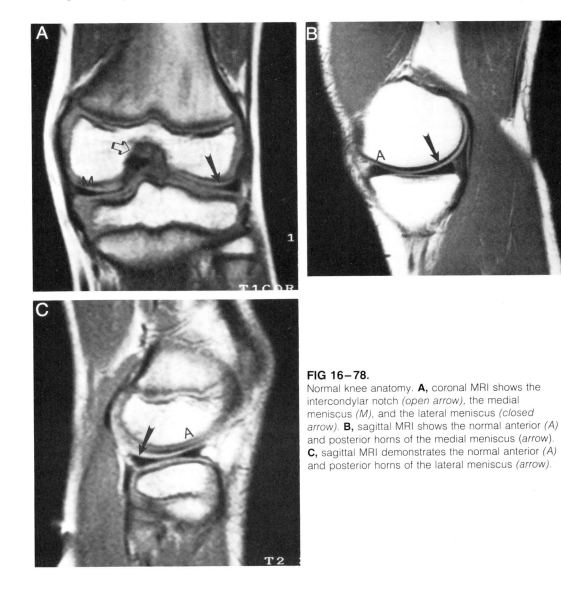

FIG 16–78.
Normal knee anatomy. **A,** coronal MRI shows the intercondylar notch *(open arrow),* the medial meniscus *(M),* and the lateral meniscus *(closed arrow).* **B,** sagittal MRI shows the normal anterior *(A)* and posterior horns of the medial meniscus *(arrow).* **C,** sagittal MRI demonstrates the normal anterior *(A)* and posterior horns of the lateral meniscus *(arrow).*

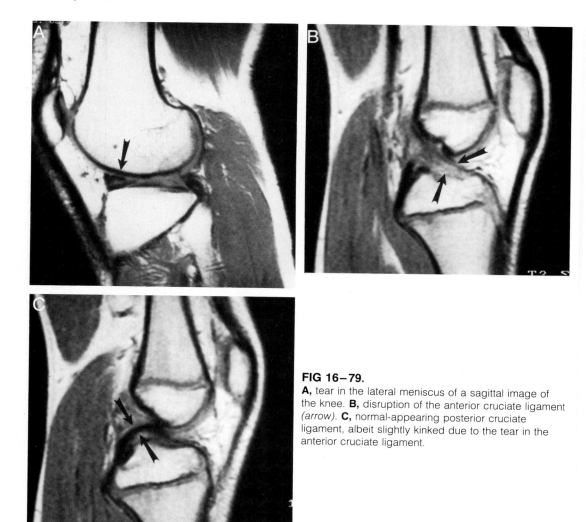

FIG 16–79.
A, tear in the lateral meniscus of a sagittal image of the knee. **B,** disruption of the anterior cruciate ligament *(arrow)*. **C,** normal-appearing posterior cruciate ligament, albeit slightly kinked due to the tear in the anterior cruciate ligament.

ing of the shoulder offer a tremendous advantage over other modalities in addition to the use of variable-pulse sequencing protocols, which can be modified to bring out or accentuate subtle findings. Degenerative changes as well as partial or complete tears of the rotator cuff are sensitive to MRI detection (Fig 16–80).

Impingement of the supraspinatus tendon as caused by an abnormal acromium process or os-

teophyte formation of the acromioclavicular joint can lead to early degenerative changes and makes the tendon more susceptible to tears. Tendinitis, bursitis, rupture of the biceps tendon, or determination of the integrity of the cartilaginous glenoid labrum also lend themselves to identification by MRI.

MRI is also helpful for assessing injuries to other regions of the musculoskeletal system. As

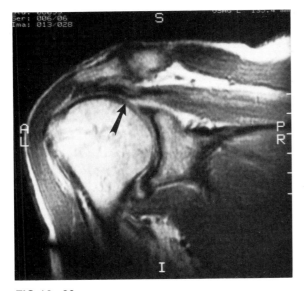

FIG 16–80.
Coronal oblique MRI of the shoulder demonstrates a rotator cuff tear *(arrow).*

will be mentioned later, aseptic or avascular necrosis of the navicular bone of the wrist is receptive to MRI detection. There are several studies available that indicate the value of MRI in assessing the carpal tunnel syndrome. In this condition, magnetic imaging can define thickening of the tendon sheaths and distortion in the outline of the median nerve.

The elbow and ankle can be appropriately analyzed for traumatic abnormalities by MRI (Fig 16–81). Tears of the Achilles tendon is a prime example, and the severity and extent of the lesion can be properly determined by the magnet. Loose bone or cartilagenous bodies on occasion can be appreciated within joints.

Examination of the temporomandibular joints is facilitated with the use of MRI. Tears and dislocations of the meniscus and whether it reduces with opening or closing of the jaw are discerned.

Acute trauma or chronic stress tenosyovitis or bursitis often lead to the production of synovial fluid as a result of inflammation. Traumatic hemorrhage into joints or bursae can also occur.

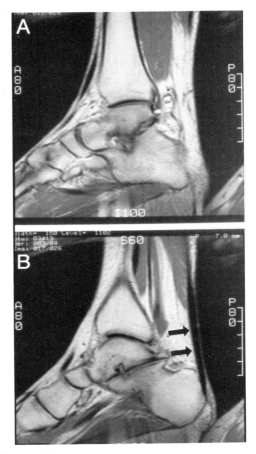

FIG 16–81.
A and **B,** normal sagittal images of the ankle. Note the Achilles tendon *(arrows).*

These abnormal fluid collections are well demonstrated by MRI.

Osteonecrosis.   There are numerous causes of aseptic necrosis or avascular osteonecrosis of bone, the most common being trauma that results in disruption of the regional vascular supply. Nontraumatic etiologies include vascular thrombosis secondary to hemaglobinopathies such as sickle-cell anemia. A commonly encountered reason for aseptic necrosis is exogenous steroids or rarely Cushing's disease. Less fre-

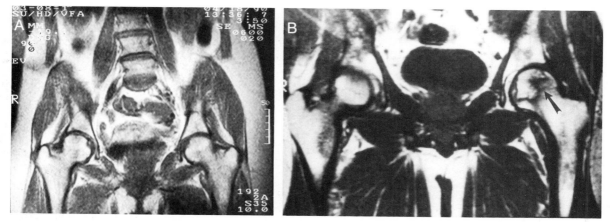

FIG 16—82.
A, normal coronal MRI of the hips. **B,** a coronal view of the hips demonstrates avascular necrosis on the left *(arrow).*

quently found diseases accounting for osteonecrosis are barotrauma, irradiation, collagen vascular diseases (vasculitis), lymphoproliferative diseases (Hodgkin's lymphoma), pancreatitis, and even some cases of gout.

The common denominator in the pathogenesis of both traumatic and nontraumatic aseptic necrosis is vascular compromise. The resultant marrow ischemia, which most often occurs in the growth centers or metaphyseal regions of long bones, provokes an inflammatory response with vascular congestion and edema of the bone marrow.

This pathophysiologic response can be detected by conventional radiographs on a delayed basis or early by the sensitive but nonspecific and poorly resolved images of a nuclear bone scan. CT can also detect the changes of avascular

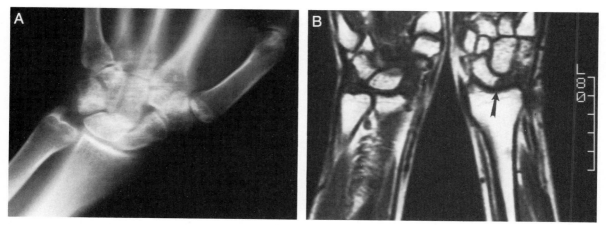

FIG 16—83.
A, a standard linear x-ray tomogram of the wrist shows the faint sclerotic line of a healing fracture. **B,** MRI of both wrists in the same patient confirms the clinically suspected avascular necrosis of the proximal carpal navicular fragment *(arrow).*

necrosis relatively early, but the findings are also nonspecific, and CT of the distal parts of extremities has been found to be very limited.

MRI of osteonecrosis has been determined to be very sensitive as well as specific early in the disease process. In the femoral head (Fig 16–82), the images will delineate subarticular areas of decreased signal intensity (dark). Injuries to the carpal navicular bone, as has been pointed out previously, can defy detection by standard imaging. Appreciation of the process of aseptic necrosis of the proximal navicular fracture fragment requires early detection for best results, and MRI provides a very accurate means to determine this abnormality (Fig 16–83). Other regions vulnerable to osteonecrosis such as the humeral head (Fig 16-84), knee, mandibular condyle, and spine are easily examined by magnetic imaging.

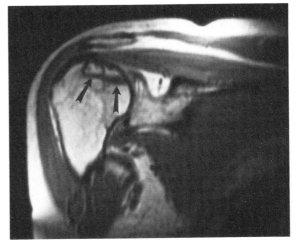

FIG 16–84.
Coronal oblique MRI shoulder image demonstrates osteonecrosis of the humeral head in a steroid user *(arrows)*.

BIBLIOGRAPHY

Aegerter E: Diagnostic radiology and the pathology of bone disease. *Radiol Clin North Am* 1970; 8:215.

Anderson RE: Practical aspects of CT imaging of the spine. *Curr Probl Diagn Radiol* 1982; 11:2.

Beabout JW, McLeod RA, Dahlin DC: Benign tumors of the spine. *Semin Roentgenol* 1970; 5:419.

Berquist TH: *Magnetic Resonance of the Musculoskeletal System.* New York, Raven Press, 1987.

Birkner R: *Normal Radiologic Patterns and Variations of the Human Skeleton.* Baltimore, Urban Schwarzenberg, 1978.

Bisese JH: *Orthopaedic MRI: A Teaching File Approach.* New York, McGraw-Hill, 1990.

Blaser SI, Berns DH: Disks, degeneration and MRI. *MRI Decisions,* 1988; 2:23.

Brodeur AE: *Radiologic Diagnosis in Infants and Children.* St Louis, CV Mosby Co, 1965.

Brodeur AE, Silberstein MJ, Graves ER, et al: The basic tenets for appropriate evaluation of the elbow in pediatrics. *Curr Probl Diagn Radiol* 1983; 12:5.

Burk DL, Mitchell DG, Rifkin MD: Recent advances in magnetic resonance imaging of the knee. *Radiol Clin North Am* 1990; 28:379.

Caffey J: *Pediatric X-ray Diagnosis,* vol 2, ed 6. Chicago, Year Book Medical Publishers Inc, 1973.

Christenson PC: The radiologic study of the normal spine: Cervical, thoracic, lumbar and sacral. *Radiol Clin North Am* 1977; 15:133.

Daffner RH: Ankle trauma. *Radiol Clin North Am* 1990; 28:395.

Dahlin DC: *Bone Tumors: General Aspects and Data on 3,987 Cases,* ed 2. Springfield, Ill, Charles C Thomas Publishers, 1967.

Dalinka MK, Zlatkin MB, Chao P, et al: The use of magnetic resonance imaging in the evaluation of bone and soft-tissue tumors. *Radiol Clin North Am* 1990; 28:461.

Djukic S, Genant HK, Helms CA, et al: Magnetic resonance imaging of the postoperative lumbar spine. *Radiol Clin North Am* 1990; 28:341.

Donovan-Post MJ, Green BA: The use of computed tomography in spinal trauma. *Radiol Clin North Am* 1983; 21:327.

Dunn AW, Morris HD: Fractures and dislocations of the pelvis. *J Bone Joint Surg* 1968; 50:1639.

Edeiken J, Cotler JM: Ankle trauma. *Semin Roentgenol* 1978; 13:145.

Edeiken J, Hodes PJ: *Roentgen Diagnosis of Diseases of Bone.* Baltimore, Williams & Wilkens Co, 1989.

Edelman RR, Siegel JB: Advances in musculoskeletal MRI. *MRI Decisions* 1988; 2:27.

Epstein BS: *Atlas of Tumor Radiology: The Vertebral Column.* Chicago, Year Book Medical Publishers Inc, 1974.

Forrester DM, Brown JC, Nesson JW: *The Radiology of Joint Disease,* ed 2. Philadelphia, WB Saunders Co, 1978.

Forrester DM, Kerr R: Trauma to the foot. *Radiol Clin North Am* 1990; 28:423.

Foster SC, Foster RR: Lisfranc's tarsometatarsal fracture dislocation. *Radiology* 1976; 120:79.

Freedman GS: Radionuclide imaging of the injured patient. *Radiol Clin North Am* 1973; 11:472.

Freiberger RH: *Bone Disease Syllabus,* Set 9. American College of Radiology Self-evaluation and Continuing Education Program. Baltimore, Waverly Press Inc, 1976.

Gelman, MD: *Radiology of Orthopedic Procedures, Problems and Complications.* Philadelphia, WB Saunders Co, 1984.

Gold RI, Seeger LL, Bassett LW, et al: An integrated approach to the evaluation of metastatic bone disease. *Radiol Clin North Am* 1990; 28:471.

Goldman AB, Freiberger RH: Localized infections and neuropathic diseases of the spine. *Semin Roentgenol* 1979; 14:19.

Greenfield GB: *Radiology of Bone Diseases,* ed 2. Philadelphia, JB Lippincott Co, 1975.

Greulich WW, Pyle SI: *Radiographic Atlas of Skeletal Development of the Hand and Wrist.* Stanford, Calif, Oxford University Press, 1959.

Harris JH Jr: Acute injuries of the spine. *Semin Roentgenol* 1978; 13:53.

Harris JH Jr, Edeiken J: Acute cervical spine trauma. *Radiol Sci Update Series* No 17, 1976.

Harris JH, Jr, Harris WH: *The Radiology of Emergency Medicine.* Baltimore, Williams & Wilkins, 1975.

Hill HA, Sachs MD: The grooved defect of the humeral head: A frequently unrecognized complication of dislocations of the shoulder joint. *Radiology* 1940; 35:690.

Jacobson HG: *Bone Disease Syllabus: Disorders of the Skeleton,* Set 2. American College of Radiology Professional Self-evaluation and Continuing Education Program. Baltimore, Waverly Press Inc, 1972.

Kaye J: Fractures and dislocations of the hand and wrist. *Semin Roentgenol* 1978; 13:109.

Kaye JJ, Nance EP: Thoracic and lumbar spine trauma. *Radiol Clin North Am* 1990; 28:361.

Keats TE: *An Atlas of Normal Roentgen Variants That May Simulate Disease.* Chicago, Year Book Medical Publishers Inc, 1988.

Kohler A, Zimmer EA: *Borderlands of the Normal and Early Pathologic in Skeletal Roentgenology,* ed 3. New York, Grune & Stratton, 1968.

Kricun R, Kricun ME, Dalinka MK: Advances in spinal imaging. *Radiol Clin North Am* 1990; 28:321.

Kursonoglu-Brahme S, Gundry CR, Resnick D: Advanced imaging of the wrist. *Radiol Clin North Am* 1990; 28:307.

Lee JKT, Sagel SS, Stanley RJ: *Computed Body Tomography.* New York, Raven Press, 1983.

Lichtenstein L: *Bone Tumors,* ed 4. St Louis, CV Mosby Co, 1972.

Littleton JT: Tomography: A current assessment. *Curr Probl Diagn Radiol* 1974; 4:3.

Lodwick GS: *Atlas of Tumor Radiology: The Bones and Joints.* Chicago, Year Book Medical Publishers Inc, 1971.

Maravilla KR, Hartling RP: Imaging decisions in degenerative spinal disease. *MRI Decisions* 1988; 2:3.

Mark AS, Atlas SW: MRI of the cervical spine and cord. *MRI Decisions* 1988; 2:23.

McLeod RA, Stephens DH, Beabout JW, et al: Computed tomography of the skeletal system. *Semin Roentgenol* 1978; 13:3.

Merrill V: *Atlas of Roentgenographic Positions and Standard Radiologic Procedures.* St Louis, CV Mosby Co, 1975.

Meschan I: *Roentgen Signs in Clinical Practice.* Philadelphia, WB Saunders Co, 1966, vol 1.

Mirvis SE, Wolf A: Emerging MRI Role: Assessing Cervical Spine Trauma. *MRI Decisions* 1990; 4:21.

Modic MT, Maszryk TJ, Ross JS: *Magnetic Resonance Imaging of the Spine.* Chicago, Year Book Medical Publishers Inc, 1989.

Moss AA, Gamsu G, Jenant HK: *Computed Tomography of the Body.* Philadelphia, WB Saunders Co, 1983.

Mounts RJ, Schloss CD: Injuries to the bony pelvis and hip. *Radiol Clin North Am* 1966; 4:307.

Murray RO, Jacobson HG: *The Radiology of Skeletal Disorders.* Baltimore, Williams & Wilkins, 1971.

Nelson SW: Some important diagnostic and technical fundamentals in the radiology of trauma with particular emphasis on skeletal trauma. *Radiol Clin North Am* 1966; 4:241.

Newberg AH: Computed tomography of joint injuries. *Radiol Clin North Am* 1990; 28:445.

Patten RM: Musculoskeletal neoplasms: Imaging approach. *MRI Decisions* 1989; 3:13.

Patten RM, Shuman WP: MRI of osteonecrosis. *MRI Decisions* 1990; 4:2.

Paul LW, Juhl JH: *Essentials of Roentgen Diagnosis of the Skeletal System.* New York, Harper & Row, 1967.

Pavlov H, Freiberger RH: Fractures and dislocations about the shoulder. *Semin Roentgenol* 1978; 13:85.

Pitt MJ, Speer DP: Imaging of the elbow with an emphasis on trauma. *Radiol Clin North Am* 1990; 28:293.

Pyle SI, Hoerr NL: *Radiographic Atlas of Skeletal Development of the Knee.* Springfield, Ill: Charles C Thomas Publishers, 1955.

Richardson ML: Magnetic resonance imaging of the musculoskeletal system. *Radiol Clin North Am* 1986; 24:2.

Rogers LF: Fractures and dislocations of the elbow. *Semin Roentgenol* 1978; 13:97.

Rogers LF: The radiology of sports injuries. *Curr Probl Diagn Radiol* 1983; 12:1.

Rogers LF, Campbell RE: Fractures and dislocations of the foot. *Semin Roentgenol* 1978; 13:157.

Rogers LF, Lowell JD: Occult central fractures of the acetabulum. *AJR* 1975; 124:96.

Ross J, Masaryk TJ, Hueftle MLG, et al: Imaging decisions in low back pain. *MRI Decisions* 1987; 1:16.

Runge VM, Wolf C, Wood ML, et al: The clinical utility of IV gadopenetate dimeglumine for MRI of the head and spine. *MRI Decisions* 1989; 3:2.

Scott JA, Rosenthal DI, Brady TJ: The evaluation of musculoskeletal disease with magnetic resonance imaging. *Radiol Clin North Am* 1984; 22:4.

Sherman RS: General principles of the radiologic diagnosis of bone disorders. *Radiol Clin North Am* 1970; 8:173.

Sherman RS: The nature of radiologic diagnosis in diseases of bone. *Radiol Clin North Am* 1970; 8:227.

Siberstein EB, Saenger E, Tofe AJ: Imaging of bone metastasis with Tc-99m EHDP and skeletal radiography. *Radiology* 1973; 107:551.

Simeone FA, Rothman RH: Clinical usefulness of CT scanning in the diagnosis and treatment of lumbar spine disease. *Radiol Clin North Am* 1983; 21:197.

Smith GR, Loop JW: Radiologic classification of posterior dislocations of the hip: Refinements and pitfalls. *Radiology* 1976; 119:569.

Subbarzo K, Jacobson HG: Fractures and dislocations around the adult knee. *Semin Roentgenol* 1978; 13:135.

Subbarzo K, Jacobson HG: Primary malignant neoplasms of the spine. *Semin Roentgenol* 1979; 14:44.

Sze G: MRI of tumor metastases to the leptomeninges. *MRI Decisions* 1988; 2:2.

Teplick JG, Hakin ME: CT and lumbar disc herniation. *Radiol Clin North Am* 1983; 21:259.

Thaggard A, Harle TS, Carlson V: Fractures and dislocations of the bony pelvis and hip. *Semin Roentgenol* 1978; 13:117.

Theros, EG: *Bone Disease Syllabus,* Set 16. American College of Radiology Self-evaluation and Continuing Education Program. Baltimore, Waverly Press Inc, 1980.

Vix VA, Ryu CY: The adult symphysis pubis: Normal and abnormal. *AJR* 1971; 112:517.

Wilkinson RH, Kirkpatrick JA: Pediatric skeletal trauma. *Curr Probl Diagn Radiol* 1976; 6:3.

Wilkinson RH, Strand RD: Congenital anomalies and normal variants of the spine. *Semin Roentgenol* 1979; 14:7.

Wiot JF, Dorst JP: Less common fractures and dislocations of the wrist. *Radiol Clin North Am* 1966; 4:261.

Yiu-Chiu VS, Chiu LC: Complementary values of ultrasound and computed tomography in the evaluation of musculoskeletal masses. *Radiographics* 1983; 3:1.

Zatzkin HR: Trauma to the foot. *Semin Roentgenol* 1970; 5:419.

Zlatkin MB, Dalinka MK, Kressel HY: Magnetic resonance imaging of the shoulder. *Magn Reson Q* 1989; 5:3.

CHAPTER 17

Maxillofacial Injuries

John J. Heieck, M.D.

Increasing violence in today's society combined with the development of local hospital emergency rooms as trauma centers have placed many emergency and primary-care physicians in the position of initial responsibility for the isolated or multicomplex injured patient. Usually, the physicians are able to recognize potential thoracic or abdominal injuries more easily than maxillofacial defects. Their ability to identify maxillofacial injuries, of course, is necessary for the complete evaluation of the condition of any trauma patient. Although not lethal per se, undiagnosed facial fractures may have potential lethal complications or may produce contour deformities or functional disabilities.

The surgical literature lists many causes for maxillofacial injuries. The automobile accident, however, is the most frequent cause overall. Other causes include motorcycle accidents, fistfights, sports, falls, bicycle accidents, and convulsive disorders. Identification of the cause is important since one third of patients with maxillofacial injury caused by motor vehicle accidents will have associated life-threatening cranial, pulmonary, or intra-abdominal injuries. About one third will also be accompanied by nonlethal injuries such as extremity fractures or eye loss. On the other hand, patients with maxillofacial injuries secondary to low-velocity causes (assaults or falls) have a markedly decreased incidence of associated injury: life-threatening (4%) and nonlethal (10%).

ASSOCIATED INJURIES

The primary physician's initial introduction to the maxillofacially injured patient may be as an isolated injury or as part of a multisystem involvement. However, the principles of treatment are similar in either case. Establishment of a patent airway should be the most immediate concern. Control of hemorrhage from open wounds or bleeding orifices by pressure dressing or packing should be accomplished next. If shock does exist, treatment should include rapid infusion of intravenous lactated Ringer's solution followed by blood administration as soon as possible. Investigation for possible cranial, thoracic, or intra-abdominal injuries should be completed before identifying the maxillofacial abnormalities.

Airway obstruction with subsequent hypoxemia can easily develop in the patient with a maxillofacial fracture. Blood clots, broken teeth or dentures, and foreign bodies such as dirt or glass can physically obstruct the airway. The posterior displacement of the tongue secondary to the patient's position or to a mandibular fracture may occlude the airway. Other potential causes include glossopharyngeal edema and expanding hematoma. In all situations, a patent airway must take immediate priority. Sweeping debris from the oropharynx and mouth by using one's finger may be a lifesaving technique. Suction, if available, will be helpful. Simple traction on a posteriorly displaced tongue by suture or towel clip may alleviate obstruction. If these methods fail, oral intubation must be instituted. If facial edema, facial fractures, or cervical spine fractures prevent oral or nasal intubation, a cricothyroidotomy can be performed through the membrane between the thyroid and cricoid cartilages. This site is a bloodless field, and the procedure can easily be done in the emergency room with only a scalpel. Later, an elective lower tracheotomy can be performed under controlled circumstances in the operating room. A low tracheotomy performed in the emergency room may be very hazardous and should be avoided.

Hemorrhage from open wounds can be controlled most easily by pressure dressings consisting of layers of gauze (Kerlix) and elastic bandages. Occasionally, an active bleeder in a facial wound can be easily clamped and ligated. However, blind clamping of possible bleeding sites is condemned due to the high incidence of iatrogenic complications such as facial nerve dysfunction. Nasal hemorrhage may require packing. Shock occurs very seldom from an isolated maxillofacial injury and is most commonly due to a thoracic or abdominal injury.

All patients should be considered candidates for cervical spine fractures, which occur in 4% to 7% of maxillofacial injuries. The initial examiner should palpate the neck for tenderness over the cervical spine and evaluate grip strength and motion in all extremities. Before other roentgenograms are taken, a cross-table lateral view of the cervical spine with all seven vertebrae visible should be examined for fracture or dislocation.

Other associated injuries in the maxillofacial patient may involve one or more systems. Subdural, epidural, or intracerebral hematoma may be present in a comatose or semilucid patient, indicating the need for skull roentgenograms and computerized axial tomographic scan. Possible chest injuries include rib fractures, pneumothorax or hemothorax, flail chest, aortic rupture, and pulmonary or cardiac contusion. Chest films and arterial gas studies may be indicated. Intra-abdominal injuries, of course, would include a ruptured spleen, transected liver, major vessel injuries, and/or perforated intestine. A pregnant woman may suffer an abortion as a result of the accident. Single or multiple extremity fractures may also be present.

All life-threatening associated injuries must receive first priority in the treatment of the multi-injured patient. After repair and/or stabilization of the associated injuries has been accomplished, reduction of the maxillofacial fractures may be performed.

EXAMINATION AND DIAGNOSIS

An accurate history should be obtained whenever possible from the patient and/or witnesses at the scene of the accident. The type of accident, the patient's position in the car, the use of safety belts, the mode of impact, and the patient's condition at the time of injury are all important considerations in the initial assessment. Since alcohol is involved in 50% of automobile accidents, a blood alcohol sample should be drawn. Ingestion of other drugs should be ruled out. A review of the patient's past history should include other illnesses, previous surgery, allergies, and all current medications.

A diagnosis of facial bone injury can be established by three methods: observation, palpation, and radiologic evaluation. Moderate to severe facial edema may mask bony irregularities and asymmetries (Fig 17–1). However, after resolution of the edema, facial asymmetry is suggestive of an underlying fracture. Light manual palpation is important in making the initial diagnosis. A systematic approach should be used routinely in ex-

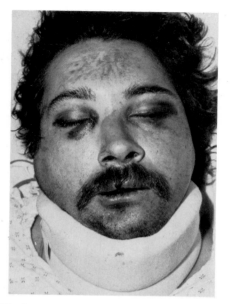

FIG 17–1.
This 32-year-old man suffered a Le Fort III maxillary fracture, nasal fractures, a displaced mandibular fracture, and an undisplaced fracture of the seventh cervical vertebra. The nasal deformity is easily recognized, but the remaining deformities are masked by facial edema.

amining all potential facial fracture patients. The clinician should palpate the boundaries of the orbit, the projection of the malar eminences and zygomatic arches, the maxillary and mandibular arches, and the nasal bones. During palpation, the physician should assess possible asymmetry by noting any depressions or step deformities as well as observing tenderness in areas of potential fracture. Evaluation of the function of the extraocular muscles may demonstrate superior gaze impairment with subsequent diplopia. Orbital ridge or floor fractures will commonly result in infraorbital nerve numbness of the cheek and the maxillary gingiva on the side of the fracture. Crepitus to light touch suggests fracture extension through the nasal airways or paranasal sinuses. Rhinorrhea confirms the involvement of the fracture through the cribriform plate. The presence of trismus may indicate a hematoma or contusion in the muscles of mastication or could

suggest either zygomatic arch or mandibular fractures. A complete examination for possible facial injuries includes a thorough evaluation of dental occlusion for any abnormality.

Radiologically, the Waters' view is the single most informative roentgenogram in evaluation of the maxillofacial patient in the emergency room (Fig 17–2). This study visualizes the floor and rims of the orbits, the walls of the sinuses, the zygomatic bones, the zygomatic arches, and the nasal septum with minimal interference of other bony structures. Opacity of a maxillary sinus suggests hemorrhage as a result of an orbital ridge and/or floor fracture. However, this view requires the cooperation of the patient and a normal cervical spine since the patient must be in the prone position during the examination. If the patient is comatose, uncooperative, or suspected of having a cervical fracture, a reverse Waters' view with the patient in the supine position is a satisfactory substitute since it gives almost the same detail of information. Other films worth consideration in the emergency room are the submental vertex view of the zygomatic arches

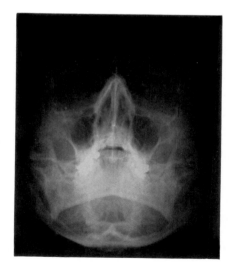

FIG 17–2.
The Waters' view is the best single roentgenographic study of the facial bones. It most clearly visualizes the rims of the orbits, the zygomatic bones and arches, and the maxilla. Note the clarity of the maxillary sinuses.

and a mandible series. More sophisticated and detailed studies can be obtained later during the hospitalization or as an outpatient for isolated facial fractures.

Until the development of computed tomography (CT scan), linear tomography and the Waters' view x-ray were the standard studies for complex facial trauma after the resolution of edema and treatment of other injuries. The CT scan, however, is a more accurate diagnostic study and allows an evaluation of complicated facial fractures before the resolution of edema. When using 1½ mm coronal cuts, a CT scan will show the various degrees of comminution of the facial bone fractures as well as the amount of displacement or rotation of the fragments. Additionally, injuries to the soft-tissue structures in the area of trauma can be better evaluated; for example, the optic nerve or orbital herniation of the orbit (Fig 17–3). Additional information can also be obtained by reformatting the data from the CT scan into a three-dimensional picture.

The only disadvantage to the use of the CT scan is seen when artifacts caused by either dental fillings or metal appliances occur. CT exposes

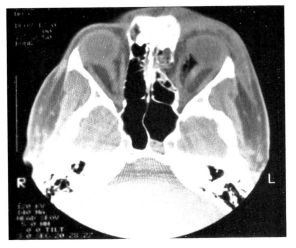

FIG 17–3.
Axial CT of the orbits clearly demonstrates the optic nerve and the extraocular muscles in maxillofacial injuries

the patient to a radiation dosage equal to the amount from linear tomography. Studies have been done that suggest that the amount of radiation from either study is less than the amount needed to cause cataracts.

MANDIBULAR FRACTURES

Although it is the thickest and heaviest of the facial bones, the mandible is the most commonly fractured, excluding nasal bone fractures. Mandibular fractures may occur as isolated injuries or as components of complex maxillary and mandibular fractures.

The most frequent cause of mandibular fractures are acts of violence that encompass simple falls, assaults, or motor vehicle accidents. Occasionally, systemic diseases such as hyperparathyroidism and osteomalacia may predispose to mandibular fractures. Infrequently, benign or malignant tumors, cysts, or osteomyelitis may precipitate such fractures.

Factors influencing the severity of the displacement of the fracture segments are multiple and interrelated. The direction and intensity of

the force of injury will cause different fractures. High-velocity injuries cause a fracture at the site of impact, whereas a slow, less violent force not only causes a fracture at the impact site but also may fracture the opposite condylar neck. A blow to the area of the symphysis may cause fractures of both condylar necks. Second, the site of the fracture may influence the amount of displacement of the segments, depending on the direction of the fracture line and the direction of the different muscle movements in the area. A fracture line that runs downward and forward from the molar area has less displacement than does a line that runs downward and backward. The muscle groups that operate the mandible include the anterior (depressor-retractor) group and the posterior (elevator) group. The anterior muscle group will displace fragments in a downward, posterior, and medial direction, whereas the posterior group displaces fragments in an upward, forward, and medial direction. Consequently, a fracture through the angle of the mandible in a downward and backward direction will have a far greater displacement due to the distracting forces of the posterior muscle group. If the fracture line, however, was in the downward and forward direction, the muscle pull of the posterior group would tend to keep the fracture segments in an anatomic position. Third, the presence or absence of teeth will influence displacement of the fractures. Teeth on the proximal segment may decrease the displacement of the fractures by meeting the corresponding teeth of the maxilla. Finally, the presence and extent of soft-tissue wounds will result in a larger displacement with larger defects.

Clinically, the patient may present with varying degrees of malocclusion. He may simply admit "my teeth don't feel right," or physical examination may demonstrate gross malocclusion. Anesthesia of the lower lip is common in fractures of the body of the mandible. Edema and ecchymosis may mask mandibular asymmetry. On examination, tenderness to palpation over the fracture site and pain with movement will be observed. Crepitation may be seen with motion. Oral excursion will be decreased. However, the principal physicial abnormality will be malocclusion.

Although the clinical examination most frequently establishes the diagnosis of mandibular fractures, roentgenographic studies more clearly define the direction of the fracture line, the relationship of the teeth to the fracture, and the degree of displacement. Posteroanterior and oblique lateral views of the mandible will demonstrate fractures of the body and the angle without difficulty. If available, a Panorex view of the mandible is an excellent study and will show fractures at any site. However, fractures of the temporomandibular joint and condylar area are sometimes difficult to demonstrate on routine mandibular roentgenograms and may require tomograms for the final diagnosis (Fig 17–4).

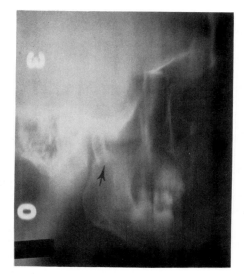

FIG 17–4.
Tomograms of the condylar process are often required to establish a fracture of the condylar neck *(arrow)*.

The most frequent fracture of the mandible is in the neck of the condyle. According to Dingman and Natvig (1964), 36% of all fractures occur in the condylar process. The frequency of fractures in this site is closely followed by that of fractures in the angle of the mandible (20%), the body (21%), and the area of the symphysis (14%). Other sites are much less frequently involved.

The principles of treatment for mandibular fracture include early anatomic reduction of the fracture, immobilization, and control of infection. An isolated mandibular fracture should be reduced at the time of injury. However, if other life-threatening injuries are present, treatment of the mandibular injury may be postponed for 7 to 10 days. All mandibular fractures are considered compound if the slightest displacement is present and consequently, preoperative and postoperative antibiotics are recommended. Immobilization will require at least the application of arch bars and intermaxillary fixation with rubber bands or wires for a minimum of 5 weeks.

Specific treatment for each mandibular fracture will vary with the site of the fracture, the degree of displacement, and the presence or absence of teeth. Whenever possible, closed reduction of the mandibular fracture with application of arch bars and intermaxillary fixation is the treatment of choice.

Significant changes in the open reduction of mandibular fractures have occurred over the last several years. Actually, the use of plating and screw fixation for mandibular fractures was introduced in 1972, but was not really accepted in the United States until the last 5 years. The advantages of using plating and lag screws for mandibular fractures include rigid stabilization and early return of function by avoiding the lengthy period of intermaxillary fixation (IMF). Consequently, the expected weight loss and the inability to maintain good oral hygiene in patients with IMF are markedly reduced. The disadvantages of the plating system are the increased operative time of the surgical procedure as well as the need for an external approach for some fractures. However, the recent introduction of instrumentation, including a right-angle screwdriver, may make the intraoral approach more feasible for all fractures.

Fractures in the region of symphysis or the angle of the mandible commonly require open reduction and internal fixation with compression plates and lag screws. An arch bar will be placed on the alveolar ridge of the mandible to act as a tension band. However, IMF is not usually needed, and the patient can return to oral intake as soon as his recovery from surgery allows. Similarly, fractures in the body of the mandible with teeth absent on the proximal side, or no teeth present on either side of the fracture, will require open reduction and internal fixation with plates (Fig 17–5).

The use of compression plates has made the treatment of edentulous patients with mandible fractures much simpler. Instead of using the patient's dentures for the application of arch bars and then suspending the dentures from the zygomatic arches, open reduction and internal fixation with compression plates are used.

Postoperatively, the care of the patient with a mandible fracture will depend on the type of treatment. If open reduction with internal fixation using compression plates or lag screws has been the method of treatment, the postoperative

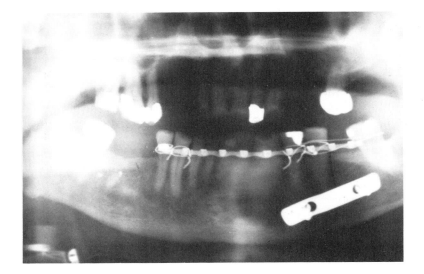

FIG 17–5.
A postoperative x-ray film of a mandibular fracture demonstrates the use of the compression plate in an open reduction and internal fixation of a mandible fracture. No IMF was needed. The arch bar acts as a tension band.

course is markedly simple. The patient is allowed a liquid to soft diet beginning almost immediately. A soft diet is continued for approximately 5 or 6 weeks postreduction. Consequently, the patient's nutritional status is maintained, and the problem of possible weight loss does not normally become a matter of concern.

On the other hand, if closed reduction using arch bars and IMF with rubber bands or wires has been the treatment, a period of immobilization of 5 weeks will be needed for solid union to develop at the fracture site, even though roentgenograms will not demonstrate healing at that time. The use of the Water-Pik is highly recommended to maintain good oral hygiene during the period of mobilization. Nutrition is maintained very simply by using a blenderizing regular diet. The patient should be seen weekly to check dental occlusion and to replace broken rubber bands to maintain immobilization. Dental wax may be applied to irritating wires. At the end of 5 weeks, the rubber bands are removed, and the patient is allowed to eat for a week. If the patient experiences no pain with oral ingestion, the arch bars are removed with the patient under intravenous sedation. However, if pain or movement at the fracture site can be elicited with eating, the rubber bands are reapplied for another 7 to 10 days of immobilization.

Occasionally, after removing the arch bars, the patient experiences a transient period of trismus due to the prolonged contraction of the muscles of mastication during the period of immobilization. By sliding an increased number of tongue blades between his teeth, the patient should be able to forcibly open his mouth over a period of time and, consequently, regain the proper use of his mandible.

Early complications of mandibular fracture may include infection, avascular necrosis, osteitis, and osteomyelitis. Predisposing factors to infection are poor oral hygiene, multiple caries, or a compound fracture. Diabetic patients are more susceptible to infections. Acute infection will be manifested as an abscess and would be reflected by pain, swelling, and erythema in the area of the abscess. Incision, drainage, and systemic antibiotics constitute the treatment of choice. Chronic infections such as osteitis and osteomyelitis usually occur when a comminuted fracture with an avascular bone segment has occurred. Pain and roentgenographic changes suggestive of osteomyelitis are usually evident. Late complications may also include malocclusion or nonunion and would require further corrective surgery.

FRACTURES OF THE MAXILLA

Fractures of the maxilla, or midface, are most commonly due to a high-velocity–type injury. Their incidence in recent years has decreased, primarily due to the lower highway speed limits and the increased use of seat belts. However, such injuries may occur in collisions at speeds as low as 30 miles per hour. The force necessary to cause fractures of the maxilla also increases the likelihood of severe injuries to other organ systems. Associated injuries of various degrees of severity more frequently involve the head but occur in the chest and abdomen as well. Skeletal injuries may be present in approximately one

third of the patients, while blindness is observed in 10%. Finally, the frequency of cervical spine injury is much higher than other types of facial fractures and is due to the effects of sudden cervical hyperflexion.

Maxillary fractures can be divided into two groups: vertical and horizontal. Vertical fractures will split the palate on either side of the septum. However, the three classic fractures of the maxilla are those horizontal defects described by Le Fort. The Le Fort I (transverse) fracture is a horizontal facture immediately above the level of the teeth. The Le Fort II fracture has the configuration of a pyramid, with the apex being the nasal bridge. It extends through the nasal bones, the frontal processes of the maxilla, the lacrimal bones, the inferior rim and floor of both orbits, and the maxillozygomatic suture line. From this last point, the fracture continues posteriorly through the lateral wall of the maxilla and the pterygoid plates and into the pterygoid maxillary fossa. The Le Fort III fracture separates the craniofacial complex and extends through the zygomaticofrontal, maxillofrontal, and nasofrontal suture lines, the floors of the orbit, and the ethmoid and sphenoid bones (Fig 17–6).

Clinically, the patient may be comatose and may require immediate neurosurgical consultation. If conscious, he may complain of the inability to "match" his teeth properly. Infraorbital nerve numbness may be present. In Le Fort II or III fractures, nasal hemorrhage is usually evident. On physical examination, facial deformities may be masked by edema and ecchymosis. Bimanual palpation along the orbital ridges may detect steplike deformities or separations and tenderness. Forward movement of the maxilla will be elicited with all three Le Fort fractures; in the Le Fort III fracture, the entire midthird of the face

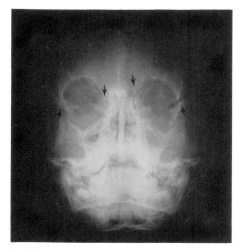

FIG 17–6.
A Le Fort III craniofacial separation *(arrows)* is evident in a Waters' view of an 8-year-old patient. The opacity of the left maxillary sinus is more severe than the right.

may move. However, occasionally these fractures may be impacted, and no movement will be evident. Malocclusion can be an initial sign and should suggest a maxillary fracture if the mandible is intact. Extraocular muscle dysfunction may be manifested by diplopia with superior gaze. Blindness is uncommon but may occur.

With extension of the maxillary fractures into the cribriform plate, rhinorrhea mixed with blood will be detected as a result of the dural defect. The patient may admit to a salty taste in the back of his mouth. Any clear fluid from the nose should be tested for glucose. If the glucose level is greater than 30 mg/100 cc, the presence of cerebrospinal fluid (CSF) has been confirmed, and a tear in the dura has occurred. Consequently, the patient's nose should not be packed despite the possible presence of depressed nasal fractures, and the patient should be instructed not to blow his nose. Prophylactic antibiotics that cross the blood-brain barrier should be instituted to decrease the possibility of the development of a retrograde infection. When meningitis has occurred in this type of injury, the most common organism isolated has been *Pneumococcus,* sensitive to penicillin.

Roentgenographically, the Waters' view is the most reliable in demonstrating maxillary fractures in the emergency room. For vertical or alveolar fractures, occlusal views are more suitable. CT scans of the facial bones will detail more accurately the full extent of the fractures (Fig 17–7). The study is usually done in the coronal view and will show the amount of the comminution, the degree of rotation, and the extent of displacement of the fracture segments. Additionally, injury to the optic nerve or fat herniation may be visible.

In those cases where the presence of rhinorrhea has persisted for more than 2 to 3 weeks after the injury or after reduction of the facial bone fractures, an intrathecal injection of metrizamide contrast by lumbar puncture before CT scanning will localize the cranial defect for the neurosurgeon. Radionuclear scans are no longer indicated for the evaluation of CSF leak.

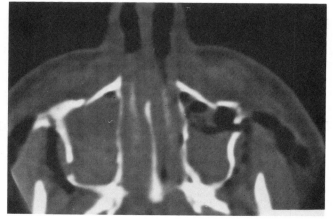

FIG 17–7.
Axial CT scan view of maxillary fractures. Bilateral maxillary clouding is evident, greater on the right. Fractures of both the anterior and lateral walls are clearly visible. (Coronal CT scan views show facial bone fractures in a more familiar orientation.)

Initially, the airway may be compromised by the posterior displacement of the maxillary fractures or by the combination with mandibular fractures. An endotracheal tube is the preferred treatment, although a cricothyroidotomy occasionally may be necessary.

After adequate resolution of facial edema, open reduction and internal fixation of the maxillary fractures will be required in order to establish the proper dental occlusion and to maintain an adequate midface projection.

The use of compression plates in craniofacial surgery for congenital abnormalities has been widely accepted for the treatment of maxillary injuries. The compression plates are placed across the fracture sites and give good stability (Fig 17–8). IMF is usually not required, although in areas of severe complex fractures elastics may be required for several weeks instead of wire fixation. The orbital floors are explored in Le Fort II or III fractures, and defects are reconstructed with either synthetic implants or cranial bone grafts. Preoperative and postoperative antibiotics are recommended.

Rarely is a tracheotomy required in the isolated midface fracture. However, maxillary fractures combined with pulmonary or thoracic injuries may require a tracheotomy to ensure proper ventilation and adequate pulmonary toilet postoperatively.

In the edentulous patient with minimal displacement of the midface, correction of the anatomic defect may be maintained by adjustment with new dentures. However, any significant displacement will require open reduction and internal fixation with compression plate fixation.

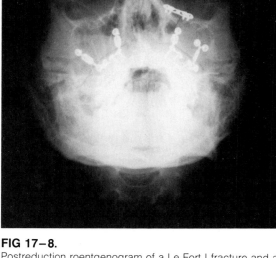

FIG 17–8.
Postreduction roentgenogram of a Le Fort I fracture and a left zygoma fracture treated by compression plates only. No IMF was needed for satisfactory reduction.

Occasionally, the patient with extensive maxillary fractures will also suffer a severe head injury with resultant coma. After stabilization of the neurologic status and with the approval of the neurosurgeon, correction of the maxillary fractures is recommended. If treated within 3 weeks of injury, adequate reduction and fixation of the fracture can be accomplished. Otherwise, months may elapse before some degree of consciousness occurs, and surgical intervention then will be markedly more difficult, will probably require osteotomies with bone grafting, and will have less satisfying postoperative results.

Usually, the presence of rhinorrhea will spontaneously cease about 5 days after injury. Alternatively, the CSF leak will cease with adequate reduction of the maxillary fractures. If rhinorrhea continues 3 weeks after injury or after reduction, a craniotomy will be required to close the dural defect.

The use of compression plates allows the airway to be easily managed and lessens the patient's stay in the intensive care unit. Postoperatively, improved oral hygiene and food intake result in the patient's quicker rehabilitation. And finally, the use of plates avoids the possible midfacial shortening and/or midfacial retrusion sometimes seen with wire fixation and craniomandibular suspension.

Late complications of maxillary fractures include nasal obstruction, chronic sinusitis, and lacrimal duct dysfunction. Anesthesia or hypoesthesia of the infraorbital nerve may persist. Malunion of the fracture may occur and, if unrecognized until 4 months after reduction, will require planned osteotomies with bone grafting for correction. If recognized within 4 months of the initial reduction, the malunion may be corrected by a second attempt at open reduction and internal fixation. Malocclusion after treatment may occur about 20% of the time. Orthodontics usually can correct this problem; only in severe cases will reconstructive osteotomies be required.

FRACTURES OF THE ZYGOMA

The zygoma or malar bone forms the prominence of the cheek and, consequently, is frequently injured. The usual cause of a zygoma fracture is the low-intensity, less violent type of injury: fistfights, falls, collisions.

The zygoma articulates with the maxilla, frontal, and temporal bones. Injury to it may cause a separation at the suture lines in an isolated injury or may be combined with fractures of the middle third of the face. If displaced, the zygoma will be depressed in the direction of the traumatic force, which most commonly is in the posterior, downward, and medial direction. Although six different groups of malar fractures have been described, fractures of the zygoma are basically either an isolated zygomatic arch fracture (Fig 17–9) or the "tripod" fracture (Fig 17–10).

Clinically, the patient may complain of pain in the area of the zygomatic arch when attempting to open his mouth. Infraorbital nerve anesthesia may be present in both the ipsilateral cheek and the maxillary gingiva (gingival numbness suggests orbital floor and rim fractures). The patient may also admit to diplopia with upward gaze.

On initial examination, the anatomic abnormalities may be masked by significant edema. Since blindness can occur with these injuries, the physician must immediately evaluate the vision of the affected eye. Ecchymosis may involve the conjunctiva and sclera as well as the eyelids. Bimanual palpation of both the orbital rims and the zygomatic arches should be done simultaneously and may elicit tenderness at the fracture site. After resolution of the edema, the clinician may be able to identify depression over the zygomatic arch, step-off deformities of the orbital rim, flattening of the malar eminence, or inferior displacement of the lateral canthus. Oral excursion

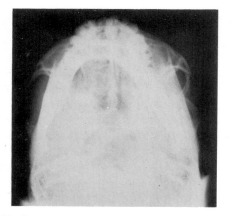

FIG 17–9.
A markedly depressed zygomatic arch fracture is demonstrated by a submental-vertex view.

may be limited to less than 2 cm. (Limitation of oral excursion can occur if the zygomatic arch is depressed 1 cm and impedes the movement of the coronoid process of the mandible.) Diplopia with superior gaze may be present if the inferior

rectus muscle is trapped by an orbital floor fracture. Enophthalmos may occur if a significant orbital floor defect is present.

The best roentgenographic studies obtainable from the emergency room are the Waters' view of the facial bones and the submental-vertex view of the zygomatic arches. Displacement of the malar fragment and/or opacity in the maxillary sinus in a tripod fracture is readily visible on a Waters' view. After resolution of the edema, a CT scan of the orbits can be obtained to further delineate the extent of the fractures (Fig 17–11).

Actual treatment depends on the type of fracture, the degree of fragmentation, and the direction and degree of displacement of the fracture sites. Resolution of the facial edema is necessary to assess the malar deformity and to ensure good symmetry with the opposite malar prominence during reduction. A nondisplaced tripod malar or zygomatic arch fracture may not need surgical intervention. Antibiotics are prescribed for tripod fractures since the maxillary sinus is usually violated and a compound fracture is created.

Surgical reduction of the isolated zygomatic

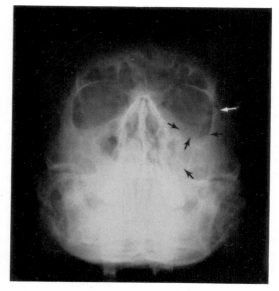

FIG 17–10.
A comminuted left tripod malar fracture is visualized on a Waters' view. A step deformity of the orbital rim can be anticipated on physical examination *(arrows)*. Note the opacity of the left maxillary sinus.

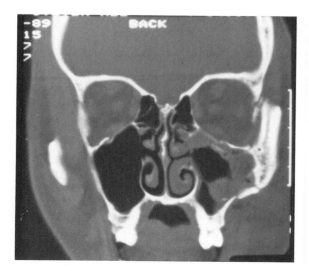

FIG 17–11.
A coronal CT scan demonstrates a displaced left malar fracture. Opacification of the left maxillary sinus is clearly evident. Also note the ability for the CT scan to demonstrate the extraocular muscles.

arch fracture can be done either intraorally or extraorally on an outpatient basis. Extraorally, an incision is made either in the lateral eyebrow or in the temporal portion of the scalp behind the hairline. The fracture is reduced by passing an instrument beneath the temporal muscle fascia to a point behind the zygomatic arch and popping the depressed segment into place. If the fracture's reduction is unstable, a circumferential wire is passed percutaneously around the zygomatic arch and tied over a metal eye shield to maintain reduction for 3 weeks. At the end of the 3-week period the wire is removed in the office. Severe comminuted arch fractures may need open reduction and plating through a coronal incision.

Treatment of displaced tripod malar fractures may be accomplished by closed or open reduction. Closed reduction consists of inserting a bone hook at the base of the zygoma and reducing the fracture with the opposite malar prominence as a reference point. However, the incidence of late complications of diplopia, malunion, and facial deformity are relatively high, and this method is not recommended.

Most surgeons prefer an open reduction of zygoma fractures. After reduction of the bone fragments, the position is maintained by compression plating. Previously, K-wire fixation to the opposite malar complex was advocated. However, such a technique can allow rotation of the segments and subsequent deformity. By use of the compression plates, solid fixation is achieved that resists the pull of the masseter muscle (Fig 17–12). Recent evidence suggests that many fractures can be fixated at two points with plates placed at the frontal zygomatic suture line and the zygomatic maxillary buttress. For severely displaced and rotated fractures, a coronal incision will be needed to allow fixation at the zygomatic arch as well. Fractures of the zygoma should be reduced within 3 weeks of injury.

The orbital floor should be examined before and after reduction of the zygoma fracture. A defect in the orbital floor may increase with satisfactory malar reduction and require reconstruc-

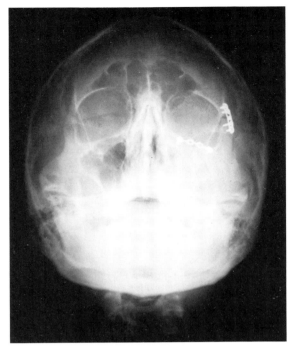

FIG 17–12.
A postreduction film of a zygoma fracture treated by compression plates. Often a third plate will be placed at the zygoma/maxillary buttress if instability is present.

tion with either a synthetic implant or a cranial bone graft.

Postoperatively, antibiotic coverage is continued for a week. A light dressing may be applied over the ipsilateral eye, but it is removed on the first postoperative day. The patient is followed weekly in the office in order to monitor both malar symmetry and extraocular muscle function.

Complications secondary to zygoma fractures are unusual but would include infection, malunion, and nonunion. Infection usually occurs in those cases requiring orbital floor reconstruction with an implant, especially if the maxillary sinus has also been packed. The infection may develop early or late with respect to the repair of the fracture and requires removal of the implant as well as antibiotics administered for systemic effect. Malunion of the zygoma may cause facial asymmetry and interference with mandibular function. Correction can be achieved by osteotomies at the zygomaticofrontal and zygomaticomaxillary suture line, elevation of the zygoma, bone grafting, and fixation. Nonunions will necessitate bone grafting and rigid fixation. Any residual contour deformity may be corrected at a later date with the use of onlay bone, cartilage, or synthetic grafts.

BLOW-OUT FRACTURES

Strictly speaking, the term "blow-out" fracture should be restricted to fractures of the orbital floor without involvement of the orbital rim. Blow-out fractures result from the transmission of a sudden increased intraocular pressure through the weakest point of the orbital floor, most commonly near the infraorbital nerve canal. A second common site of fracture is the medial orbital wall.

The most frequent cause of blow-out fractures is the automobile accident. A third of the cases usually result from blunt trauma secondary to fist blows, ball injuries, falls, and other forms of assault. Although the orbital rim protects the eyeball itself against direct injury from objects greater than 5 cm in size, ocular injury must be ruled out in all blow-out fractures. The incidence of ocular injury with orbital fractures varies widely in the literature, but the incidence of hyphema and retinal hemorrhage appear to be the most common. However, more severe injuries such as decreased vision or blindness may also occur. Direct ocular injury is more common in low-velocity injuries (14%) than in auto accidents (0.6%).

During examination, the patient may volunteer the presence of diplopia, infraorbital nerve numbness, and possibly, decreased vision. Clinically, periorbital edema and ecchymosis may handicap the initial examination. However, the eyelids can usually be pried open to allow a gross examination of vision and light perception. Diplopia may occur as a result of limitation of superior gaze (Fig 17–13). As the periorbital edema resolves, diplopia may lessen in severity. If the periorbital edema is minimal, enophthalmos may be present.

The most common cause of diplopia in blow-out fractures is entrapment of the inferior rectus muscle, inferior oblique muscle, or a periorbital fat herniation. Other causes of immediate diplopia include injury to cranial nerves III, IV, and VI; direct injury or hemorrhage into the extraocular muscles; or displacement of the eyeball into the maxillary sinus. The "traction test" will simplify the differential diagnosis. Topical anesthesia is applied to the conjunctiva. The eyeball is pinched with a fine forceps at the insertion of the inferior rectus muscle and rotated. If rotation of the eyeball cannot be accomplished, entrapment of the inferior rectus muscle is demonstrated. If rotation of the eyeball is achieved, then the diplopia is due to one of the other causes.

Enophthalmos may be evident on the initial examination or masked by the periorbital edema. With subsequent resolution of the edema, enophthalmos will become more apparent. The

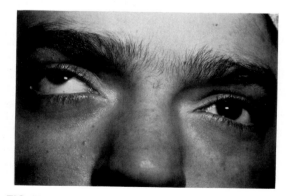

FIG 17–13.
Impairment of superior gaze occurred after a blow to the left eye. A traction test confirmed entrapment of the inferior rectus muscle.

mechanism of enophthalmos includes herniation of the orbital fat into the maxillary sinus, posterior position of the ocular globe due to entrapment of the inferior rectus muscle, or the downward displacement of the ocular globe through a large orbital floor fracture. Additionally, enophthalmos may develop as a result of orbital fat necrosis secondary to the injury, to pressure from an orbital hematoma, or to a low-grade inflammatory process.

The most pertinent roentgenographic studies are a Waters' view initially, followed by orbital floor tomograms or a CT scan. Coronal views by CT scan may be the most accurate in diagnosing this defect. However, its use may be limited by the positioning requirements of the patient or by the presence of multiple dental fillings. Abnormal findings would include lowering of the orbital floor, orbital fat entrapment in the maxillary sinus (Fig 17–14), or massive orbital contents displacement into the maxillary sinus.

Treatment of blow-out fracture is twofold. If definite ocular injury is demonstrated on initial examination, an ophthalmologic consultation must be obtained immediately for evaluation. If no ocular injury is present, surgical considerations are postponed until the resolution of periorbital edema. The two primary indications for surgical correction of a blow-out fracture include diplopia confirmed by a positive traction test or enophthalmos. Usually, roentgenographic evidence will support the diagnosis of a blow-out fracture, but a normal study should not postpone surgery if there is a positive traction test or enophthalmos present.

The surgical procedure should be performed within 2 weeks after injury since the incarcerated contents become more difficult to release after this period. If surgery is postponed more than 2 or 3 weeks, motility problems and enophthalmos may appear as late complications. The surgical procedure consists of exploration of the orbital floor through a lower eyelid incision, release of the entrapped inferior rectus muscle, retrieval of the herniated orbital contents, and reconstruction of the orbital floor with either a synthetic implant or a cranial bone graft.

Antibiotics are recommended both preoperatively and postoperatively due to the involvement with the maxillary sinus. An eyepatch is usually applied at the completion of the operation and removed on the first postoperative day. The patient is followed as an outpatient for persistence of either diplopia or enophthalmos.

Useful binocular vision at the end of 3 months commonly occurs. However, if diplopia is not improved by that time, an ophthalmology consultation will be required for further evaluation and possible prescription of glass prisms to allow useful vision. After 6 months, extraocular muscle surgery may be necessary to correct the persistent diplopia. The persistence of enophthalmos presents a very difficult problem. Recent work has shown that enophthalmos may be corrected by osteotomies and reconstruction with a cranial bone graft. However, this surgical procedure is a major effort to correct a deformity that might have been prevented at the initial surgical repair.

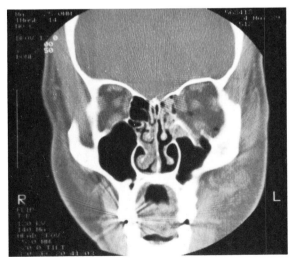

FIG 17–14.
A coronal CT scan demonstrating a left blow-out fracture. Soft-tissue entrapment can be seen. Note the artifacts created by the dental fillings on the right side.

NASAL FRACTURES

Fractures of the nasal bones are the most common of all facial bone fractures. Early treatment will allow easy reduction with satisfactory postoperative results. Neglect of treatment, however, may produce both a physiologic and a cosmetic deformity much more difficult to correct.

The types of nasal fracture may vary from a simple displacement of the nasal pyramid from a lateral blow to a more complex comminuted fracture with a resultant "smashed"-nose appearance from a frontal force. Associated injuries include fractures extending through the cribriform plate, medial canthal ligament displacement, or lacrimal gland or duct injuries. Sequelae of the comminuted nasal fracture include traumatic telecanthus, dacryocystitis, and epiphora.

Clinical evaluation plays the most important role in making an accurate diagnosis. The presence of pre-existing disease, nasal deformity, or a previous nasal operation should be investigated at the time of the initial examination. On physical examination, nasal and periorbital edema are common. Nasal obstruction may be present secondary to either edema, clots, or displaced nasal bone fractures. Movement of the nasal bone fragments may be elicited by palpation. Subcutaneous emphysema may be present. The possibility of a telescoping-type injury should be considered if the nasolabial angle is greater than 100 degrees (especially in a man) or if a step deformity is noted dorsally at the junction of the nasal bone with the septum.

The importance of identifying a hematoma of the septum at the time of the initial examination cannot be stressed too strongly. If overlooked, a septal hematoma can progress either to a partial nasal obstruction or to a septal perforation. Topical application of 10% cocaine will shrink the nasal mucosa and allow examination of the nasal passageways by a speculum. The presence of a septal hematoma should be treated immediately by incision and drainage.

Very often, the posteroanterior and lateral roentgenographic views of the nasal bones are not very helpful in supporting the clinical impression of a nasal fracture. A Waters' view may better demonstrate fractures of either the nasal septum or the bony pyramid. However, the clinical impression is much more meaningful in diagnosing this fracture.

Ideally, the treatment of a nasal fracture should be done when initially seen. Usually, however, the presence of nasal edema does not permit immediate reduction. At the end of 3 to 5 days, the edema will resolve sufficiently to allow satisfactory reduction of the nasal fracture. Most simple fractures are treated by closed reduction. However, complicated fractures that result from a frontal impact are more likely to be treated by an open reduction. The fragments are reduced under direct vision and wired together. Medial canthal ligament injuries are repaired. Bone grafting may be done.

Although the procedure can be performed with the patient under either general anesthesia or a combination of local and topical anesthesia, general anesthesia is recommended to protect the airway from posterior nasal bleeding. After satisfactory reduction, a nasal speculum should be used to demonstrate the patency of the airways and to evaluate the position of the nasal septum. A displaced septum should be returned to its position in the vomerine groove. Nasal packing is inserted to maintain the nasal bone reduction. A nasal splint is applied for further stabilization.

Postoperatively, the nasal packing will be left in place for approximately 5 days and the nasal splint for 7. During the second week, the nasal splint is usually worn only at night. Any activity that would endanger the nasal reduction (for example, contact sports) should be avoided for 6 weeks. During the interval of packing, nasal decongestants and antibiotics are used.

Late complications of nasal fracture include nasal deformity or airway obstruction. The nasal deformity may be secondary to malunion of the nasal bones or to a septal injury. Malunion usually occurs as a result of the patient's failure to seek early medical attention. Correcting a nasal fracture after 14 days past the injury is rarely successful and will require rhinoplasty to correct the deformity. Persistent nasal deformity or airway obstruction may be due to a septal injury and will also require rhinoplasty and possible sub-mucous cartilage resection for correction. In the pediatric age group, rhinoplasties are normally postponed until the age of 15 years to avoid any possible growth disturbances with the development of the nose. In the adult, rhinoplasty can be performed after satisfactory wound healing has occurred, usually about 3 months after the injury.

FRONTAL SINUS FRACTURES

Frontal sinus fractures are not common (6%), but they do warrant special considerations. Such injuries are usually accompanied by fractures of other facial bones and may be associated with an intracranial injury.

On clinical examination, anesthesia of the forehead and scalp may be present as a result of soft-tissue injury to the supratrochlear and su-praorbital nerves. If a depressed supraorbital ridge fracture is present, diplopia will be demonstrated as a result of dysfunction of the superior rectus and superior oblique muscles. Periorbital ecchymosis and edema will be present, which may mask the frontal depression secondary to the fracture. Tenderness and crepitation to palpation may be elicited. Rhinorrhea may also be noted.

Roentgenographic studies should include a skull series and a Waters' view of the facial bones. Occasionally, there may be difficulty in demonstrating a frontal sinus fracture since fractures of the posterior wall are difficult to see roentgenographically, even with good tomographic studies. A CT scan is very useful in diag-nosing posterior wall fractures. However, the presence of an intracranial aerocele is pathognomonic for a dural tear and would implicate a fracture of the posterior wall of the frontal sinus.

Treatment of a frontal sinus fracture depends on the extent of the fracture and the amount of fragmentation present. Antibiotic coverage should begin on the day of injury. Surgical correction of a depressed or compound anterior wall fracture requires elevation and wiring of the bony fragments. Treatment of posterior wall fractures is controversial and involves open exploration with sinus obliteration by any variety of ways. In the presence of a dural tear, a transfrontal craniotomy with repair of the dura should be done in conjunction with reduction of the fracture.

Potential complications of frontal sinus fractures can be life-threatening. A posterior wall fracture with a dural tear may develop either a retrograde meningitis or brain abscess. Frontal sinus infections may also extend into the orbital cavities. The frontal sinus duct may be obstructed with the subsequent development of a mucocele.

FACIAL FRACTURES IN THE PEDIATRIC PATIENT

The incidence of facial fractures in the pediatric age group varies in reported series from 1.4% to 10%. In the author's experience, the most common fractures involve the nose and mandible. Maxillary fractures are very uncommon since the bones are small and the sinuses are not well pneumatized. If a maxillary fracture does occur, it is usually a LeFort III fracture associated with other severe facial injuries, especially blindness. Most fractures are greenstick in nature due to the resiliency of the facial bones in this age. Although the principles outlined for treatment of facial fractures do not change with age, several important considerations should be noted.

Clinical and roentgenographic evaluation may be more difficult to obtain. The child may not understand or answer questions about his injury. Cooperation in the physical examination may be difficult to obtain, but tenderness to palpation usually can be elicited. Roentgenographic studies may require sedation to ensure films of good detail. The presence of unerupted teeth may mask the site of a fracture.

In general, the treatment of maxillofacial injuries in the child is basically similar to the treatment described in the previous pages. Difficulty sometimes arises in maintaining IMF since the ligation of arch bars to the short roots of deciduous teeth is difficult and precarious. Care also must be used to avoid injury to the unerupted teeth with application of the arch bars by wire ligatures. The extent of immobilization by IMF is shorter when the fractures are the greenstick type.

Mandibular fractures confined only to the condyle are treated more conservatively. If the child has a good occlusion on physical examination, then observation, early motion, and a liquid diet are the appropriate treatment. If occlusion cannot be demonstrated, then immobilization with IMF for 3 weeks is indicated.

Late complications of a facial fracture would also include the loss, delay, or maleruption of developing teeth; malocclusion; and facial deformity. Facial deformity may be the result of abnormal development secondary to a growth center disturbance at the time of injury. Consequently, the parents should be alerted to this possibility and the child should be observed throughout adolescence for any evidence of growth abnormality.

SOFT-TISSUE INJURY MANAGEMENT

Soft-tissue injuries are commonly seen in any emergency room on a daily basis. The appropriate management includes not only evaluation of the wound itself but also evaluation for any deeper injury and repair by the appropriate methods. Complicated wounds require the expertise of a surgical specialist. However, many wounds are simple and can be treated by either the emergency room or primary-care physician.

The general principles of wound repair apply to injuries occurring in any region of the body. However, for the purpose of discussion, most of the examples will be confined to the head and neck area. Before any local anesthesia is administered, evaluation of facial nerve function can be simply done by asking the patient to raise his eyebrows, close his eyelids, and smile. If any weakness is present, then a nerve injury should be considered. Vertically oriented lacerations across the cheek have a potential underlying parotid duct injury, especially if the laceration appears to extend into the parotid gland. Oftentimes, cannulating Stensen's duct opposite the second maxillary molar can be done in the emergency room. Injection of methylene blue solution will allow the diagnosis to be made. If either a parotid duct or facial nerve injury is identified, the patient should be referred to a surgical specialist for management in the operating room.

Commonly, most soft-tissue injuries are isolated and can be managed in the emergency room. Such wounds range in severity from simple lacerations to dog bite injuries to more complicated soft-tissue wounds. For those lacerations that do not require the expertise of a surgical specialist, simple general principles may guide the emergency room or primary-care physician in a prompt and satisfactory repair.

Surgical Technique

Local infiltration with plain xylocaine or xylocaine with epinephrine is the most common choice of anesthesia. In facial wounds, 1% xylocaine with epinephrine, 1:200,000, is the more appropriate choice since the head and neck area is extremely vascular. The use of epinephrine decreases the amount of bleeding, prolongs the duration of anesthesia, and allows for greater volume of infiltration if necessary. However, epinephrine may cause cardiac irritability. Large amounts should be avoided in patients with cardiac disease, arrythmias, or hypertension. Epinephrine should not be injected in wounds that have a high risk for infection or in wounds with marginally viable tissue.

Proper administration of local anesthesia may avoid some patient discomfort. Direct wound infiltration through the wound margin by using a 25- or 27-guage needle is better tolerated than is injection through the intact skin. The injection should be done as a slow, steady application of anesthesia in contrast to the sudden, painful injection of a bolus of the local solution.

After the wound is anesthetized, it should be treated with an appropriate solution such as povidone-iodine (Betadine) and draped. If any foreign material is still present or suspicion of bacteria seeding is high, local irrigation of the wound is performed. Such irrigation provides mechanical cleansing of the wound. The choice of the solution for irrigation is not as important as the actual cleansing of the wound. The simplest technique for irrigation is the use of a 25-cc syringe with a 22-guage needle. The amount of irrigation necessary to clean the wound, of course, depends on the contamination and tissue injury of the wound. The irrigation may also be supplemented by using a toothbrush or scrub brush to remove any embedded particles.

Any bleeding point should be coagulated. Most emergency rooms now have battery-operated disposable cauteries that can be used. Thus, coagulation will help minimize the chance of postclosure bleeding with a subsequent increased risk of infection or development of hematomas.

Most simple lacerations do not require much surgical manipulation. Occasionally, there may be an area of questionable tissue on the wound margin that would require debridement. Conser-

vation should be the primary goal whenever debriding edges of such wounds. However, the nonviable tissue should be removed in order to provide optimal results for wound healing. If the extent of the debridement is of concern to the physician, then surgical consultation should be obtained.

Lacerations that extend through the dermis into the subcutaneous tissue will require a two-layer closure. Closure of the dermal subcutaneous junction with an absorbable suture is the first step and provides the strength in wound repair. The choice of absorbable suture can be either 5-0 Dexon or Vicryl. The sutures are placed in such a manner that the knot is inverted. The needle is first passed through the subcutaneous tissue into the dermis on one side of the wound and passed through the dermis into the subcutaneous tissue on the other side of the wound where it is tied. Such a technique allows the knot to be covered by the full layer of the skin and thus minimizes the changes for "spitting" of the suture.

In small lacerations, the physician can proceed from one end of the wound to the other. However, for longer wounds, it is easier to divide the wound into quarters with placement of the first three sutures. This approach allows for more accurate closure and avoids the appearance of "dog ears."

After the dermal layer is approximated, closure of the skin layer should be completed. Using small interrupted sutures of 6-0 nylon placed at short intervals is an acceptable technique. (Slightly more demanding is the subcuticular suture, which may present a better outcome by avoiding the chances of crosshatching seen occasionally with interrupted suture repair.) The interrupted skin sutures should not strangulate the skin. Sutures should be removed before the sixth day to avoid crosshatching or "railroad tracks". The application of sterile strips can be done at the time of suture removal.

Wounds to the lower eyelids are usually closed with 6-0 silk to minimize the possible irritation of sutures on the ocular globe. Nylon sutures are stiff and can cause corneal abrasions.

Anatomic Considerations

The technique described will allow the emergency room or primary-care physician to handle all wounds with confidence that optimal wound healing can occur. However, wounds at various anatomic sites do require special attention and will be discussed briefly.

Many physicians do not consider scalp wounds to be significant and simply close them with staples or large sutures. However, in men, male-pattern baldness may develop, and thus the scar may become visible at some time in the future. Therefore, closure of such wounds should be done with care. If possible, one should close the galea with a 4-0 absorbable suture (Dexon or Vicryl) or one of the newer, longer-lasting sutures such as Maxon. Then interrupted sutures with 4-0 nylon can be used to complete the skin closure.

Eyelid wounds that are superficial and do not involve the underlying tarsal plate or levator musculature can be closed with simple sutures. Normally, lacerations to the upper eyelid are closed with 6-0 nylon, whereas 6-0 silk would be used for lower eyelid wounds.

Repair of small through-and-through lacerations of either the nose or ear can be accomplished in the emergency room. Sometimes infiltration of local anesthesia is not well tolerated for nasal wounds, but repair of wounds at either site is done in a similar manner. In nasal wounds, repair is done by placing 5-0 absorbable sutures for the nasal mucosa repair and a 6-0 nylon suture in the skin layer. For ear lacerations, 6-0 nylon sutures are used for both the preauricular and postauricular skin closure. Sutures are not placed in the cartilage of either the ear or the nose.

Lip lacerations are common and may completely split either the upper or lower lip. Such injuries will require layer closure for optimal results. The labial mucosa closure can be accomplished with a 5-0 absorbable suture. The orbicularis oris muscle should be approximated with a 4-0 absorbable suture such as Dexon. The dermis is closed with the 5-0 absorbable suture and the skin with a 6-0 nylon suture. For the vermilion portion of the wound, 6-0 silk sutures would be appropriate. If the laceration violates the vermilion cutaneous border, careful approximation of the border should be done in order to avoid a notching defect. The closure can be accomplished by placing a stitch either just above or below the vermilion cutaneous junction and approximating this point first. Subsequent interrupted sutures can then be placed for final closure.

Postoperative care for the wounds is important for optimal results. Antibiotics are prescribed for dog bites and wounds that extend into the oral cavity. No dairy products are allowed for two days in wounds involving the oral cavity. Since most wounds will develop some edema after closure, a light compression dressing should be applied and maintained for several days postrepair.

On the second or third day after injury, the dressing is removed and the wound examined for any sign of inflammation that may suggest an early infection. For wounds that are close to the eye or on the lip, an antibiotic ointment is usually applied for the first several days after repair. The patient is advised to clean the wound with a 50% mixture of peroxide and water and to reapply a light coating of the antibiotic ointment.

The sutures of facial wounds should be removed by the fourth to sixth day depending on the type of wound and type of closure. Steristrips can be applied after suture removal.

After the sutures are removed, the patient should be seen in 3 weeks for follow-up. The patient is instructed in the general principles of wound healing and followed every 3 months for the first year after injury until the maturation of the wound is complete. If the physician or the patient is unhappy with the final results of the scarring, then the patient should be referred to a surgical specialist for possible revision.

BIBLIOGRAPHY

Converse JM, Dingman RO: Facial injuries in children, in Converse JM (ed): *Reconstructive Plastic Surgery,* ed 2. Philadelphia, WB Saunders Co, 1977.

Converse JM, Smith B, Wood-Smith D: Orbital and naso-orbital fractures, in Converse JM (ed): *Reconstructive Plastic Surgery,* ed 2. Philadelphia, WB Saunders Co, 1977.

De Marino DP, et al: Three-dimensional computed tomography in maxillofacial trauma. *Arch Otolaryngol Head Neck Surg* 1986; 112:146.

Dingman RO, Converse JM: Clinical management of facial injuries and fractures of facial bones, in Converse JM (ed): *Reconstructive Plastic Surgery,* ed 2. Philadelphia, WB Saunders Co. 1977.

Dingman RO, Natvig P: *Surgery of Facial Fractures.* Philadelphia, WB Saunders Co, 1964.

Finkle DR, et al: Comparison of the diagnostic methods used in maxillofacial trauma. *Plast Reconstr Surg* 1985; 73:32.

Kawamoto HK Jr: Late post-traumatic enophthalmos: A correctable deformity? *Plast Reconstr Surg* 1982; 69:423.

Luce EA, Tubb TD, Moore AM: Review of 1,000 major fractures and associated injuries. *Plast Reconstr Surg* 1979; 63:26.

McCoy FJ, et al: An analysis of facial fractures and their complications. *Plast Reconstr Surg* 1962; 29:381.

Milaukas AT, Fueger GF: Serious ocular complications associated with blow-out fractures of the orbit. *Am J Ophthalmol* 1966; 62:670.

Morgan BDG, et al: Fractures of the middle third of the face: A review of 300 cases. *Br J Plast Surg* 1972; 25:147.

Mulliken JD, et al: Management of facial fractures in children. *Clin Plast Surg* 1977; 4:491.

Murray JAM, et al: Open vs. closed reduction of the fractured nose. *Arch Otolaryngol* 1984; 110:797.

Natvig P, Dootzbach RK: Facial bone fractures, in Grabb WC, Smith JW (eds): *Plastic Surgery,* ed 2. Boston, Little, Brown & Co, 1973.

Nohum AM: The biomechanics of maxillofacial trauma. *Clin Plast Surg* 1975; 2:59.

Noyek AM et al: Contemporary radiologic evaluation in maxillofacial trauma. *Otolaryngol Clinic North Am* 1983; 3:473.

Parker MG, Lehman J Jr: Management of facial fractures in children. *Perspect Plast Surg* 1989; 3:1.

Reynolds JR: Late complications vs. methods of treatment in a large series of mid-facial fractures. *Plast Reconstr Surg* 1978; 61:871.

Sataloff RT, et al: Surgical management of the frontal sinus. *Neurosurgery* 1984; 15:593.

Schaefer SD, Diehl JT, Briggs WH: The diagnosis of cerebrospinal fluid rhinorrhea by metrizamide CT scanning. *Laryngoscope* 1980; 90:871.

Schneider RC, Thompson JM: Chronic and delayed cerebrospinal rhinorrhea as a source of recurrent attacks of meningitis. *Am J Surg* 1957; 145:517.

Schultz RC: Facial injuries from automobile accidents: A study of 400 consecutive cases. *Plast Reconstr Surg* 1967; 40:45.

Schultz RC: Supraorbital and glabellar fractures. *Plast Reconstr Surg* 1970; 45:227.

Spiessl B: Rigid internal fixation of fractures of the lower jaw. *Trauma Reconstr Surg* 1972; 13:124.

Steidler NE, et al: Incidence and management of major middle third facial fractures at the Royal Melbourne Hospital: A retrospective study. *Int J Oral Surg* 1980; 9:92.

Steidler NE, et al: Residual complications in patients with major middle third facial fractures. *Int J Oral Surg* 1980; 9:259.

Stranc MF, Robertson GA: A classification of injuries of the nasal skeleton. *Ann Plast Surg* 1979; 2:468.

CHAPTER 18

Special Topics

REFLEX SYMPATHETIC DYSTROPHY

Reflex sympathetic dystrophy is a syndrome of unknown cause that often follows a relatively minor injury. It has been called by several names: Sudeck's atrophy, causalgia, shoulder-hand syndrome, post-traumatic dystrophy, and others. The pathogenesis of the disorder is unclear, but a disturbance in the sympathetic nervous system apparently develops that leads to the characteristic symptoms and signs of pain and vasomotor disturbances.

Clinical Features

Persistent pain that develops after an injury is the characteristic feature. It is frequently severe and often out of proportion to the amount of trauma. Initially, the pain is localized to the area of the injury, but gradually it spreads throughout the extremity. Hypersensitivity to light touch is also a frequent symptom. The extremity appears swollen and warm, and excessive perspiration may be present. Later, motion in the affected joints becomes restricted, and the involved area becomes cool and atrophic. The skin appears dry and glossy. Stiffness and intractable pain may persist for several weeks or months.

The roentgenogram often reveals patchy osteoporosis (Fig 18–1). The bone scan often shows increased vascularity.

Treatment

Reflex sympathetic dystrophy is best treated by prevention. All injuries should have immediate attention, and pain and swelling should be controlled. Early use of the extremity is also important. Once reflex sympathetic dystrophy develops, it is very difficult to treat. The most important aspect of therapy is restoration of motion by exercise. Active use of the extremity should be encouraged in spite of the pain. The edema may be controlled by elevation. Physical therapy in the form of passive range-of-motion exercises may be helpful but should not replace home treatment by the patient. Smoking should be discouraged. Repeated sympathetic blocks are frequently necessary. The treatment is often prolonged, but most patients eventually improve.

ROTATIONAL DEFORMITIES OF THE LEGS IN CHILDREN

Developmental abnormalities of the lower extremities are common and are frequently a source of concern to parents. The cause of these deformities is unknown, but hereditary and per-

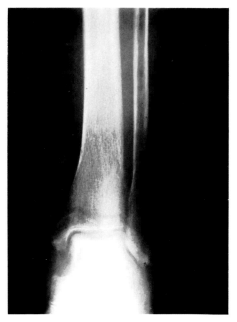

FIG 18–1.
Roentgenogram of the ankle several weeks following a relatively minor sprain. Severe osteoporosis (Sudeck's bone atrophy) of the lower portions of the tibia and fibula are present.

sistent postnatal malpositioning play important roles. Most correct themselves spontaneously.

In-toeing

The in-toeing gait pattern seen in young children is the most common rotational deformity and is usually secondary to one or more of the following causes: (1) internal rotation deformity of the hip secondary to contracture or excessive femoral anteversion, (2) internal (medial) torsion of the tibia, or (3) metatarsus varus (adductus) of the foot.

All three of these deformities are aggravated by positions or postures that are frequently assumed by the child or infant. Lying in the prone position with the legs extended and the feet internally rotated is often associated with in-toeing deformity. Sitting in the "reverse-tailor" position with the feet internally rotated beneath the but-

tocks is directly related to persistent tibial rotation and adduction of the forefoot (Fig 18–2). Children may assume these positions for extended periods of time while sleeping, playing, or watching television.

Children with internal rotation deformities have a high incidence of bowing of the lower extremities. This is frequently more apparent than real because the lower limb is never visualized in the true anteroposterior plane but rather in the oblique plane. The gait is often clumsy, and the appearance may be unsightly.

Internal Femoral Torsion

The diagnosis is made by clinical examination. It is helpful to mark the patellae and observe their position as the child walks. If the child toes in and the patellae face medially, excessive femoral anteversion or an internal rotation contracture of the hips should be suspected. If the child toes in and the patellae face straight forward, then the deformity is distal to the knee, either internal tibial torsion or metatarsus varus. Internal femoral torsion can also be measured with the patient prone, the hips extended, and the knees flexed 90 degrees (Fig 18–3). External and internal measurements of hip motion are then made, with the tibia acting as a pointer. An internal rotation deformity exists at the hip when internal

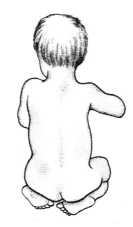

FIG 18–2.
The reverse-tailor position.

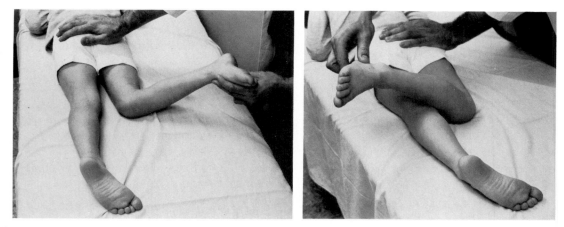

FIG 18–3.
Measuring femoral torsion. The tibia can act as a pointer. Internal femoral torsion is present when internal rotation *(left)* is 30 degrees greater than external rotation *(right)*. External femoral torsion exists when external rotation exceeds internal rotation by the same amount.

rotation exceeds external rotation by greater than 30 degrees.

Internal Tibial Torsion

An approximate measurement of tibial torsion can be obtained by having the patient sit on the examining table with the knees flexed 90 degrees over the side. The tibial tubercle is palpated and directed straight forward. The malleoli are then grasped with the thumb and index finger, and the position of the axis of the ankle joint is determined (Fig 18–4). Normally, approximately 20 to 30 degrees of external tibial torsion is present in adults, and the lateral malleolus will be posterior to the medial malleolus. In children with internal tibial torsion, the lateral malleolus will be anterior to the medial malleolus.

Metatarsus Varus

With the child in the same sitting position, the foot is examined for deformity. If metatarsus varus is present, the lateral border of the foot is convex, and the medial border is concave (Fig 18–5).

Treatment

The treatment of internal rotation deformity of the hip is first directed at developing proper

sleeping and sitting habits. The child is encouraged to sleep on the side rather than in the prone position. The reverse-tailor position should be avoided. A stool or chair should be used for sitting rather than the floor. Passive

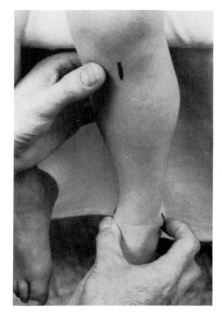

FIG 18–4.
Measuring tibial torsion.

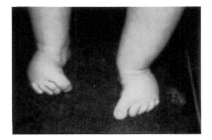

FIG 18–5.
Metatarsus varus (adductus). The lateral border of the foot is convex.

stretching exercises of the hips are performed several times daily in the direction opposite the deformity, and the family is reassured that internal rotation deformity of the hips usually corrects itself spontaneously by the age of 6 years. Although of questionable benefit, the Denis Browne splint may be useful in these cases, but it should be employed with some caution (Fig 18–6). Overaggressive atempts at correction of the hip deformity can result in ligamentous instability and angular deformity at the knee. Little actual corrective force can be applied to the hip by a device attached only to the feet. The splint

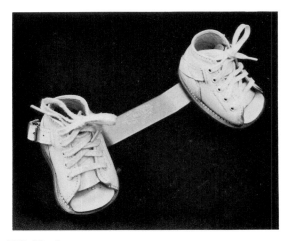

FIG 18–6.
The Denis Browne bar. It should not be wider than the width of the pelvis. Regular shoes may be used unless treatment is necessary for a deformity of the foot. The bar may be used full-time in the infant or at night only.

should be used primarily to hold the feet in a neutral position. It may be used up to the age of 3 years, but it is usually not tolerated very well after that age. Initially the splint is worn full-time in the infant. After correction is obtained, it is used during naps and at night for several weeks to maintain the proper neutral alignment and prevent recurrence. Roller skating is an excellent exercise for these children. The rare severe case that does not correct itself by the age of 8 years may require surgery.

Tibial torsion is best treated by observation and reassurance until the age of 18 months. Sponaneous correction usually occurs with growth. Improper sitting and sleeping habits should be corrected. Stretching exercises are of no value. The Denis Browne may be tried. Shoes with corrective wedges or torque heels appear to be of no benefit in the treatment of any of these problems.

The treatment of metatarsus varus will depend on whether the deformity is fixed or not. If the foot is flexible and the deformity easily overcorrectable, passive stretching exercises and a straight or reverse-last shoe are usually effective (Fig 18–7). If passive correction of the forefoot is not possible, early treatment with corrective casts is indicated. The correction should begin shortly after birth. When the disorder is seen after the age of 1 or 2 years, operative intervention is occasionally necessary. Early diagnosis is therefore important.

Out-toeing

External rotation deformity of the lower extremities is usually caused by the following: (1) external rotation of the hip secondary to soft-tissue contracture or femoral retroversion (external femoral torsion), (2) external tibial torsion, or (3) calcaneovalgus or flatfeet. Out-toeing is often associated with a genu valgum deformity and may be aggravated by sleeping in the prone position (Fig 18–8). The use of wide diapers or a children's "walker" with a wide pad will also potentiate an externally rotated gait.

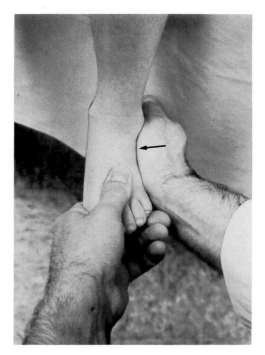

FIG 18−7.
Stretching exercises for metatarsus varus. The heel is firmly grasped. The forefoot is then passively manipulated into the corrected position and held for 10 seconds. The exercise is repeated two to three times at regular intervals during the day.

If femoral retroversion is the cause, examination will reveal that external rotation of the hips is significantly greater than internal rotation. Ex-

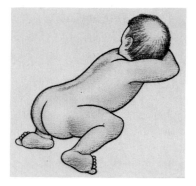

FIG 18−8.
The prone sleeping position, which frequently potentiates external rotation deformities.

ternal tibial torsion is diagnosed by the marked posterior position of the lateral malleolus as compared with the medial. The flatfoot deformity is frequently associated with eversion of the heels (see Chapter 12).

Treatment

Observation and reassurance are indicated. Improper postural habits should be corrected. Wide diapers and walkers with wide canvas slings are avoided. Stretching exercises are begun for any hip deformity. The Denis Browne bar may be used for external femoral and tibial torsion, but only to hold the feet in the neutral position. Surgery is rarely necessary.

ANGULAR DEFORMITIES OF THE LEGS IN CHILDREN

Genu Varum (Bowed Legs)

Genu varum with mild internal tibial torsion is a common, almost normal finding in early childhood. With growth and weight bearing, this developmental bowing spontaneously corrects itself in over 95% of patients. There is even a normal physiologic "swing" to a knock-knee deformity between the ages of 18 months and 3 years in many cases. The knock-knee deformity will then usually correct itself between the ages of 4 and 7 years.

The child is commonly seen because of the wide space between the knees and the mild in-toeing gait. Other possible causes of bowing (rickets, Blount's disease, and so on) can generally be ruled out by the child's history. Roentgenograms may be necessary. There is usually no evidence of any intrinsic bone disease. The amount of genu varum can be determined by measuring the distance between the medial femoral condyles with the child standing and the medial malleoli touching.

Developmental genu varum is usually not severe and rarely requires any treatment. The family can be reassured that spontaneous correction will usually occur by the age of 3 years. Any associated metatarsus varus or tibial torsion should be appropriately treated, however. If improvement fails to take place by the age of 3 or 4 years, corrective braces may be necessary. Severe cases should be referred to rule out Blount's disease.

Genu Valgum (Knock-Knee)

Knock-knee may be due to a variety of disorders, including injury and metabolic disease. Most genu valgum, however, is present as one stage in the normal physiologic "swing" between developmental genu varum and normal alignment. It is usually bilateral and is most common between the ages of 2 and 4 years.

The severity of the deformity can be determined by measuring between the medial malleoli or Achilles tendons with the child standing, the medial femoral condyles touching, and the patellae facing forward (Fig 18–9).

Most patients need only reassurance and follow-up. Children with knock-knee who are under the age of 7 years usually require no treatment as long as the intermalleolar distance is less

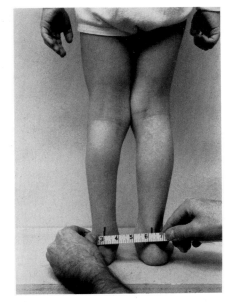

FIG 18–9.
Measuring genu valgum.

than 8.75 cm. The rare case that persists beyond the age of 7 years may require brace correction. If the deformity is excessive or unequal, a thorough search should be made for the underlying abnormality.

LEG LENGTH INEQUALITY

Limb length discrepancies in the lower extremities may result from several causes. The most common are fractures, osteomyelitis, neuromuscular disease, and vascular anomalies. Usually the affected limb is shorter, but occasionally the inequality is the result of overgrowth due to epiphyseal stimulation by inflammation or injury. Frequently, no cause is found. The inequality may cause a mild limp and compensatory scoliosis.

In children, a thorough search should be made to determine the cause. If any is found, the appropriate treatment is instituted. If no cause is noted and the difference is less than 1 cm, the child is followed by repeated careful measure-

ments until mature to determine whether the inequality is static or increasing. Both types of inequality require specialized care, and surgical correction of the asymmetry may be indicated. In children with growth remaining, equalization of the discrepancy may be accomplished either by lengthening the shortened extremity or by partially stopping epiphyseal growth on the longer extremity.

In the adult, the amount of leg length discrepancy that is clinically significant is controversial, but it would appear that up to 2.0 cm of shortening is well tolerated. Chronic low back pain that may be accompanied by a leg length discrepancy should probably be treated with a shoe lift, however, to compensate for the difference. It is not known whether the leg length discrepancy actually causes the low back pain, but occasionally the pain will be relieved by the lift.

BRACES

Braces are appliances that allow partial movement of a joint. They perform several functions, including protection and stabilization. They are most commonly used to temporarily support and restrict motion in the treatment of painful disorders of the spine. The patient should also be encouraged to exercise and develop proper muscular tone, however, so that dependence on the support is avoided.

Cervical Collars

Cervical collars extend from the head to the thorax and are usually soft, although semirigid collars are also available (Fig 18–10). The soft collar is usually more comfortable but restricts motion less than the other collars. These appliances are all used in the treatment of degenerative disc disease and minor ligamentous or muscular injuries of the cervical spine.

Taylor Brace

This is a fundamental back brace useful in dorsal and lumbar spine disease (Fig 18–11). It is a high, semirigid brace that may be modified. Degenerative disc disease and minor factures may be treated with this brace or one of its modifications (long Taylor, modified Taylor, short Taylor).

Knight Spinal Brace (Chairback)

This is a rigid lumbar orthosis that is very useful in treating chronic low back pain when more support is required. It is also used in the treatment of disc disease and spondylolisthesis.

Jewett (Hyperextension) Brace

This three-point brace provides pressure over the lumbar spine, sternum, and symphysis pubis.

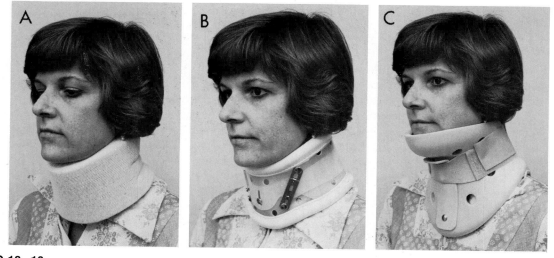

FIG 18–10.
Cervical collars. **A,** the soft foam collar. **B,** the adjustable collar. **C,** the Philadelphia collar.

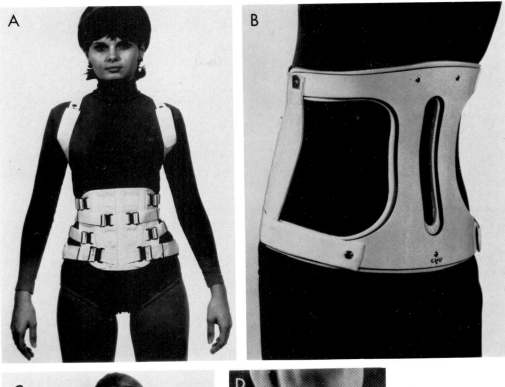

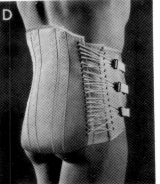

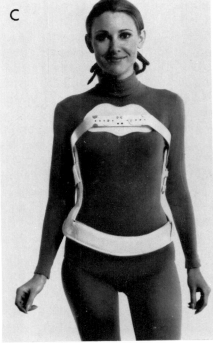

FIG 18–11.
Spinal braces. **A,** the Taylor brace. **B,** the Knight spinal (chairback) brace. **C,** the Jewett hyperextension brace. **D,** the lumbosacral support. (From Camp International, Inc, Jackson, Mich. Used by permission.)

It is used in minor fractures of the dorsal spine when extension is desired. It is also useful in the treatment of epiphysitis.

Knight-Taylor Spinal Brace

This is a rigid high back brace used for fractures of the spine above L3. It may also be used for degenerative disc conditions throughout the entire spine.

Light Lumbar Supports

These supports are usually made of canvas and may be reinforced with metal stays. They are commonly used in the treatment of lumbar disc disease and chronic low back pain syndromes. They also function to increase the intra-abdominal pressure that aids in the support of the lower portion of the back. They are more comfortable than the Knight spinal brace but provide less support.

DISABILITY RATING

The physician is frequently called upon to determine the amount of disability that is present as the result of musculoskeletal disease or injury. This determination is frequently used as the basis for settlement in workmen's compensation cases as well as personal injury litigation. It is usually, however, the "physical impairment rating" expressed as a percentage rather than "disability" that must be determined. It is not the duty of the physician to determine how this impairment affects the patient socially or economically. Frequently, however, it is the impairment rating that is used as the sole basis for the determination of disability by those administrators responsible for it.

Disability may be defined in various ways and is not a medical but rather an administrative term. Medically, it is physical impairment that prohibits the performance of normal physical function. Under Social Security, it means the inability to do any work for at least 12 months because of a physical impairment. Legally, it means permanent bodily injury for which restitution may be judged necessary. Under workmen's compensation statutes, disability is frequently divided into (1) temporary total disability during which period of time the patient is under care and unable to work, (2) temporary partial disability during which time recovery is sufficient that some employment may be begun, or (3) permanent disability, which is permanent loss of function after maximum recovery.

Physical impairment can usually be measured accurately on the basis of the loss of physical function. A careful clinical history and physical examination are mandatory. Laboratory and roentgenographic analysis may also be necessary. In the evaluation of pain that may be present by history or during the examination, it is generally accepted that when no organic findings or clinical manifestations are found to substantiate its presence, it contributes little, if anything, to a physical impairment rating.

For the determination of specific ratings for each impairment, the following manuals are excellent: *Manual for Orthopedic Surgeons in Evaluating Permanent Physical Impairment,* "A Guide to the Evaluation of Permanent Impairment of the Extremities and Back," and *Disability Evaluation Under Social Security.*

JOINT REPLACEMENT SURGERY

Great advances have been made in the past 15 years in the surgical treatment of degenerative and rheumatoid arthritis. These advances have been due primarily to improvements in the techniques of joint arthroplasty. This procedure is most commonly used for conditions of the hip and knee, but devices have been developed for use in almost every joint (Fig 18–12).

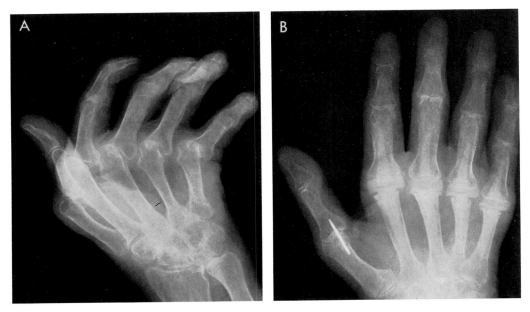

FIG 18–12.
A, severe rheumatoid arthritis of the hand with dislocations of the metacarpophalangeal joints. **B,** postoperative roentgenogram following metacarpophalangeal replacement. The alignment and function are markedly improved. The thumb has also been fused.

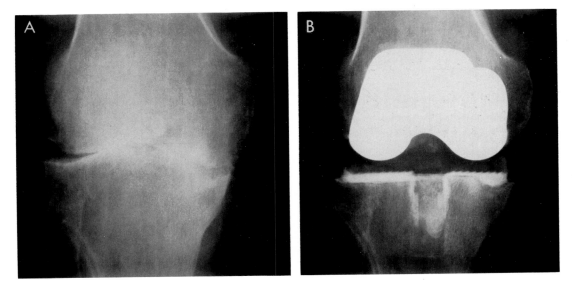

FIG 18–13.
A, degenerative arthritis of the knee. **B,** postoperative roentgenogram following total knee replacement. Because of the occasional problem of loosening, newer procedures have been developed for use in the knee and hip that do not require the bonding cement.

The basic purpose of these techniques is to implant a device into the joint that replaces the degenerated articular surfaces. Most of the procedures utilize a hard plastic, high-density polyethylene for the socket (Fig 18–13). This articulates with a metallic component, both components usually being fixed to the bone by a cementing compound, methylmethacrylate.

The goal of joint replacement surgery is to eliminate the disability that results from pain, loss of motion, and malalignment. The operation is indicated in adults with osteoarthritis and patients with rheumatoid arthritis at any age. It is suitable in patients with bilateral disease, and advanced age is no contraindication. It has been used successfully in almost every age group. Re-habilitation following a joint replacement is usually rapid. Motion and partial weight bearing are started within 2 to 4 days after surgery on the lower extremities. Progressive ambulation is allowed for the remainder of the hospitalization, which normally lasts 7 to 10 days. A home exercise program is continued for 2 months after discharge, and a cane or crutches may be necessary for that period of time.

Mechanical problems following total knee replacement are slightly more common than those following total hip replacement, but the results are uniformly good in both procedures. Over 90% of patients undergoing arthroplasty have excellent relief of pain and improvement in motion.

COMPARTMENT SYNDROMES OF THE LOWER PORTION OF THE LEG

Compartment syndromes are disorders of the extremities in which increased tissue pressure compromises the circulation to the muscles and nerves within the space (see Chapter 15). These conditions are most common in the lower part of the leg, where four natural compartments exist (anterior, lateral, deep posterior, and superficial posterior). The anterior compartment is most commonly involved.

The disorder may be acute or chronic in nature. Chronic cases may be confused with stress fractures, tendinitis, and other forms of "shin splints." The acute case is associated with significantly greater morbidity.

Clinical Features

The acute form may follow exercise, burns, trauma, or vascular injury. Excessive pain, numbness, and weakness are the most common complaints. The pain is often very severe because of muscle and nerve ischemia. The chronic case is usually related to exercise, and symptoms are generally mild.

Weakness, hypoesthesia, and pain on passive stretch of the involved muscle are usually present. The affected area may also be swollen and tense. The peripheral pulse is often diminished. There is usually an increase in intracompartmental tissue pressure that can be measured directly.

Roentgenographic findings are usually normal (except in fractures) but should be obtained in the chronic case to rule out stress fracture.

Treatment

The chronic case usually subsides with rest, but fasciotomy is occasionally performed to prevent recurrence. The acute form requires immediate surgical decompression. Without treatment, necrosis of muscle and nerve may occur and result in permanent weakness, contracture, and nerve dysfunction similar to Volkmann's ischemic contracture in the upper extremity.

INJECTION AND ASPIRATION THERAPY

Locally injected analgesics and steroids are frequently used in the treatment of musculoskeletal diseases. Their use in many specific affections has been described in previous chapters. This section will deal with their usage in other common conditions.

In general, these compounds are used to relieve pain and improve the function of inflamed joints, tendons, and bursae. The exact mechanism by which this is accomplished is unknown. An increase in local blood flow and improvement in local tissue metabolism are common explanations. A placebo effect is undoubtedly present in some cases. Systemic absorption is less following their use than it is with oral administration. Some minor absorption does occur, nonetheless, and 2 to 3 weeks should pass before reinjecting large joints.

A variety of materials is available but the most commonly used is 1% plain lidocaine, usually mixed with equal amounts of various corticosteroids, either short acting or long acting. Many of these steroids are offered in different strengths, although the more concentrated solutions may offer no advantage over the less concentrated ones. The stronger forms should definitely be avoided in superficial injections because they cause significant subcutaneous atrophy. The lidocaine and steroid may be injected separately or together. The use of a small amount of lidocaine alone for skin and soft-tissue infiltration may be necessary in the apprehensive patient. If a joint is to be entered that has a thick capsule, it may also need to be infiltrated because passing a larger needle through the capsule may be uncomfortable. The anesthetic is best injected with a 25-gauge needle (5/8 in. or 1 ½ in.). This needle size may also be used to inject the steroid/lidocaine mixture, especially if the injection is superficial. A 22-gauge, 1½-in. needle is sometimes necessary in deeper injections. A "giving" sensation usually occurs as the needle penetrates the tough fibrous capsule, especially in the knee. The needle should not be advanced once the joint has been entered to avoid joint trauma.

The volume of fluid injected will depend on the size of the joint or soft-tissue area. A total mixture of 4 to 5 mL is often used in the knee; 2 to 3 mL in the shoulder bursa, and 1 to 2 mL in the treatment of tennis elbow.

If aspiration is necessary, which is sometimes the case in the knee, an 18-gauge needle works best. It is less apt to be occluded by joint debris or synovium. As much fluid is removed as possible by expressing the fluid toward the needle. Aspiration may be preceded by a local soft-tissue injection of lidocaine for comfort. Aspiration of some fluid also ensures proper needle placement for the injection of large joints such as the knee. If aspiration is performed, the needle may simply be left in position, and the syringe is exchanged for the one containing the medication.

A mild postinjection inflammation occurs in 5% of the cases following the injection and may last 12 to 24 hours. It is characterized by increased local pain and begins several hours after the injection. It usually responds to ice, rest, and analgesics.

If there is no response to the first injection, it may be repeated in 2 to 3 weeks, but further injections are probably not indicated if there is no improvement.

When employing these compounds, it is important not to rely solely on their use in the treatment of any disorder. They are used only as an adjunct to the appropriate treatment of the underlying abnormality. Sufficient knowledge of the relevant regional anatomy is also essential, and no more than four to six injections should be given over a 6-month period.

General Principles

1. Maintain strict sterile technique.

2. Avoid injection and aspiration in the presence of local infection. A needle passed into a joint through an area of cellulitis may spread the infection into the joint.

3. Avoid the injection of major weight-bearing tendons (patellar tendon, Achilles tendon) and joints. Such injections may mask the normal symptoms and allow a level of activity that could be locally harmful. An exception is for temporary relief of the degenerated joint.

4. Avoid injecting previously infected joints.

5. Avoid injecting markedly unstable joints.

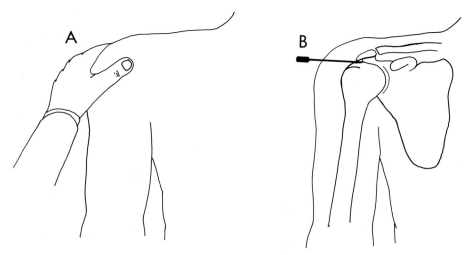

FIG 18−14.
Injecting the subacromial space and rotator cuff. **A,** the sulcus between the acromion and humeral head is palpated. The finger may be kept in position and used as a guide for the needle, or the site may be marked with the fingernail. **B,** the needle is passed into the space, and it is injected. Fluid should flow freely. The tendon is not directly injected. The bicipital groove anteriorly and the acromioclavicular joint may also require injection.

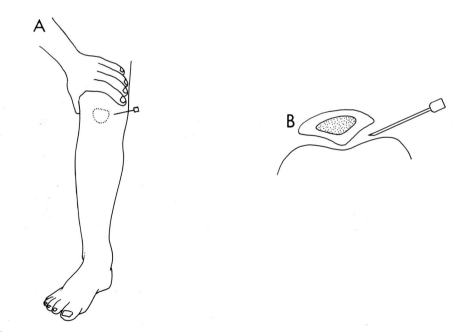

FIG 18−15.
Knee joint injection. The knee should be placed in extension. **A,** the knee is injected in the groove between the patella and femur medially. The finger is used to establish the line of needle placement. **B,** the patellofemoral space is usually wider medially because of a slight tilt to the patella.

Soft-Tissue Injection

Painful disorders of the soft tissue include such conditions as bursitis, tendinitis, tenosynovitis, trigger points, and so-called fibrositis (Fig 18–14). Most of these conditions have been previously described. Trigger points, fibrositis, and other similar syndromes are poorly understood disorders that present with pain and localized tenderness. A common site for the development of these tender areas is the spine, especially the interscapular and lumbosacral areas.

The depth of the injection varies from 1.25 to 5 cm, and it may be necessary to inject several areas. The best relief is obtained when the area is well defined. If the area to be infiltrated lies directly over bone, it is usually safe to insert the needle until it touches bone. Fluid may be injected at this point, and the needle is then retracted for further infiltration. Particular care should be exercised, however, when the injected area does not lie over bone but rather over soft structures such as viscera.

Joint Injection

There are occasional instances where intra-articular aspiration and injection are helpful. These are more easily performed when an effusion is present. Except for the shoulder and hip, most joints are entered on their extensor aspect (Fig 18–15). The major neurovascular bundle is usually found on the flexor side. Fluid will also usually distend the joint most in the direction of the extensor side, which makes entrance easier.

The knee is the joint most commonly entered. If fluid is present in the suprapatellar pouch, the joint may be entered through the area of maximum swelling. Otherwise, the medial or lateral surface is used so that the needle passes between the patella and femur with the knee extended. Relaxation of the extensor mechanism is necessary. Other joints, including the smaller joints, are entered in a similar manner.

FROSTBITE

The severity of injury produced by exposure to cold will depend upon many factors. The most important are the duration of exposure and the degree of temperature. High humidity and wind also increase the amount of damage. Moisture also has a negative effect because it allows for more rapid cooling of the involved part. In addition, previous cold injury and pre-existing peripheral vascular disease increase the susceptibility to future injury. Frostbite will usually require several hours unless the exposure occurs at high altitudes.

Although any area can be affected, the nose, ears, hands, and feet are the most common sites of involvement. The signs and symptoms will depend upon the amount of damage. Mild injury may cause only hyperemia and edema. Soft flesh is usually palpable beneath the frozen, stiff skin. Upon recovering from this degree of involve-

ment, the part often becomes bright red and very painful. Vesicles may appear later.

With more severe injury, the part never recovers, and necrosis of varying degrees begins to appear after thawing. A sign that gangrene may develop is the appearance of heat, edema, and pain in the surrounding tissues. Even after recovery, the part often remains susceptible to cold, and permanent paresthesias and discomfort are often the end result.

Treatment

Cold injury can be prevented by avoiding tight-fitting clothing and by wearing loosely fitted clothing that is relatively windproof but not completely impervious to moisture. Long periods of immobility should be avoided, and socks and gloves should be kept dry.

Treatment depends on the severity of involvement. Mild exposure is treated by removing all wet and constricting clothing in a sheltered area. The part is warmed by applying gentle pressure or, as in the case of the hands and feet, by placing the part under an armpit or on the abdomen beneath the clothing of another individual. The part should never be rubbed or massaged.

More severe degrees of acute injury are treated by rapid warming. Smoking is not permitted. Use of the part should always be avoided, and after transfer to the appropriate facility, the extremity is placed in warm water that is kept at 40°C to 42°C (104°F to 108°F) for 20 to 30 minutes. Higher temperatures or prolonged time are unnecessary and may even be harmful. The extremity should be temporarily removed whenever more warm water is being added. Touching the sides or bottom of the vessel should be avoided. The affected part should never be exposed to an open fire, excessive dry heat, or hot water. The extremity is insensitive and may be burned. Exercise should be avoided. Rewarming is often painful, and the patient may require narcotics. Injuries over 24 hours old are not rewarmed.

Following rewarming, the extremity is elevated to control the edema, and the area is exposed to the air. Blisters should be left intact. Daily whirlpool baths at body temperature are begun with an antibacterial solution, and the injured part is observed for tissue demarcation that may take several weeks. Early debridement should be avoided because actual tissue loss is usually much less than initially estimated. Only the onset of infection with wet gangrene requires immediate surgery with removal of the site of sepsis. Antibiotics and tetanus prophylaxis are given as necessary.

Postfrostbite sequelae such as sensitivity, paresthesias, and edema may benefit from sympathectomy.

DISORDERS OF TREATMENT

Several musculoskeletal problems develop with some frequency during treatment for other conditions. They often occur during hospitalization and can usually be prevented by simple means.

Ulnar Neuritis

This condition may develop in the hospitalized patient and usually results from sleeping in the supine position with the elbows slightly flexed and resting on the bed. It often develops when the elbows are used to push up from the bed. Pain and numbness along the ulnar nerve distribution are typical symptoms, and the nerve is tender to palpation at the elbow. The condition is often bilateral.

The disorder is prevented by having the patient wear soft pads strapped to the elbow to prevent pressure. The patient is not allowed to lie with the elbows in slight flexion, and a trapeze should always be available so that the patient will not have to use the elbows for propping up. Once the symptoms occur, surgical treatment is occasionally necessary.

Crutch Palsy

Crutch palsy may occasionally result from the improper use of crutches. The patient often supports the weight of the body with the axillary portion of the crutch and may develop variable degrees of pain and paresthesias in the arm with prolonged usage. The symptoms are most frequently caused from pressure on the lower portion of the brachial plexus, and the ring and small fingers are typically affected.

The condition is easily prevented by instructing the patient to apply pressure on the hand portion of the crutch and not on the axillary portion.

Trochanteric Bursitis

Bursitis over the greater trochanter is occasionally seen in the hospitalized patient as a result of prolonged recumbency in the lateral position. Pressure over the trochanter results in inflammation of the bursa. Ultrasound, hot packs, anti-inflammatory medication, and a local steroid injection are usually curative.

Frozen Shoulder

Inactivity of the shoulder, frequently in association with cardiac or pulmonary disorders, may lead to stiffness in the shoulder and reflex sympathetic changes in the upper extremity. The etiology of this condition, sometimes called shoulder-hand syndrome or adhesive capsulitis, is unclear. The stiffness, similar to that seen in frozen shoulder from other causes, is progressive, but fortunately, full, pain-free motion is the eventual outcome. The sympathetic component is manifested as pain, edema, osteoporosis, and dystrophic skin changes.

The most important aspect of treatment is prevention. The patient is encouraged to move the shoulders as frequently as possible, and passive range of motion is also performed.

PAGET'S DISEASE

Paget's disease is a nonmetabolic bone disease of unknown origin that causes excessive bone destruction and repair with associated deformities. Up to 3% of patients over the age of 50 years may show localized lesions, but clinically important disease is much less common.

Bone pain is usually the first symptom. Kyphosis, bowed tibias, large head, waddling gait, frequent fractures, and neuropathies may also be seen. Serum calcium and phosphate levels are normal, and the alkaline phosphatase level is elevated. Roentgenograms usually show dense expanded bones (Fig 18–16). This disease must be differentiated from primary bone lesions, such as osteogenic sarcoma or multiple myeloma, and secondary bone lesions, such as metastatic carcinoma and osteitis fibrosis cystica.

Overall, the prognosis of the mild form of this disease is good, and the most frequent complications are sarcomatous changes or renal complications secondary to hypercalciuria. Treatment generally consists of a high-protein diet with adequate vitamin C intake; a high calcium intake is generally desirable, and the use of antimetabolic hormones for osteoporosis should be considered. Salicylate analgesics usually are helpful in controlling the bone pain, and sodium fluoride has been tried in refractory cases. For progressive disease with symptomatology, thyrocalcitonin and mithramycin have recently been investigated and used.

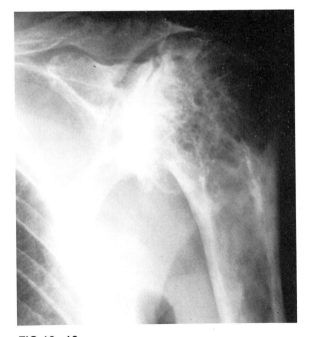

FIG 18–16.
Paget's disease of the humerus. Osteoarthritis of the glenohumeral joint is also present.

MISCELLANEOUS NEUROMUSCULAR DISORDERS

A variety of neuromuscular problems may present as "orthopedic" conditions with weakness, numbness, and/or pain. Among the more common are the following:

Peripheral Nerve Compression Syndromes

Localized injury or compression of peripheral nerves are common problems. The more frequent disorders have been previously discussed. Other syndromes are similarly caused by trauma or inflammation (Table 18–1). Early recognition is the key to effective treatment. Frequently, only the distal sensory portion of the nerve is involved. If superficial, Tinel's sign is usually positive. Minor sensory deficits are commonly present.

Postpolio Sequelae

Many victims of polio were left with varying degrees of weakness and deformity. Most of these patients are now over 50 years of age, and in recent years, some of them have begun to experience new symptoms, mainly increased fatigue, weakness, and joint pain. Most of the time, their musculoskeletal complaints can be attributed to arthritic changes (wrist and knee especially) or other expected disorders such as carpal tunnel syndrome. Sometimes, the symptoms have no clear etiology, and the weakness and fatigue may even follow the same pattern as the original infection.

This "syndrome" has received a great deal of media attention, sometimes alarming many patients. Among the possible causes advanced for these symptoms are (1) "burnout" or overuse of a few surviving motor units; (2) progressive anterior horn cell loss; (3) age-related muscle and ligament weakness, which further compromises marginal muscle function; (4) improper or inappropriate braces and orthotics; and (5) an ALS-like syndrome. The most likely factors involved are overuse, age-related progression, and the use of poor or outdated prosthetic devices.

Management

Reassurance and understanding are the most important. Very few patients who have had polio have any serious progression of their weakness. The role of exercise has not been clearly established, but excessive physical strain should be avoided, and these patients will probably benefit from a careful, *nonfatiguing,* resistive exercise program. Braces, orthotics, and other assistive devices should be evaluated and updated or modified as necessary.

Herpes Zoster

This is a common condition also known as "shingles." It develops from the activation of a varicella (chicken pox) virus, which often resides asymptomatically in dorsal root ganglia. As a result, the affected nerve root becomes painful, and a typical skin eruption develops along the distribution of the root.

The skin rash may not develop for several days, which makes an early diagnosis difficult. The pain is usually quite severe. The skin later becomes reddened, and eventually, clusters of vesicles appear. These, too, are painful and last for 1 to 2 weeks.

Multiple Sclerosis

Multiple sclerosis (MS) is a demyelinating neurologic disorder of unknown etiology that presents with recurrent episodes of neurologic dysfunction. (Patients with pain in the legs will frequently worry that their symptoms are from MS.) The early diagnosis is very difficult due to the variability of presenting symptoms. Pathologically, the lesions of MS are those of patchy loss of

TABLE 18–1.

Miscellaneous Peripheral Nerve Syndromes

Nerve	Common Cause	Symptoms	Treatment/Prognosis
Proximal Radial (Saturday night palsy)	Pressure from arm over chair (or person). Fracture midhumerus	Wrist drop. Sensory loss on dorsum of wrist or first dorsal web space	Cock-up splint. Spontaneous recovery likely in 6–12 wk. Surgical exploration occasionally required if due to fracture
Superficial radial nerve at wrist	Tight watchband or glove. Swelling due to de Quervain's disease	Sensory loss in first web space, thumb, index finger	Remove, treat cause. Spontaneous recovery is usual
Femoral nerve	Hemorrhage in groin due to anticoagulation. Iatrogenic due to stretching from retractor during abdominal surgery	Weakness of knee extension, stair walking. Anterior thigh atrophy, numbness	Exercise to maintain strength. Spontaneous recovery is likely
Peroneal nerve at fibular head	Cast rubbing, keeping leg crossed. Fracture of fibular neck	Foot drop or weak great toe. Numbness on dorsum of foot, first web space	Remove cause. Drop foot brace if needed. Recovery usual but sometimes incomplete if due to fracture
Infrapatellar branch of saphenous nerve (crosses patellar tendon from medial to lateral)	Kneeling, surgical incision, prepatellar bursitis	Numbness, lateral to patellar tendon. Pain over nerve at patellar tendon	Remove cause. Recovery likely. Permanent if due to surgical incision
Spinal accessory nerve	Iatrogenic loss due to biopsy of node in posterior triangle. Trauma (contusion)	Trapezius paralysis and atrophy	Occasional recovery if due to closed trauma. Permanent if iatrogenic
Long thoracic nerve	Direct trauma, traction? Backpacking, weight lifting	Scapular winging (serratus anterior paralysis)	Recovery is common but variable. No effective treatment
Superficial peroneal nerve on dorsum of foot	Tight laces on shoes. Swelling due to extensor tenosynovitis	Variable numbness on dorsum of foot, first web space.	Remove cause. Treat inflammation. Recovery is usual

myelin in the white matter. Inflammation and edema may be present in the acute stage, and scarring occurs in the chronic phase.

The disease usually presents in the third decade, and females are more commonly affected than males. Paresthesias, disturbances in sensation and gait and visual and bladder dysfunction are the most common initial symptoms. Many of these mimic other disorders, which makes a diagnosis difficult to establish. While the diagnosis is ultimately based on clinical evidence (objective neurologic findings such as ataxia, incoordination, hyperactive reflexes, positive Babinski sign, visual loss, and Lhermitte's sign—tingling paresthesias with neck flexion), a number of laboratory and imaging tests are helpful.

Special Studies

Magnetic resonance imaging (MRI) is the preferred imaging modality. Typical abnormalities (periventricular plaques) are found in the majority of cases and, when combined with a positive history and neurologic examination, usually establish the diagnosis without further testing.

The cerebrospinal fluid (CSF) usually has elevated protein and leukocyte levels. The gammaglobulin level is often increased (70% of cases), and agar gel electrophoresis of concentrated CSF often shows migration in a typical pattern called oligoclonal bands.

Evoked potentials (electrical responses to sensory stimulation recorded by surface electrodes) are often abnormal although, like most other tests, are not specific for MS.

Prognosis

The long-term outcome is variable although many (one third) patients have a relatively benign course. Predicting the prognosis for an individual patient is difficult.

EXERCISE AND GOOD HEALTH

Regular exercise is the key to good health. People who are physically fit have more energy, sleep better, and are less depressed. They suffer fewer illnesses and pains than average and enjoy a more positive sense of well-being. Exercise is just as important for the person who does heavy labor all day as it is for those who do desk work. Doing hard work does burn some calories and strengthen muscles, but it does very little to make patients fit and may even cause chronic pain to muscles and back. Most patients need some kind of regular exercise, and the best is known as "aerobic" (literally "with air"). Before starting, a general physical examination may be needed if there is any indication of chronic illness.

Aerobic Exercise

In order for the exercise to be considered aerobic, it must be fast enough to improve cardiovascular fitness. The heart rate is usually used to determine whether the exercise is sufficient to develop the aerobic effect. To be effective, the activity simply needs to raise the pulse to what is known as the "target heart rate" (THR) and *sustain* the THR during the exercise for at least 15 to 20 minutes.

The individual's THR is determined by first subtracting the patients age from 220 to obtain that individual's maximum heart rate (MHR). That figure is then multiplied by 0.60 to 0.80 to determine the target heart rate zone (Table 18–2). Exercise performed in this zone improves aerobic conditioning.

Walking and Jogging

These are certainly the simplest of aerobic exercise, and because it is "low impact" (no excessive jumping or pounding), brisk walking is easier on the back and legs and provides about the same benefits as jogging. Walking is also the least risky exercise for those individuals with chronic medical problems. In addition to improving cardiovascular function, walking may also (1) help slow bone loss, especially in women, (2) extend life (walking 12 to 20 miles per week will decrease the annual death risk by about 27%), (3) help control cholesterol levels, and (4) help control weight.

As with all exercise, the activity should be begun slowly. Eventually, the patient should walk at least four times per week for about 45 to 60 minutes while pausing from time to time to check the heart rate. Usually, walking at a rate of 120 steps per minute is adequate. For walking, warming up is not necessary, but a "cool-down period" after finishing running is better than stopping abruptly.

Once the patient is comfortable walking, jogging may be tried. A slow pace is more than adequate.

TABLE 18–2.

Target Heart Rates (Measured at 60% to 80%)*

Age (yr)	25	30	35	40	45	50	55	60	65
Target heart range	117–156	114–152	111–148	108–144	105–140	102–136	99–132	96–128	93–124

*Notes:
1. The level of exertion required to exercise in the THR zone correlates well with the individuals' maximum oxygen capacity (VO_2 max), which is the best measurement of aerobic fitness.
2. Brisk walking or similar activity that burns 2,000 calories per week can protect against heart disease.
3. Patients should be encouraged to climb stairs rather than ride elevators. Even short bursts of exercise such as this are helpful.
4. If knee pain occurs, patients may have to avoid hilly areas or stairs, activities that place the extensor mechanism under flexion load.
5. It should take about 2 months of gradually increasing exercise for the patient to reach the THR.
6. Walking burns about 80 calories per mile.
7. After jogging or other vigorous exercise, patients should "cool down" by walking slowly for 5 to 10 minutes.
8. Hand-held or ankle weights may be used when walking but are not necessary.
9. With regular exercise, the resting pulse decreases, a sign of more effective cardiovascular function.

Other Exercises

Swimming, cycling, rowing, cross-country skiing, and jumping rope are also excellent activities. Swimming removes the body weight and may be better in patients with painful joints. Swimmers should avoid any stroke that requires that the neck be extended and the chin raised because this can irritate cervical disc disease. Swimming at a THR for 20 to 30 minutes three times per week is sufficient. If cycling is tried, the bike needs to fit properly so that the lower portion of the back will not become strained.

Stretching exercises may be good before any vigorous exercise. Stretching should be done after warming up for 5 minutes by walking (see Chapter 15). Cold muscles should not be stretched.

LOCAL SOFT-TISSUE TREATMENT

All musculoskeletal problems involve the soft parts at least to some degree. For purposes of discussion, they are divided into acute and chronic disorders.

Treatment of Acute Injuries

These injuries are generally those of muscle strains of varying degrees, contusions, and ligamentous sprains. They are all accompanied by hemorrhage and swelling. For the first 24 to 72 hours, ice is applied for 30 minutes every hour. Rest, elevation, and soft compression are also used ("RICE"). Crushed ice in a plastic bag is preferred to the chemical cold packs. These packs can cause blistering and severe chemical burns. After 3 days, gentle range-of-motion and stretching exercises are begun several times a day while cold is applied. Cold is maintained for about 5 minutes after the exercise.

Protected use of the part is allowed as tolerated. Heat in any form, vigorous stretching, massage, or exercise are avoided in order to prevent further injury. Hematomas that may form usually do not require aspiration. In the majority of cases, they absorb spontaneously over the course of several weeks.

(**Note:** Ice is also very helpful in cases of

chronic "overuse" problems such as tendinitis. It is usually applied for 5 minutes after the offending activity.)

Treatment of Chronic Disorders

Among the forms of "therapy" available for patient care are occupational and physical therapy and other rehabilitation services. In referring patients for these services, consultation with the therapist or physiatrist may be helpful. The diagnosis should be included as well as specific instructions regarding the treatments and their frequency. In addition, a maximum time limit (usually 2 to 4 weeks) should be set to determine whether or not the treatments are truly being effective. If the patient is hospitalized, the treatments are often prescribed twice a day. As an outpatient, they are usually given once a day or every other day. In order for the therapy to be continued, the patient should show more than just temporary improvement. If not, the treatment should be stopped and the patient re-evaluated.

Most therapeutic modalities have developed over the years on a purely empiric basis, and various treatments have been in vogue at various times. All of these treatments are expensive, and patient improvement is often anecdotal and short-lived. A placebo effect due to the "hands-on" aspect of the care undoubtedly plays a considerable role. Among the more commonly used treatments available at this time are the following: (1) heat therapy for pain relief, (2) massage, (3) therapeutic exercises, and (4) traction.

Heat Therapy

Whether to use ice or heat therapeutically in the treatment of pain is arbitrary. Heat remains the most popular. Heat treatment is either superficial or deep. The theories behind thermotherapy are that it increases blood flow, helps resolve edema and inflammatory products, and increases the extensibility of collagen, thus producing pain relief and diminishing stiffness.

Superficial heat (1 to 5 mm) can be delivered at home as well as in a therapy office. Paraffin baths (usually for hands), infrared lamps, hot packs (hot water bottles, heating pads, etc.), and various forms of whirlpool "hydrotherapy" are available. Perhaps the simplest, least expensive is "moist heat" at home. A small towel is dampened and any excess moisture removed (many heat pads come with soft pads designed for this purpose). A plastic sheet is placed between the towel and heat source. Heat is then applied to the affected area for 1 to 2 hours one to two times a day or more as needed. Care should be taken not to raise the temperature level too high and cause a skin burn.

Deep heat is usually available as (1) shortwave diathermy, (2) microwaves, and (3) ultrasound. Diathermy and ultrasound are more commonly used. The type must be specified.

The following points should be remembered when using any form of heat: (1) patients should not fall asleep with their heating pad, (2) heat before exercise (stretching especially) often enhances the effect of the exercise, (3) heat should not be used in areas of cancer or near the gonads or a developing fetus, and (4) heat should be avoided in tissues without pain sensation or adequate circulation. The increased temperature increases the metabolic demand without the tissue's ability to respond with increased vascular supply. Necrosis may then occur.

Massage

A number of various techniques are used for "spasm" or "nodules". They are usually types of kneading and stroking and are most commonly used in spine pain.

Therapeutic Exercise

In general, if stiffness is present (for example, frozen shoulder), stretching or gentle manipulation (sometimes preceded by deep heat) are recommended. If weakness is present, resistive exercises are taught to the patient so that they can be performed at home.

Traction

Various forms of spinal "stretching" are used, generally in the treatment of chronic spine pain. There is little evidence that any real distraction of disc or facet joints ever occurs, although patients sometimes report improvement with cervical traction.

Others

Trigger point injections, phonophoresis (ultrasound with cortisone cream), dimethyl sulfoxide (DMSO, investigational), acupuncture, biofeedback, electrotherapy, ice massage, and manipulation are all available. Transcutaneous electrical nerve stimulation (TENS) seems to be helpful in some chronic pain problems with localized pain, although its effect seems to decline with time. TENS may alter pain perception by stimulation of certain afferent fibers in order to inhibit spinal cord transmission of painful stimuli. For a more complete discussion of occupational therapy and other rehabilitation services, the reader is referred to the bibliography.

BIBLIOGRAPHY

Bennett RL, Knowlton GC: Overwork weakness in partially denervated skeletal muscle. *Clin Orthop* 1958; 12:22.

Bloomberg MH: *Orthopedic Braces.* Philadelphia, JB Lippincott, 1964.

Charnley J: The long-term results of low-friction arthroplasty of the hip performed as a primary intervention. *J Bone Joint Surg [Br]* 1972; 54:61.

DiBenedette V: Keeping pace with many forms of walking. *Phys Sports Med* 1988; 16:145.

Disability Evaluation Under Social Security. Chicago, American Medical Association, 1969.

Ekelund LG, et al: Physical fitness as a predictor of cardiovascular mortality in asymptomatic North American men: The lipid research clinics mortality followup study. *N Engl J Med* 1988; 319:1379.

Epperson LW: The late effects of poliomyelitis. *Ala J Med Sci* 1988; 25:173.

Gross RH: Leg length discrepancy: How much is too much. *Orthopedics* 1978; 1:307.

A guide to the evaluation of permanent impairment of the extremities and back. *JAMA* 1958; 166 (special issue).

Johnson RM, et al: Cervical orthoses: A study comparing their effectiveness in restricting cervical motion in normal subjects. *J Bone Joint Surg [Am]* 1977; 59:332.

Knight R: Developmental deformities of the lower extremity. *J Bone Joint Surg [Am]* 1954; 36:521.

Kottke FJ, Stillwell GK, Lehmann JF: *Krusen's Handbook of Physical Medicine and Rehabilitation,* ed 3. Philadelphia, WB Saunders Co, 1982.

Ladd AL, et al: Reflex sympathetic imbalance: Response to epidural blockage. *Am J Sports Med* 1989; 17:660.

Leon AS, et al: Leisure-time physical activity levels and risk of coronary heart disease and death: The multiple risk factor interventional trial. *JAMA* 1987; 258:2388.

Manual for Orthopedic Surgeons in Evaluating Permanent Physical Impairment. Chicago, American Academy of Orthopedic Surgeons, 1959.

Matsen FA, Clawson DK: The deep posterior compartmental syndrome of the leg. *J Bone Joint Surg [Am]* 1975; 57:34.

Matsen FA, Winquist RA, Krugmire RB: Diagnosis and management of compartment syndromes. *J Bone Joint Surg [Am]* 1980; 62:286.

Maynard FM: Post-polio sequelae. Differential diagnosis and management. *Orthopedics* 1985; 8:857.

McCauley RL, et al: Frostbite injuries: A rational approach based on pathophysiology. *J Trauma* 1983; 23:143.

Morley AJM: Knock-knee in children. *Br Med J* 1957; 2:976.

Nickel VL: *Orthopedic Rehabilitation.* New York, Churchill Livingstone, 1982.

Owen RR, Jones D: Polio residual clinic: Conditioning exercise program. *Orthopedics* 1983; 8:882.

Payne R: Neuropathic pain syndromes with special reference to causalgia and reflex sympathetic dystrophy. *Clin J Pain* 1986; 2:59.

Poplawski WB, Wiley AM, Murray JT: Posttraumatic dystrophy of the extremities: A clinical review and trial of treatment. *J Bone Joint Surg [Am]* 1983; 65:642.

Rusk HA: *Rehabilitation Medicine,* ed 4. St Louis, CV Mosby Co, 1977.

Salenius P, Vankka E: The development of the tibiofemoral angle in children. *J Bone Joint Surg [Am]* 1975; 57:259.

Schutzer SF, Gossling HR: The treatment of reflex sympathetic dystrophy syndrome. *J Bone Joint Surg [Am]* 1984; 66:625.

Sheridan GW, Matsen FA: Fasciotomy in the treatment of the acute compartment syndrome. *J Bone Joint Surg [Am]* 1976; 58:112.

Sherman M: Physiologic bowing of the legs. *South Med J* 1960; 53:830.

Slattery MR, Jacobs DR, Nichaman MZ: Leisure time physical activity and coronary heart disease death. The railroad study. *Circulation* 1989; 79:304.

Swanson AB: Flexible implant arthroplasty for arthritic finger joints. *J Bone Joint Surg [Am]* 1972; 54:435.

Swanson JW: Multiple sclerosis: Update in diagnosis and review of prognostic factors. *Mayo Clin Proc* 1989; 64:577.

Tachdjian MO: *Pediatric Orthopedics.* Philadelphia, WB Saunders Co, 1972.

Wagstaff P, Wagstaff S, Downey M: A pilot study to compare the efficacy of continuous and pulsed magnetic energy (short wave diathermy) in the relief of back pain. *Physiotherapy* 1986; 72:563.

Weiner DS: The natural history of "bow legs" and "knock knees" in childhood. *Orthopedics* 1981; 4:156.

Index